ATI TEAS®

Study Manual

2020-2021

FOR THE TEST OF ESSENTIAL ACADEMIC SKILLS

Contributors/Reviewers

Susan Keiffer-Barone, Ed.D
Curriculum & Instruction, NBCT

Nancy Geldermann, MS
Curriculum & Instruction, NBCT

Matthew R. Leach CAGS
Mathematics Education

Alicia Sussman, M.Ed.
Secondary Mathematics
Education

Melissa O'Connor, MS English
Education

Pamela Wagner, M.Ed. Science
Education, NBCT

Bonnie C. Walter, M.Ed
Secondary Education

Karen Lee Banks, EdD
Educational Technology &
E-Learning

Angela Broaddus, PhD

Curriculum & Instruction

George Christoph, M.Ed.
Mathematics, NBCT

Shauna Hedgepeth, MS
Science Education

Deidre Meyer, MS Instructional
Design

Joe Meyer, BS Mathematics,
NBCT

Suzanne Myers, MS Curriculum
& Instruction

Derek Prater, MS Journalism

Vidya Rajan, PhD Genetics

Kris Shaw, MS Education

Charlotte Waters, MS Science
Education

Manager of content development: Ron Watson, Integra Software Services

Project management: Joanne Manning, Integra Software Services

Layout: Integra Software Services

Illustrations: Randi Hardy, Ascend Learning
                 Integra Software Services

Cover design: Jason Buck, Ascend Learning

Interior book design: Emily Friel, Integra Software Services

Table of Contents

Introduction   1

ATI TEAS Preparation Strategies   5

Unit 1: Reading   11

Unit 2: Mathematics   127

Section: Number and Algebra

Section: Measurement and Data

Unit 3: Science   235

Section: Human Anatomy and Physiology

Unit 4: English and Language Usage   373

ATI TEAS Comprehensive Practice Test 425

Introduction

Welcome to the ATI TEAS® Study Manual, your guide to successful preparation for the Test of Essential Academic Skills (TEAS). This book provides you with an overview of the content and skills included on the TEAS and suggestions for effectively preparing for the test. First, this guide will outline the parts of the test. The TEAS covers a broad range of essential skills in reading, mathematics, science, and English and language usage that you have developed over the course of your academic career. Next, this guide will help you create a study plan for success in each subject area. Finally, this study guide provides a full chapter of instruction on each objective of the TEAS. Each chapter includes examples, diagrams, and graphic organizers to help you review key ideas. Each chapter ends with questions similar to those on the TEAS to help you practice for the exam. A detailed explanation of the correct answer for each question is also included to ensure you understand key concepts that will appear on the TEAS.

TEAS Subject Areas

The TEAS test was developed for health science schools to evaluate the academic preparedness of prospective students. Questions on the TEAS assess student knowledge of 65 objectives that address topics presented in grades 7 to 12. The objectives describe skills and concepts that health science educators believe are most important for success in health science programs. The objectives cover the academic subject areas of:

- Reading
- Mathematics
- Science
- English and Language Usage

The 65 chapters of this manual provide instruction for each of the 65 objectives of the TEAS. Keep in mind that the examples provided in the manual are not comprehensive. They do not include all of the possible content appropriate for that objective. The chapters do, however, provide a clear overview of the content and skills you will encounter on the TEAS.

TEAS Questions

The TEAS is composed of 170 items that include 20 unscored pretest items, all of which are four-option, multiple-choice questions. The test is available in both paper-and-pencil and computer-administered formats. Questions from the four subject areas are grouped in separate sections, and each has a separate, individual time limit. The following table provides the number of questions and time limits for each section of the TEAS.

Subject Area	Number of Questions	Time Limit
Reading	47 questions (6 pretest items)	64 minutes
Mathematics	32 questions (4 pretest items)	54 minutes
Science	47 questions (6 pretest items)	63 minutes
English and language usage	24 questions (4 pretest items)	28 minutes
Total	**170**	**209 minutes**

Questions in each subject area are organized by the key topics being assessed. There are a set number of questions for each key topic. The following table shows the number of scored questions for each key topic.

Subject Areas and Key Topics	Number of Scored Items
Reading	**47**
Key ideas and details	22
Craft and structure	14
Integration of knowledge and ideas	11
Mathematics	**32**
Number and algebra	23
Measurement and data	9
Science	**47**
Human anatomy and physiology	32
Life and physical sciences	8
Scientific reasoning	7
English and language usage	**24**
Conventions of standard English	9
Knowledge of language	9
Vocabulary acquisition	6

Taking the TEAS

The TEAS is administered in a standardized environment overseen by a proctor. The proctor will ensure that all testing protocols are strictly enforced.

What to Bring

- **Photo ID:** To be admitted to your testing session, you will need to present proper photo identification, such as a driver's license, passport, or green card. You will not be admitted or be able to take the test if your ID does not meet the following requirements: government-issued, current photograph, examinee signature, and permanent address. A credit card photo or a student ID does not meet the criteria.

- **Writing instrument:** Be sure to bring two sharpened No. 2 pencils with attached erasers. No other writing instruments are allowed.

- **ATI log-in information:** If you are taking the online version of the test, you will need to create a student account at www.atitesting.com prior to your test day and remember to bring your log-in information with you.

What Not to Bring

Plan ahead and leave the following items at home or in your car because they are not permitted in the exam room:

- **No additional apparel is allowed**, including but not limited to jackets, coats, hats, and sunglasses. Discretionary allowances are made for religious apparel. All apparel is subject to inspection by a proctor.

- **No personal items** of any sort **are allowed,** including but not limited to purses, computer bags, backpacks, and duffel bags.

- **No electronics** of any kind are allowed, including but not limited to cell phones, smartphones, beepers/pagers, digital watches, and smartwatches.

- **No food or drink is allowed**, unless it is documented as a medical necessity.

What to Expect

- Testing staff will check your photo ID, admit you to your test room, and direct you to a seat.

- Proctors in the room will monitor any odd or disruptive behavior. This should not include you, but if it does, you will be dismissed, and your exam will not be scored.

- A four-function calculator will be provided by the testing center. Personal calculators will not be allowed. Calculators provided do not have built-in functionalities or other special features.

- The proctor will provide scratch paper for use during the test. Scratch paper cannot be used before the exam or during breaks. All paper, in its entirety, must be returned to the proctor at the end of the testing session.

- After the mathematics section, you may take a 10-minute break. During the break, do not access any of your personal items.

- If you need to leave your seat at any time other than during the break, raise your hand and the proctor will guide you. Note that timing for that section of the exam will not stop, and any time lost as a result cannot be made up.

- During the exam, if you have a technical issue with your computer or need the proctor for any other reason, raise your hand for assistance.

- Any challenges that arise during testing or any testing room complaints should be reported to the proctor before leaving the room on the day of your exam.

The TEAS Study Guide

This guide is organized to help target your studies in preparation for your success on the exam.

- There is a unit for each subject area and a chapter for each objective.

- Each chapter provides an overview of an objective that includes an outline of important concepts along with examples of the specific knowledge and skills that pertain. Chapters also include key terms and definitions, practice questions, and study exercises.

- An answer key for the practice questions is provided at the end of each key topic section. Both answers and explanations are provided so that it is clear why the correct answer is right and why the incorrect answers are wrong. This will help you develop a deeper understanding of test-taking skills and provide thoughtful strategies to use when taking the actual test.

- There is a quiz at the end of each section that matches the number of scored items in the test plan. The quizzes provide an excellent practice opportunity because they have been developed using the same guidelines as the TEAS itself.

- A key with detailed explanations of the correct answers to each question immediately follows after each quiz.

Using this study manual to familiarize yourself with each of the TEAS objectives, to practice answering TEAS-style questions, and to guide study of the additional concepts covered on the test will pave the way to your success on the TEAS. Keep in mind, though, that this is a study guide; it should not be the only resource you use in your preparations. The TEAS covers a broad range of knowledge, and this study manual does not detail every concept that could possibly covered on the exam itself.

Online Practice TEAS

Two online practice versions of the TEAS are available for purchase. These practice versions were developed using the same test plan used for the actual proctored versions. They provide an opportunity for additional practice answering TEAS-style questions and also for assessing readiness for success on the TEAS. Each of these tests contains 150 items, all of which are scored. The testing interface is similar to that of the online proctored version, except that rationale for each question and answer are provided to further your learning and understanding. On completion of the online practice test, a score report will appear with both your results and a list of topics for review. The list of topics for review will correspond to the objectives in the test plan and study manual and will indicate the areas in which you should focus additional study.

TEAS Scoring

The online version of the test is scored on completion. Your TEAS score report will be posted immediately and can be viewed at that time. Paper-and-pencil versions of the TEAS will be scored by ATI within 48 hours of their receipt from the testing site. The score report will include both the total overall score and the individual content area scores. In addition, the report will identify any specific topic areas deemed challenging for you along with references to specific places in the study manual where content can be reviewed to improve your skills.

Your ATI TEAS score report can be accessed at any time through your ATI account under My Results. In that same area, next to the score report, there is an option to create a Focused Review. A Focused Review is an online e-tool that aligns missed question topics with relevant study guide pages that will be helpful for your review.

You can also submit your TEAS score to your health science program. If you tested on-site at the program you are applying to, your TEAS transcript will already be available to them. If you want to send your transcript to a different program, visit www.atitesting.com/ati_store/ to purchase and send an official TEAS transcript to the program of your choice.

ATI TEAS Preparation Strategies

When should you start studying for the test? Evidence shows that studying should begin well ahead of the time you will take the tesr so that by continuously reviewing the material, you will be able to store new information in your long-term rather than your short-term memory.[1] Planning to review your notes, writing mock exams, and developing concept maps are just a few strategic ways to ensure effective study time.[2] Research suggests that plans containing clear study goals, repeated study over time, and self-regulated learning (keeping track of what you do) result in improved performance[3] on exams. Studying collaboratively with peers and asking questions such as, "How could I explain this to someone else?" or "How does this apply to my life or something else that I have learned?" can also help you learn and understand the material.[4]

Preparing for the Test

Time Management

One of the most effective ways to study for a test is to create a personal time-management system. Like an athlete or a musician, you need to set aside "practice time." Start taking control by doing an assessment of what actual free time you have. Plot it out. You may be surprised how a few small changes to eliminate minor distractions that steal your time will open up more time that you can then set aside for studying. With a little planning, you will find that within what appears to be a very busy day, week, or month, there is almost always a way to find a time for practice.

Tips

- **Set your priorities.** Decide how much time you will need for each part of the test. Review each section and think about which subjects need more of your attention. Plan to spend more time on those that you need to learn and less on those that just need your review.
- **Make a schedule.** Use a weekly planning tool, something you are already comfortable with, and set up a schedule. First, list things that are constant, such as work, sleep, and social obligations, and then look for blocks of time you can reserve for studying. These blocks should be planned for the time of day when you are most alert and able to concentrate rather than times when you are tired or easily distracted.

Goal Setting

Once you have organized your time, you will need to decide how to use it effectively. Use your priority list to determine what you will need to do to guarantee success in each subject area and how much time that will take. Make a list of what is required for each so you can check off both major and minor goals as they are reached.

---

[1]Kornell, 2009; Kitsantas, 2002; Terry 2006
[2]Tinnesz, Ahun, & Kiener, 2006
[3]Kistantas, 2002
[4]van Blerkom, van Blerkom, & Bertsch, 2006; Roberts, 2008; Weinstein, Ridley, Dahl, & Weber, 1988

Tips

- **Be realistic.** Set goals that are achievable. Do not expect to complete a challenging section of review in the same amount of time it will take for some subject with which you are more familiar.
- **Be consistent.** Once you have set your goals and your schedule, go to work and follow your plan. Planning ahead, setting goals, and consequently reaching them will give you confidence to achieve the success you are aiming for on the exam.

Reality Checks on Progress

Assign a specific time in your weekly schedule for review and reflection. Did you meet your weekly goal? If not, what adjustments can you make for the next week? Be objective and honest about what worked and what did not. Revise accordingly, check off your accomplishments, and then congratulate yourself!

Avoiding Test Anxiety

Sometimes, even with the best organization and planning, underling stress and apprehension can lead to test anxiety. Worrying about what-ifs can get in the way of success during test preparation and when actually taking the exam. Being prepared is the best way to alleviate test anxiety. Organizing your time, setting goals, and checking off your progress are the best ways to build confidence and to avoid unnecessary tension that may pop up and get in the way of your success.

Tips

- **Balance your schedule.** When creating your study schedule, build in regular times for leisure activities, exercise, eating, and socialization along with your plans for learning.
- **Maintain a positive attitude.** Be optimistic about your success. Develop a method of reassuring yourself with a slogan or a saying, even a gesture or a song, to avoid any naysaying and to reinforce an affirmative outlook.
- **Get plenty of rest.** The more rested you are, the more you will be able to focus on your work and accomplish both your long- and short-term goals.
- **Be flexible.** Even the best made plans can change. If something unexpected interrupts your schedule, be flexible. Adjust accordingly and get back on track the next day.
- **Talk to others.** Do not keep everything to yourself. Talk to your friends, family, and fellow test takers about what you are experiencing as you prepare for the test. Sharing your feelings with others may be away to relieve the stress and help build your confidence.

Use the following worksheet to help prepare for the test. Adapt it to meet your individual needs.

The TEAS test is on the following date and time:	
The most important areas for me to study are:	
My top four goals for studying are:	I can find or create practice questions at the following places or with the following people:
1.	1.
2.	2.
3.	3.
4.	Days and times I have set aside exclusively for studying for this test
Resources I will use for studying	
1.	Mondays:
2.	Tuesdays:
3.	Wednesdays:
4.	Thursdays:
Concepts or examples I don't understand and need to ask someone about	Fridays:
	Saturdays:
1.	Sundays:
2.	
3.	
4.	

Where and When to Study

Different people prefer different places and times to study. You might prefer a quiet library, the comfort of your own home, or perhaps a bustling coffee shop. In addition to choosing a place that is comfortable, it is equally important to choose a study site that is effective. A balance between preference and practicality must be struck when deciding where to study. A similar balance should be considered when deciding when to study. Select a time when you are most alert and least distractible.

Tips

- **Check the lighting.** Adequate lighting will prevent you from struggling and straining while you read and will also help you stay awake and focused.
- **Check the temperature.** Your study environment should not be too hot or too cold, although a cooler room is preferable to one that is excessively warm. Warm temperatures can make you sleepy.
- **Check your posture.** Find a place with a supportive chair and working surface that encourage you to sit upright and attentive rather than slouching or too relaxed.
- **Have plenty of space.** Your study area should allow you to spread everything out in an orderly manner. Materials should be organized so that they can be accessed without a great deal of maneuvering. A plus would be to have a dedicated space where you could leave your things arranged safely and protective over time.
- **Avoid distractions.** Choose a study area in a place with few distractions. The more focused you are when studying, the more productive and effective the studying will be.
- **Study during your alert times.** If you are a morning person, schedule your studying early in the day. If you are an evening person, study at night. In either case, be sure to schedule your study time in way that does not interfere with your sleep.

Using Reading Strategies

Developing strategies for reading texts is the key to test preparation. It is especially important in using this study manual because of the large amount of information you will be reviewing. To retain more information, research suggests it is helpful to connect new content to prior information[5] as you read. Research also suggests that scanning for key words and taking notes will add to overall retention.[6] The more organized your study plan is, the more successful you will be at remembering what you have read.

Tips

- **Preview the text.** Before delving into the reading, read the introduction, summary, key terms and definitions, and any stated learning objectives.
- **Outline the text.** Outlining the text on a separate sheet of paper as you read keeps you focused on the content, helps you synthesize and internalize the material, and encourages your anticipation of what will come next in the text.
- **Underline topic sentences.** This will help you focus while you are reading and also identify key concepts to revisit when you go back through each section for review.
- **Annotate in the margin.** Note vocabulary words, key concepts, and your comments and questions in the margin of the text as you read. Interactive annotating keeps you engaged, helps you remember, and allows you to highlight key concepts and ideas as they are identified.

Test-Taking Strategies for Multiple-Choice

Remember that the TEAS is a multiple-choice test. There are specific test-taking strategies that can be used to improve your score on a multiple-choice test by helping to eliminate incorrect response choices.[7] For example, if a question has four potential answer options (i.e., A, B, C, or D), and only one of them is correct, there is an automatic 25% chance for you to select the right one. If you can eliminate one of those options, your chance of being right increases to 33%. If you can eliminate two wrong choices, your chance of being right increases to 50%.

Tips

- **Rule out wrong answers.** Use existing knowledge and what is presented in the text to identify obvious incorrect answers. Eliminate those and focus on those that remain.
- **Cover up the choices and answer the question yourself.** Given choices sometimes causes you to second-guess yourself. If you read the question first, there is a chance you might be able to answer it without looking at the answer choices. If that happens, when you do read the choices, you will be able to choose the option closest to your answer without being put off by the distractors, which are purposely included to meant to mislead you.
- **Recognize opposite response options.** Often, when two response choices oppose each other, it is an indication that one of them is probably the correct answer. Watch for these.
- **Look for absolute words.** Look for words that tend to make statements incorrect (e.g., "always," "never," "all," "only," "must," and "will"). Answer choices containing absolute or definitive words tend to be incorrect because they are limited and can only apply in specific situations or under certain circumstances.

---

[5]Raphael & Au, 2005
[6]Peverly et al., 2007; Raphael & Au, 2005; Terry, 2006; Titsworth & Kiewra, 2004; Williams & Eggert, 2002
[7]Paris et al., 1991

- **Look for absolute words.** Look for words that tend to make statements incorrect (e.g., "always," "never," "all," "only," "must," and "will"). Answer choices containing absolute or definitive words tend to be incorrect because they are limited and can only apply in specific situations or under certain circumstances.
- **Make educated guesses.** If you cannot decide which response choice is best, make an educated guess based on background knowledge, logic, and reasoning.
- **Work backward.** Sometimes, it helps to look at the answer options first and then read the question to see if any of the answers makes sense. This technique is especially useful for math questions.

Improving Your Score

Did you achieve the score you wanted on the practice test? If so, congratulations! If not, reevaluate your study approach and test-taking strategies. Which ones worked? Which ones did not? Research suggests that the more active strategies you incorporate into your studying, the better your performance will be in the long term.[8] Consider the following hands-on strategy tips to improve your study habits or your test score.

Tips

- **Implement new study strategies immediately.** If you are unhappy with your results, try a new study strategy right away.
- **Join a study group.** If you normally study alone, consider studying with others. Collaboration helps everyone.
- **If you are in a study group, assess how the group uses the study time.** Is the group mainly on task, or are there distractions, interruptions, or side conversations?
- **Seek other sources, including nontext sources.** If you need greater insight into a specific topic, seek out additional information online, consult with a tutor, or find supplemental texts to enhance your understanding.
- **Ask yourself questions that reinforce your learning.** For example, "If I had to teach this concept to another individual, how would I explain it?" or "If someone asked me to summarize this concept, what would I say?"
- **Consult an academic advisor if you are experiencing test anxiety and cannot manage it.** If you are experiencing extra tension or stress as a result of your time dedicated to test preparation, an advisor might be able to provide you with some extra tips to alleviate it.
- **Reevaluate your work and extracurricular schedule.** If you work or have extracurricular activities that interfere with your study schedule, consider reducing or rearranging your hours focused on these activities so that you can spend more time studying. Alternatively, try looking for additional opportunities to add studying time such as during a long commute, in place of watching television, or on a weekend afternoon when you have nothing else planned.

---

[8]Gettinger & Seibert, 2002

Reading

The following 19 chapters cover the tasks from the ATI TEAS test plan for the Reading unit. These are focused on assessment of functional literacy skills and are organized into three sections:

- Key ideas and details
- Craft and structure
- Integration of knowledge and ideas

The Reading unit tests your knowledge of reading concepts and your ability to apply those concepts. You will be required to read various types of reading passages – including fiction, nonfiction, informational, and graphical – and those passage will be of various lengths. Some passages will have as many as seven questions based on them. Your ability to synthesize the information you've read and to think critically will be essential to your success on the Reading unit of the ATI TEAS.

Each chapter in this unit introduces knowledge, skills, and abilities relevant to the Reading task and provides an overview of some essential topics, along with specific examples to highlight important concepts. Practice questions at the end of each chapter will allow you to test your knowledge of select concepts. In addition, there are key terms included at the end of each section and a practice Reading quiz at the end of the unit. This unit quiz includes the same number of questions as the Reading unit on the ATI TEAS and matches the test plan task allocations (shown below). The quiz will give you a good idea of the number and types of sources you will encounter and the questions that will accompany those sources. Keep in mind that these chapters are a great starting point and guide to your studies, but they are not an exhaustive review of all concepts that might be tested in the Reading unit of the ATI TEAS. You should use other sources (textbooks, online resources, etc.) for additional study and practice in areas that you haven't mastered.

The key ideas and details section includes items related to the comprehension of reading selections, complex text, printed communications, and graphical representations of information. The craft and structure section includes items related to evaluating an author's purpose and point of view, as well as interpreting the meanings of words phrases. Also included are items related to recognizing the structure of texts, distinguishing between fact and opinion, and identifying biases and stereotypes. Finally, the integration of knowledge and ideas section includes items assessing a student's ability to compare and contrast themes from different sources and to evaluate an argument and its specific claims. Students will also encounter items requiring them to use evidence from the text to make predictions and inferences and draw conclusions about a piece of writing, as well as integrate data from multiple sources.

There are 47 scored Reading items on the TEAS. These are divided as shown below. In addition, there will be six unscored pretest items that can be in any of these categories.

Section	Number of scored items on the ATI TEAS
Key ideas and details	22
Craft and structure	14
Integration of knowledge and ideas	11

CHAPTER

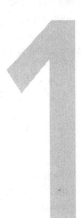

Summarize a complex text

 This objective includes, but is not limited to, the following examples of knowledge, skills, and abilities.

- Identify the topic.
- Identify key points.
- Rephrase key points.

Reading comprehension is a vital skill in all subject areas, and the ability to summarize a complex text is an important way to demonstrate comprehension. In order to comprehend a text, you must identify the topic and key points about the topic.

Identifying the Topic and Central Idea

The topic of a complex text is the subject of the entire piece of writing. The topic of a passage is often found at the beginning of the text in a topic sentence. Examples of topics in a nursing text might include blood poisoning, body organs, or blood pressure. Once you have identified the topic, you can then identify the main idea or purpose of the passage. To do this, answer the questions "What is the writer saying about the topic?" and "What is important to know about the topic?" For example, if the topic of a text is blood pressure, the main idea of the text could be how to measure blood pressure.

Identifying Key Points

In addition, the author will include key points, or supporting details, that support the main idea. For example, if the main idea is how to measure blood pressure, the key points will be steps to take to complete the measurement. Steps would include securing the blood pressure cuff and then tightening it.

Rephrasing Key Points

Once you have identified the topic, main idea, and key points, it is important to put those ideas in your own words. This will help you understand and remember what you've read. Practice reading a passage and describing its topic, main idea, and key points in one to three sentences. By rephrasing these key ideas in a shorter form, you are summarizing a complex text. For questions on this TEAS task, you will need to identify topics and key points and use that knowledge to summarize complex texts.

Summarizing a Complex Text

Read the following passage. Think about the topic and key points you would describe in order to summarize the passage.

 Sepsis occurs as a result of an infection. When the body is fighting an infection, it releases chemicals into the bloodstream, and if the body's response to these chemicals is unbalanced, sepsis can occur. This becomes potentially life-threatening because multiple organ systems can sustain damage. A further concern is the progression of sepsis into septic shock. This can result in dramatic drops in blood pressure, with the final outcome being possible death.

First, identify the topic and main idea. Because the topic is the general subject of a passage, it helps to practice asking the following question about the topic sentence: "What am I reading about?" Ask yourself that question about the following topic sentence.

 Sepsis occurs as a result of an infection.

The following box shows how the topic can be retrieved from asking the question.

Question	Topic
What am I reading about?	Sepsis

Next, ask the second question: "What is important to know about the topic?"

Question	Main Idea
What is important to know about the topic?	Sepsis can happen after an infection.

Once a reader has identified the topic and main idea, it is essential to be able to identify and rephrase the key points. A key question to ask is "What are the key points about the topic, and how do these points illustrate the topic sentence?"

The key points in the passage illustrate the topic sentence by describing what sepsis is and how it affects the body.

Next, a reader must be able to identify the key points about the topic and then notice the details about those key points.

Key Points	Details
body fighting an infection	body releases chemicals into bloodstream
body has unbalanced response	sepsis can occur
life-threatening	damage to multiple organ systems
septic shock, drops in blood pressure	possible death

Finally, it is time to rephrase the key points to help you understand the topic and main idea. This will result in a summary of a complex text. Evaluate the key points and rephrase. Following is one summary of the example passage that rephrases the main idea and key points.

Sepsis occurs when the body fights an infection by releasing chemicals into the bloodstream, causing the body to have an unbalanced response. Sepsis can become life-threatening when organ systems sustain damage, further resulting in septic shock and possibly death.

CHAPTER 1 PRACTICE PROBLEMS

Read the following passage. Then answer the questions.

Many jobs can be dangerous, and accidents can result in serious injury, infection, and sepsis. Consider this case: Clement is a welder and metal fabricator, and about a week ago, a large, hot metal chip landed in his lap. It burned through his pants and embedded itself in his thigh. Although he was able to remove the metal from his leg, his boss took him to the emergency room for treatment of the burn injury to his upper thigh. A couple days later, however, Clement didn't feel well when he woke up; he had a fever and was sweating. The injury from the burn seemed to be infected, as it was swollen, painful, and hot to the touch. Because Clement felt light-headed and experienced shortness of breath and a faster-than-normal heart rate, his wife took him back to the ER, where the doctor determined that Clement's burn had indeed become infected, resulting in sepsis. The doctor applied additional treatment to the burn while also administering intravenous fluids and monitoring his blood pressure, which had dropped lower than normal. In addition, Clement had to begin a course of antibiotics to battle the sepsis to ensure that he would recover fully.

1. Which of the following titles best describes the topic of the passage?
   A. The Dangers of Welding
   B. A Case Study of Sepsis
   C. Burns and Infection
   D. How to Avoid Septic Shock

2. Which of the following is the central idea of the passage?
   A. Welding safety tips
   B. Going to the ER
   C. Symptoms and treatment of sepsis
   D. Characteristics of sepsis

3. Which of the following is a key point describing a symptom of sepsis?
   A. Burned skin
   B. Slow heart rate
   C. Shortness of breath
   D. High blood pressure

4. Which of the following is a key point describing the cause of sepsis?
   A. Infection
   B. Hot metal
   C. Fever
   D. Burned skin

5. In one to three sentences, write a summary of the complex text above.

Notes:

_____

_____

_____

_____

_____

_____

_____

_____

_____

_____

_____

_____

_____

_____

_____

_____

_____

_____

_____

_____

_____

_____

CHAPTER

Infer the logical conclusion from a reading selection

This objective includes, but is not limited to, the following examples of knowledge, skills, and abilities.

- Use inferences based on information given.
- Identify key terms justifying the events selected.
- Assemble events identified and associated with the inferred information to draw a conclusion.

Whether you are reading an informational text, procedure, news article, or story, having the ability to infer logical conclusions based on what you've read is a true test of your comprehension. To prepare for this TEAS task, use key points that provide information about the topic and events described. Then practice asking yourself, "What can I infer or decide about the topic based on what I've just read?"

Inferences

An inference is an idea about a topic based on evidence and reasoning. In order to make an inference about a topic, you need to pay attention to the key points and key terms used to describe the topic. Critical readers make sense of passages by evaluating the information provided. Strong readers also use individual experiences, in addition to the text, to construct meaning. In order to use the text, the reader must observe facts, delineate arguments, and discern valid information provided by the author. Then the reader must combine what the author has provided with individual experiences to draw an inference or idea about the passage. An inference is reading between the lines of what is stated. In other words, it is applying logic and experience to facts and evidence in a passage to build an idea about the topic.

Key Terms

Identifying key terms is critical to understanding the content and context of a given passage. Key terms include those that provide sequence or chronology, descriptive words and phrases, and words that convey value judgments and opinion. These key terms can provide both explicit information and the implicit information that allows the reader to make inferences. Take this example:

 In the past, hospital nurses could only check patient vital signs by hand, which required precision and more frequent checks. Today, however, there are a variety of monitors that can help nurses ensure that patients are stable constantly.

We can infer from the passage that previously nurses had to perform procedures on hospital patients more often to check vital signs based on the key terms related to chronology. We can also infer that today technology makes monitoring patients much easier and more efficient. We can conclude from these inferences that monitoring patients in hospitals has improved because nurses have a variety of tools to assist them.

Conclusions

Many readers assume that making an inference and drawing a conclusion are the same. Each activity demands that a reader fill in some blanks. However, there is a subtle difference between the two. An inference is suggesting an idea based upon details and evidence that are not directly stated in the passage. A conclusion asks the reader to analyze the passage and make a judgment based on details, evidence, and inferences. Following is an example of using inferences (**clues in bold**) to **draw a conclusion**.

 The boxer stood in the corner of the ring, looking out over the **roaring crowd** and eyeing her **tenacious** opponent, who at that very moment pointed to her with a **snarl**. **As she waited for the sound of the bell to signal the final round, sweat stung her eyes, and her muscles tensed.**

Conclusion: The boxer is in the final round of a difficult match. We can infer that her opponent is tough and angry because of key terms such as "tenacious" and "snarl." One conclusion is that the boxer is exhausted but ready to begin the final round as she is sweating and her muscles are tense. We can also conclude that it is an exciting match because of the "roaring crowd"!

CHAPTER 2 PRACTICE PROBLEMS

Read the following passage. Then answer the questions.

After graduating from high school, Danielle decided that she wanted to follow in her grandmother's footsteps and become a nurse. Her grandmother had been a pioneer in caring for premature babies. She had developed many of the procedures used in neonatal care. Danielle enrolled in her community college's associate degree in nursing program. She worked hard and completed the program in four semesters. As Danielle approached her graduation date, she learned about the nursing residency program at a nearby hospital. Danielle was especially intrigued by the "transition to practice" philosophy of the nursing residency program. This would allow her to gain professional experience and develop real hands-on nursing skills. The next enrollment period for the program would begin soon after graduation. This meant she would be eligible to apply. However, she would also need to complete cardiopulmonary resuscitation (CPR) and basic life support (BLS) training as another requirement for joining the program. As she applied for the program, she reviewed the list of specialized areas of nursing offered. She dreamed of the day she could become a nurse in neonatal intensive care.

1. Based on key points in the passage, when could Danielle apply for the nursing residency program?

   A. After enrollment in an associate degree in nursing program
   B. After graduation from nursing school and completion of CPR/BLS training
   C. After demonstrating understanding of the "transition to practice" philosophy
   D. After choosing a specialized area of nursing in the program

2. Which of the following phrases helps the reader understand the order of events in this passage?

   A. after graduating from high school
   B. follow in her grandmother's footsteps
   C. transition to practice
   D. become a nurse

3. Using key terms, infer how long it took Danielle to complete her degree in nursing.

   A. Four years
   B. Three years
   C. Two years
   D. One year

4. Which patients would Danielle care for as a neonatal intensive care nurse?

   A. Elderly men and women
   B. Premature or critically ill newborn infants
   C. Adults requiring surgery
   D. Children with severe burns or missing limbs

5. Using evidence from the passage, draw a conclusion about the philosophy of "transition to practice." Then explain the evidence used to draw that conclusion.

Notes:

_____

_____

_____

_____

_____

_____

_____

_____

_____

_____

_____

_____

_____

_____

_____

_____

_____

_____

_____

_____

_____

_____

CHAPTER

3

Identify the topic, main idea, and supporting details

 This objective includes, but is not limited to, the following examples of knowledge, skills, and abilities.

- Determine the topic.
- Determine the main idea.
- Explain how supporting details support the main idea.

Critical reading demands that you become a selective consumer of text. Just like comparing essential versus nonessential ingredients when shopping for healthy foods, a reader must identify the topic and the author's main idea and then delineate the author's key points that support the topic. Ultimately, the reader must demonstrate comprehension of a text by explaining how supporting details clarify the main idea.

To succeed on this TEAS task, practice asking yourself, "What is the topic, and what is the author's main idea about that topic?" Then examine the supporting details provided by the author and determine how they relate to the main idea.

Determining the Topic and the Main Idea

To prepare for this section of the exam, locate the topic sentence and identify the main idea. The topic answers the question "Who or what is this paragraph about?" The topic should appear near the beginning of the paragraph and include the main idea. A topic sentence must not be too specific or too general.

 With its numerous specializations, nursing is an important career to pursue, especially in light of the current nursing shortage.

Notice that this topic sentence is not too specific (does not describe the specializations) nor too general (addresses nursing as a career rather than all medical careers).

To identify the main idea, read the entire passage. Then locate the sentence(s) that emphasize, elaborate, or clarify this information.

Explaining How Supporting Details Support the Main Idea

Supporting details develop—through explanation, elaboration, or clarification—the main idea of a text. One way to identify the supporting or key ideas is to ask the following of the topic sentence: who, what, when, where, why, and how?

 In the following example, the combination of key ideas clarifies which specializations nurses may choose that best help fill the nursing shortage.

Registered nurses (RNs) are the first and most in demand among nursing careers. They are the most flexible because of their ability to specialize in many areas and to work in various medical settings. For instance, RNs may become travel nurses to fill in wherever their services are required. They can work for different periods of time, ranging from weeks to years. Intensive care unit (ICU) nurses, also called critical care nurses, are essential providers of care in general hospitals as well as specialty units, such as neonatal intensive care units (NICUs).

Just as important as identifying the key ideas is discerning between relevant and irrelevant details. The relevant details relate back to the topic sentence and support the main idea of the text. Irrelevant statements are unrelated and, at times, random.

The **bolded** statements in the following example are irrelevant to the topic of the duties of a NICU nurse.

 NICU nurses provide specialized care for either premature infants or newborns who are critically ill. These compassionate and specially trained nurses provide both required medical attention and comfort for these tiny patients. **Some nurses may choose to work instead with children or teens.** But NICU nurses who desire to work with these newborns, the most vulnerable patient population, must earn additional certifications. **Still other nurses may choose to work in labor and delivery with pregnant mothers to help bring newborns into the world.**

CHAPTER 3 PRACTICE PROBLEMS

Read the following passage. Then answer the questions.

> The heart and cardiovascular system operate in the body in a similar way that the engine does in a car. Just as a car engine requires regular tune–ups, so does the human body. Regular exercise provides numerous benefits for optimal heart health. Among these are lower blood pressure, reduced inflammation in the body, and a healthier body weight. Most importantly, a lifestyle that includes regular, consistent exercise can help reduce the chance of cardiac events. For instance, exercise helps blood circulate more effectively so the heart does not need to work as hard to pump blood to the muscles. To keep the heart healthy, the most effective exercise routine should include both aerobic activities and resistance training with moderate weights.

1. What is the topic of this passage?
   A. Car engine tune-ups
   B. Cardiovascular system
   C. Exercise for heart health
   D. Cardiac events

2. Which sentence summarizes the topic?
   A. Regular exercise provides numerous benefits for optimal heart health.
   B. To keep the heart healthy, the most effective exercise routine should include both aerobic activities and resistance training with moderate weights.
   C. Most importantly, a lifestyle that includes regular, consistent exercise can help reduce the chance of cardiac events.
   D. For instance, exercise helps blood circulate more effectively so the heart does not need to work as hard to pump blood to the muscles.

3. How does the summary sentence support the main topic?
   A. It explains the similarity between car engines and the human heart.
   B. It defines cardiac events that can occur without proper care.
   C. It illustrates the function of the cardiovascular system.
   D. It describes types of exercises to keep the heart healthy

4. Reread the passage. Which phrase is a supporting detail?
   A. exercise helps blood circulate more effectively
   B. a car engine requires regular tune-ups
   C. reduce the chance of cardiac events
   D. reduced inflammation in the body

5. In one to two sentences, explain how the supporting detail you chose supports the main idea.

Notes:

_____

_____

_____

_____

_____

_____

_____

_____

_____

_____

_____

_____

_____

_____

_____

_____

_____

_____

_____

_____

_____

CHAPTER

4
Follow a given set of directions

 This objective includes, but is not limited to, the following examples of knowledge, skills, and abilities.

- Recognize the relationship among steps in a procedure.
- Identify key terms that signify order.
- Follow question directives, such as "choose all that apply."

Readers and writers encounter procedural documents in all areas of learning. Procedural documents are sequential, and they involve step-by-step guidance for certain tasks. For example, engineering students read procedural programs, nursing students read pain management procedures, and biology students read laboratory procedures. All readers, in daily life, should be prepared to read and properly follow procedures. Procedures can be found in any text, from recipes to vehicle manuals to do-it-yourself articles. This genre of sequential information offers readers the ability to safely, efficiently, and effectively complete activities. For the TEAS, you will need to demonstrate the ability to follow directions by identifying important terms and recognizing the relationships among delineated tasks.

Recognizing the Relationship Among Steps in a Procedure

Procedural texts are composed of specific language features and structures. These help create the organization and comprehension procedural texts require. The language features include signal words that assist the reader in recognizing the relationship among steps, and simple, objective language. Objective language is impartial, nonjudgmental, nonpersonal, and nonemotional.

For instance, when you decided to pursue a nursing degree, you had to follow certain steps in a specific order to get enrolled in a nursing program. The following words are terms that indicate order and sequence.

Procedural Signal Words			
first	second	next	last
then	finally	while	before
second	now	when	after

Read the following paragraph, and look for the words that signify order in **bold**.

When you are considering enrolling in a nursing program, your **first** step would include doing some research into which schools offered nursing degrees as well as the nursing specializations of interest to you. **Next** you might contact a few of the schools to ask questions and get clarification **before** applying to the program of your choice. **While** filling out program applications, you might have also filled out your Free Application for Federal Student Aid (FAFSA). **Then** you would wait **before** receiving responses from each school. **Finally**, you would make a choice about which school to attend.

Following Question Directives

Once a reader identifies all signal words and steps of a procedure, it is important to follow all directions. Directions are very specific, using language that tells how to accomplish the steps.

Some examples of these are listed in the following box.

From top to bottom	Carefully and with
After you have completed	Choose all that apply
Simultaneously, you can	Before moving on

Following the example of filling out applications, you might see instructions such as these: "Read the form **from top to bottom** before filling it out. Then **carefully and with** attention to detail, fill out the form. From the courses listed, **choose all that apply** to your nursing specialization."

The most common types of procedural texts include steps in an activity and steps in operating a system or object. The most common features of procedural writing include headings/subheadings; numbering/alphabetizing steps; and charts, diagrams, and photographs for clarification of steps.

For example, when filling out the FAFSA, you will see headings and subheadings such as these.

Create an ID

Gather Application Documents

    Social Security number

    Driver's license number

    Federal income tax information

CHAPTER 4 PRACTICE PROBLEMS

Read the following passage about a procedure a nurse must complete. Then answer the questions.

1. First, explain the intravenous (IV) catheter insertion procedure to the patient.

2. Next, determine if the patient has needle phobia, and if so, keep the needle out of sight until the last minute.

3. While using a soothing tone, encourage the patient to not watch the procedure.

4. Before inserting the IV catheter, follow infection control protocol by wearing gloves and swabbing the injection site with an alcohol pad.

5. When preparing to insert the catheter, look for a suitable vein in the patient's nondominant hand.

6. If a vein is not immediately visible, carefully use your fingers to locate a suitable vein.

7. Next, advance the needle slowly and carefully until you feel resistance.

8. Finally, upon successful insertion of the IV catheter, secure it with medical tape.

1. Which procedure is described in the passage?

A. Infection control protocol
B. IV catheter insertion
C. Location of suitable veins
D. Assessment of needle phobia

2. How are the steps in the passage related?

A. They all describe steps in IV catheter insertions.
B. They address patients with needle phobias.
C. They provide step-by-step directions.
D. They include procedural signal words.

3. What are key terms in the passage that signify order?

A. first, when, before
B. follow, insert, look
C. carefully use, secure it
D. advance the needle slowly

4. Which key term identifies a step occurring along with another step in a procedure?

A. next
B. before
C. while
D. finally

5. List one direction given in the procedural steps.

Notes:

_____

_____

_____

_____

_____

_____

_____

_____

_____

_____

_____

_____

_____

_____

_____

_____

_____

_____

_____

CHAPTER

5 Identify specific information from a printed communication

 This objective includes, but is not limited to, the following examples of knowledge, skills, and abilities.

- Use printed communications (e.g., memos, posted announcements, classified ads).
- Find relevant information.
- Recognize various parts of printed communications.

The word "communication" is based on the Latin root "communis." This root means to make common, impart, inform, and share. And that is exactly what you do when you communicate with someone. You share information!

Printed communication, such as memos, announcements, and advertisements, fulfills this definition. Many types of printed communication inform people about needed information. This information is shared with the people who need it. It is beneficial to understand how to discern relevant information and recognize the text structures of printed communication. The TEAS will test how well you can find the information you need from these types of communications.

Using Printed Communications

A memo is a type of informal and concise printed communication. Even though it is informal, it still must be grammatically correct. The formal format results from the audience usually being internal (business staff members, school colleagues, etc.). Correct conventions are important because the information is usually business oriented.

See the following sample memo and descriptions.

Memorandum

To: Recipient(s)

From: Author of the memo and title

Date: Date memo is shared

Re: The subject of the memo

Introductory: Informs the readers of the specific context of the memo.

Each body section should start with a strong, concise statement (claim) that informs the reader of the important information. Readers only want the important information and nothing extra.

Concluding Section: Includes strong rephrased takeaway information. This section can also include where to address any questions or concerns. There is no need to mention the author's name. The author is mentioned in the heading.

Finding Relevant Information and Recognizing Various Parts of Printed Communications

Printed Public Announcements

Memos are one way to get information to a group of people. Another way to do this efficiently is by posting announcements, such as public announcements. You've probably seen examples around your school or neighborhood. These come in various forms, but they have a few key basic elements.

Public announcements inform the public about organizations, upcoming events, and services. The message must be short, the design simple and appealing, and the important information easily accessible. The content should include a link to information access, information about the supporting organizations, and supporting details. The supporting details should be in images and short phrases if possible.

See the example and descriptions.

IT'S FLU SEASON!

Protect yourself and others. [The message]

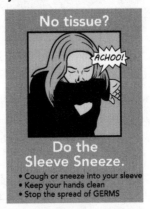

Sneeze into your sleeve. [Supporting detail]

For more tips, visit https://www.cdc.gov/flu/prevent/actions-prevent-flu.htm [Link for more info]

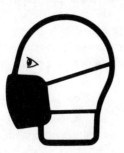

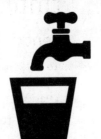

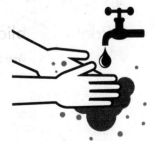

Wear a mask when in large groups. [Supporting detail]

Drink plenty of water. [Supporting detail]

Wash your hands. [Supporting detail]

Classified Advertisements

The classified advertisement is a short, detailed text offering items and services. Print and online newspapers, magazines, blogs, and forums usually charge by the word or line. Therefore, a reader can find the following information within a very small space.

- A headline that grabs the reader's attention (can be a rhetorical question, bold statement, or exclamation)
- An item or service offered to the audience (mentions the benefits of the item or service)
- A call to action (includes how to get the item or service)

 See this sample and description of an online classified advertisement.

Need a new profile picture for your nurse ID badge? [*Heading to attract specific audience*]

Sign up for a time slot convenient for you. [*Benefits to customers*]

Choose from a variety of settings. [*Benefits to customers*]

Please email NursePhotog@ID-Badges.org. [*Call to action provides information about next step*]

CHAPTER 5 PRACTICE PROBLEMS

Read the following memo. Then answer the first three questions.

Memorandum

To: NICU Nurses

From: Rena B., RN, Nursing Supervisor

Date: January 1, 2020

Re: New Year Handwashing Reminder for Proper Infection Control

Introductory: Happy 2020 to all! As we begin this new year—and we have many new NICU nurses and nursing students among us—let's review proper handwashing procedures that we are all required to follow.

Our patients are among the most vulnerable population in the hospital, and they deserve our utmost attention to proper infection control. There are no excuses for not abiding by this rule. Handwashing is the first and most important step we can take to prevent the spread of pathogens or the transfer of infections to our patients.

Handwashing is one essential part of proper hand hygiene. You must use running water in a sink, rather than a basin, and use soap, either regular or antibacterial. For at least 30 seconds, rub your hands with your palms together, and then wash around the tops of your hands and between your fingers. Keep your fingernails short to avoid having bacteria gather under them. If you wear rings, keep them on and wash them at the same time you wash your hands. Use disposable paper towels to dry your hands and then to turn off the faucet.

Concluding Section: Remember, proper handwashing is absolutely essential to avoid transferring infections or spreading pathogens among our vulnerable patients. This is NOT an option, and I expect everyone to diligently follow proper handwashing procedures.

If you have any questions or concerns, please review the handwashing poster available in the break room or contact me or your shift nurse.

Thank you.

1. What is the main point of this memo?

    A. It welcomes new nurses and nursing students.
    B. It informs nurses of their patient population's needs.
    C. It announces the handwashing poster and steps.
    D. It reminds nurses that they must wash their hands properly.

2. How long should nurses wash their hands?

    A. At least 1 minute
    B. At least 30 seconds
    C. More than 45 seconds
    D. More than 2 minutes

3. What patient population resides in the NICU?

    A. Elderly men and women with cancer or other debilitating diseases
    B. Pregnant women and those who have just given birth
    C. Infants born prematurely or who have serious illnesses
    D. Children with severe burns, deformities, or other physical challenges

Read the items listed in the table about elements included in different types of communication. Then answer the questions.

Email to schedule photo session for nurse ID tag	Reminder of handwashing procedures
Steps for inserting an IV properly	Details supporting an upcoming emergency drill
Directions for completing a patient profile	Benefits of following HIPAA regulations

4. Which item would be included in a public announcement?

    A. Steps for inserting an IV properly
    B. Details supporting an upcoming emergency drill
    C. Directions for completing a patient profile
    D. Benefits of following HIPAA regulations

5. Which item would be included in an online classified advertisement?

    A. Reminder of handwashing procedures
    B. Steps for inserting an IV properly
    C. Details supporting an upcoming emergency drill
    D. Email to schedule photo session for nurse ID tag

Notes:

_____

_____

_____

_____

_____

_____

_____

_____

_____

_____

_____

_____

_____

_____

_____

_____

_____

_____

_____

_____

_____

_____

CHAPTER

6 Identify information from a graphic representation of information

 This objective includes, but is not limited to, the following examples of knowledge, skills, and abilities.

- Read a graphic representation (e.g., map, pictograph).
- Identify relevant information.
- Recognize visuals, graphics, and figures within the text.
- Locate the important information from a graphic representation.

Graphic representations, such as maps, are important features for many texts. Graphic and pictorial images allow readers to comprehend important verbal and written ideas quickly and easily. Most graphic representations include titles and subheads that summarize complex information. Graphics can also assist readers in selecting important information that might otherwise be missing by portraying the key parts that make up a whole. Graphic representations include bar, pie, and flow charts; graphs; maps; and illustrations. When you take the TEAS, you will likely be tested on your knowledge of these tools and your ability to interpret the information they provide.

Reading a Graphic Representation and Identifying Relevant Information

Graphic representations can illustrate diverse topics and designs, but common features include titles, subheads, keys/legends, and scales. As you learn how to read maps, pictures, and graphs, you will sharpen and replicate the skills needed to read information.

Look at the following table to identify the relevant degrees needed for each type of nursing position.

Nursing Positions	Degrees Required
Registered nurse (RN)	ADN or BSN
ICU nurse	BSN preferred CCRN certification
Home health nurse	Nursing diploma or ADN or BSN
Nurse case manager	BSN or MSN
Clinical nurse specialist	MSN or PhD

Recognizing Visuals, Graphics, and Figures Within the Text

One must be able to identify the features in graphic representations just as readers must identify elements when reading informational texts.

Look at the following map of a college campus. Then refer back to it for the remainder of the lesson.

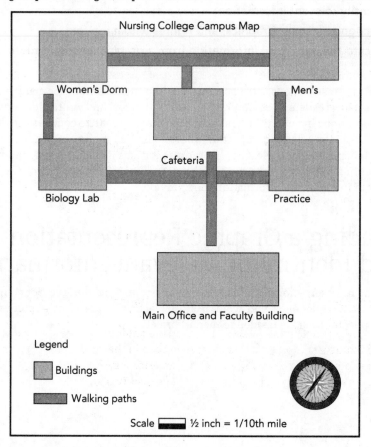

Features of Graphic Representations

Maps come in many sizes and shapes, but most include the common elements of titles, legends, and scales. The title communicates the purpose of the map. The legend clarifies what each symbol, color, or shape represents. Lastly, the scale represents the distance between points. The nursing college campus map provides an example of map features.

Locating the Important Information from a Graphic Representation

The features on the map tell readers that the length of the scale ruler is 1/10th mile. The legend combined with the title tells the reader that the map illustrates the location of buildings on the nursing college campus. The features on the legend—buildings, walking paths—demonstrate the accessibility of each building via the walking paths.

Practice

Which of the following statements is accurate based on the map?

A. The compass indicates that the practice clinic is southeast of the main office and faculty building.
B. The men's dorm is southwest of the cafeteria.
C. The women's dorm is northeast of the cafeteria.
D. The biology lab is northwest of the men's dorm.

Rationales

Option A is correct because the main office and faculty building are at the south end of the map and the practice clinic is accessible by traveling in a southeastern direction.

Option B is incorrect because the men's dorm is northeast of the cafeteria.
Option C is incorrect because the women's dorm is northwest of the cafeteria.
Option D is incorrect because the biology lab is southwest of the men's dorm.

Pictorial Representations

Pictorial representations come in many designs that depend on the purpose and content. Interpreting these involves many of the same skills required in reading informational writing. For example, a pictorial graph usually includes a combination of titles, subheads, summaries, descriptions, images representing ideas, content vocabulary, steps in a process, and data. Sometimes, this information will already be analyzed for the readers. But more likely, the representation requires a reader's understanding and analysis.

The following is an example of some of the features of pictorial representations.

Practice

Which of the following is indicated by this illustration?

A. The coracoclavicular ligament is seen in the anterior view of the shoulder.
B. The thoracoacromial artery and vein are seen in the posterior view of the shoulder.
C. The suprascapular nerve is seen in the anterior view of the shoulder.
D. The coracohumeral ligament is seen in the disarticulated view of the shoulder.

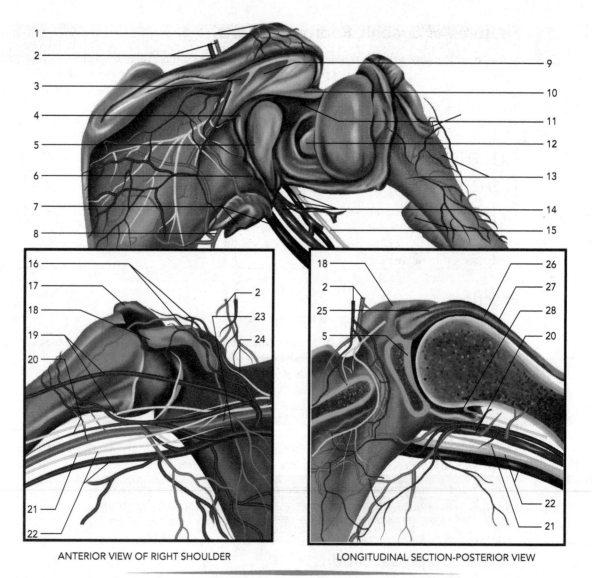

ANTERIOR VIEW OF RIGHT SHOULDER

LONGITUDINAL SECTION-POSTERIOR VIEW

1 Acromial branches of thoracoacromial artery and vein
2 Transverse scapular artery and vein
3 Coracoelavicular ligament (conoid portion)
4 Glenoidal lip: branch of supraseapular nerve
5 Glenoid cavity
6 Cut edge of articular capsule
7 Long head of triceps brachii: basilic vein
8 Scapular cireumflex artery and vein

9 Coracoclavicular ligament (trapezoid portion)
10 Cut edge of coracohumeral ligament
11 Tendon of long head of biceps brachii: anterior humeral circumflex artery and vein
12 Tendon of subscapularis
13 Posteror humeral circumflex artery and vein: teres minor muscle
14 Acillary nerve: brachial artery and vein
15 Radial nerve: teres major muscle
16 Thoracoacromial artery and vein
17 Acromion

18 Coracoid process
19 Cephalic vein: museculoeutaneous nerve
20 Brachial artery and vein
21 Median nerve
22 Ulnar nerve: basilic vein
23 Axillary artery and vein
24 Suprascapular nerve
25 Coracohumeral ligament
26 Tendon of long head of biceps brachii
27 Intertubercular mucous sheath
28 Articular capsule

Rationales

Option C is correct because the illustration shows that the suprascapular nerve is labeled number 24 in the anterior view of the shoulder.

Option A is not correct because the illustration shows the coracoclavicular ligament is labeled numbers 3 and 9 in the posterior view of the shoulder.

Option B is not correct because the illustration shows the thoracoacromial artery and vein are labeled number 16 in the anterior view of the shoulder.

Option D is not correct because the illustration shows the coracohumeral ligament is labeled number 25 in the posterior view of the shoulder.

CHAPTER 6 PRACTICE PROBLEMS

Use the information on the infographic to answer the questions.

Occupational Outlook for Registered Nurses

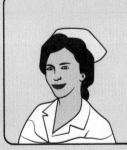

Career Projections
*Projected to grow
12 percent
from 2020 to 2028,
much faster than the
average for
all occupations,
from 3 million to
3.4 million

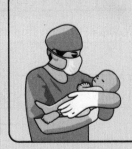

Education requirements
Minimum: Associate
Degree in Nursing (ADN)
Preferred: Bachelor of
Science in Nursing (BSN)

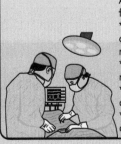

Areas of Greatest Demand
for RNs
*Aging population in need
of home health care or
residential care facilities
*Patients in long-term care
rehabilitation facilities
*Patients in outpatient
care centers
*Patients in ambulatory
care settings

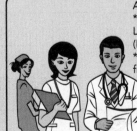

Additional Requirements
*Pass the National Council
Licensure Examinations
(NCLEX-RN)
*Receive nursing license
from state board of nursing

*Statistics from US Bureau of Labor Statistics

1. What does the number range "3 million to 3.4 million" represent?

   A. Increase in nursing graduates by 2028
   B. 12% projected growth in nursing careers
   C. Increase in nursing licenses awarded
   D. 10% projected nurse career openings

2. Which is the preferred nursing degree?

   A. ADN
   B. NCLEX
   C. MSN
   D. BSN

3. Which patients will demand greater nursing care in residential care facilities?

   A. Youth population
   B. Patients requiring rehabilitation
   C. Aging population
   D. Patients requiring ambulatory care

4. What is the NCLEX?

   A. Nursing Committee Licensing Exam
   B. National Council Licensure Examination
   C. Nursing Coalition for Licensing Expertise
   D. National Corporation Licensure Excellence

5. From which organization does a nurse receive a nursing license?

   A. State nursing board
   B. Local hospital
   C. Medical facility
   D. Healthcare nursing board

Notes:

_____

_____

_____

_____

_____

_____

_____

_____

_____

_____

_____

_____

_____

_____

_____

_____

_____

_____

_____

_____

_____

_____

CHAPTER

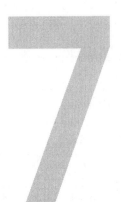

Recognize events in a sequence

 This objective includes, but is not limited to, the following examples of knowledge, skills, and abilities.

- Understand the concept of sequence.
- Locate the words or phrases that indicate sequence of events (e.g., "first," "second," "third").
- Identify language that indicates time (e.g., "today," "tomorrow")

Sequence refers to order and pattern. Recognizing sequence is beneficial because it helps with remembering information, understanding a text, and analyzing information for better comprehension. One thing to consider is the subtle difference between sequential and chronological ordering within text.

Sequential refers to a fixed order in which there is a consistent, logical pattern. Pages in a book, for example, are sequential, as are steps in a process. Chronological refers to time order where events are ordered in the way they happen. For this TEAS task, you will need to understand these concepts and be able to interpret the words and phrases that create sequence.

Understanding the Concept of Sequence

In order to find meaning in text, it is crucial to understand how to find and order the events or ideas. Each event or idea must follow a predetermined order or sequence to ensure the desired outcome is achieved. For instance, onboarding a patient involves a process and sequence of steps that begins with registration and ends with discharge and, finally, billing.

Signal words assist a reader with fitting smaller parts of the text into a larger context. This means it is easier to understand and follow the correct sequence of events by paying attention to the signal words.

Locating the Words or Phrases That Indicate Sequence of Events

Sequential order is signaled by words such as the following.

first	second	next	last
then	finally	while	before
second	now	when	after
at the beginning	prior to	afterward	subsequently

Following is an example of a passage with sequential order words **bolded**.

Marcus, an RN at a children's hospital, offered to work a shift for a fellow nurse, Roberta. **First**, Marcus asked what hours Roberta needed to have him cover. **Then** Marcus got approval from their nursing supervisor to cover the shift for Roberta. **Prior to** working that shift, **Marcus** learned about Roberta's patients. **Subsequently**, Marcus was able to effectively meet the needs of those patients.

Due to the use of sequence signal words, there is no question about the logical order of Marcus's preparations to cover Roberta's shift.

Chronological Signal Words

Chronological signal words describe when one event occurs and ends and when another event begins. Readers must be aware of these terms, which function as adverbs. They refer to when something happened, how often an event occurs, or for the length time an event occurs.

The following is a list of adverbs that signal the above chronological events.

When	How Often	Length of Time
today	always	all month
tomorrow	frequently	all season
earlier	occasionally	all week
now	never	since
last month	seldom	two hours

Following is an example of a passage with chronological order words **bolded**.

Since the beginning of the new year, the senior class of nurses had looked forward to their spring pinning ceremony that **always** accompanied the graduation ceremony. Over the **last year**, they had wrapped up their final courses and completed their practicums. They **often** thought about how they would **one day** work in their respective nursing fields. **Finally**, graduation day had arrived, and **now** the nurses could celebrate their success and eagerly look forward to beginning their nursing careers.

Chronological signal words are essential in assisting readers in keeping track of occasions in narratives and informational texts, such as passages relaying historical events. In the preceding passage, you learned about an event that the graduating class of nurses was anticipating. The time signals help keep all the events in sequential order and make more sense.

CHAPTER 7 PRACTICE PROBLEMS

Read the following passage. Then answer the questions.

> Prior to graduating from high school, Tim knew he wanted to become a registered nurse (RN). In fact, he often imagined himself working as a nurse practitioner one day like the healthcare professional who cared for him and his family. Tim then talked to his nurse practitioner to determine the path he needed to take to fulfill his career goal. He learned that he must first choose one of three ways to become a registered nurse: a nursing diploma program, an associate degree in nursing (ADN), or a bachelor of science in nursing (BSN). Tim also learned that nursing students often begin with the diploma or ADN. They can then later participate in an RN-to-BSN program, known as a bridge program, while they gain experience working as nurses. This seemed to be a good plan, since he could start his career sooner. Finally, Tim learned that he would subsequently need to earn his master of science in nursing (MSN) degree in order to become a nurse practitioner.

1. Which words or phrases from the passage indicate sequential order?

   A. one day
   B. prior to
   C. later
   D. often

2. Which words or phrases from the passage are chronological signal words?

   A. since
   B. subsequently
   C. prior to
   D. then

3. Which phrase appears to be out of sequence?

   A. Tim then talked to his nurse practitioner
   B. he must first choose one of three ways
   C. he could start his career sooner
   D. later participate in an RN-to-BSN program

4. Which is the correct sequence of degrees needed to become a nurse practitioner?

   A. Nursing diploma, MSN, BSN
   B. MSN, BSN, ADN
   C. ADN, nursing diploma, MSN
   D. ADN, BSN, MSN

5. What is the bridge program?

   A. Nursing diploma to MSN
   B. RN to BSN
   C. BSN to MSN
   D. RN to DSN

Notes:

CHAPTER

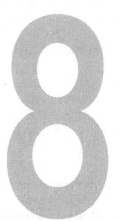

Distinguish between fact and opinion, biases, and stereotypes

 This objective includes, but is not limited to, the following examples of knowledge, skills, and abilities.

- Recognize factual writing as supported by evidence.
- Recognize author's point of view (POV) in a text (fact, opinion, biases, stereotypes).
- Recognize author's tone.
- Define stereotype and bias.
- Compare and contrast fact and opinion.

One of the challenges readers face is to understand a writer's point of view. To identify point of view, readers need to recognize fact and opinion, biases, and stereotypes. Word choice develops a tone or feeling toward a topic. Becoming aware of the tone, word choice, biases or stereotypes, and the use of fact or opinion allows a reader to evaluate critically an author's point of view. In this TEAS task, you will analyze these aspects of various pieces of writing.

Recognizing Factual Writing

Presenting facts in writing requires providing evidence to support those facts. This is especially important when making an argument. The evidence must be credible and appropriate to the topic. Evidence can be found in reliable sources and incorporated in a number of ways.

Review the following table to consider the types of sources that can provide evidence for your ideas. This table also provides methods that can be incorporated as evidence in your writing.

Types of Sources	Methods of Citing Sources
Print and electronic sources	Quotations
Observation	Paraphrasing
Interviews	Summarizing
Surveys	Statistics and data
Experiments	Charts and graphs
Personal experience	Photographs and illustrations

Recognizing Point of View and Tone

Point of view is an author's opinion or beliefs about a topic. It is important to understand the author's point of view to understand a text and how different writers approach the same topic. There are several ways to identify point of view. First, locate the topic of a text. Next, determine what ideas and evidence the writer presents about the topic. Last, consider the ideas and evidence to determine the writer's opinion. That is the writer's point of view.

An author's tone in writing is similar to the tone of voice a person may use when speaking. "Tone" is the writer's attitude toward a topic or general feeling about a topic. Point of view is an opinion, and tone is the way the writer speaks about that opinion. Tone is usually described by an emotive word, such as joyful, ominous, or detached. To determine tone, take into consideration the context, the event or circumstance, and the audience for the particular piece of writing. Then read the text carefully, looking for terms that have to do with emotions. Watch for punctuation, such as exclamation points and question marks, that expresses emotion. Determine how a writer feels about a topic by examining whether their ideas are serious, sarcastic, or show another emotion. These steps will lead you to the tone of a text.

Detecting Stereotype and Bias

It is important to recognize stereotypes and bias in what you read. Stereotypes and bias can present ideas as facts, as shown in the following table:

	Stereotype	Bias
Definition	A generalized belief that characterizes each person of a group in the same category	An unfair or close-minded opinion for or against an idea, person, group of people, or a belief
Example	All tall people are good at basketball.	Rigorous, sustained cardiovascular exercise is the only way to improve health.
Characteristics	The writer makes general statements about groups of people or uses evidence from unreliable sources about groups.	The writer uses emotionally charged words to describe a topic or purposefully omits facts that contradict ideas about an issue.

How can readers avoid stereotypes and bias regarding topics? One way is to read multiple texts about a topic. This allows the reader to compare how ideas are presented and to evaluate the evidence for ideas. Another way to avoid stereotypes is to imagine an author's side and the opposing side in a debate. This allows the reader to see a topic from multiple points of view. Review the preceding table again for ways you can recognize stereotypes and bias and how this will help you to read critically.

Fact and Opinion

Another aspect of reading critically is to determine whether a statement is a fact or opinion. To identify a fact, a reader must first evaluate whether a statement can be proven true. Next, the reader must decide whether the evidence that supports the statement is credible and reliable. If a statement is supported by multiple reliable sources and evidence, it can be considered a fact. If a statement describes an author's beliefs and is an idea that reasonable people can disagree about, it is an opinion. Opinions can be used to mislead or persuade a reader.

Consider the following examples of a fact and an opinion about nursing degrees.

Fact	Opinion
According to Rasmussen University, nurses with associate degrees earn around $67,000 a year, whereas those with master's degrees earn more than $90,000 a year.	The best way to increase your earning potential as a nurse is to earn an advanced degree. The best way to increase your earning potential as a nurse is to earn an advanced degree.

The first statement is a fact that can be checked through research. This university's data about average nursing salaries can be studied and validated. In addition, universities are usually considered reliable sources. Conversely, the second example is an opinion. The writer's belief is that an advanced degree is the best way to increase earning potential. Although earning an advanced degree may increase earning potential, reasonable people can disagree about whether this is the best way to do so. When a writer claims that an idea is the best or worst of several options, it is likely that the statement is an opinion. To compare facts and opinions about a topic, read multiple texts about that topic. This will help you to detect facts that can be checked and the differing opinions people have about that topic.

CHAPTER 8 PRACTICE PROBLEMS

Read the following passage. Then answer the questions that follow.

There are many reasons to consider making physical education (PE) mandatory in schools. According to the National Institutes of Health, regular physical activity improves cardiovascular health and promotes a healthier lifestyle. It can also help students build strength, can reduce the risk of certain illnesses, and can even improve mental health. Some studies suggest that students who participate in daily PE improve their grades. PE in school can also help students reach the daily recommended 60 minutes of physical activity. It is likely that many students will not achieve the goal of 60 minutes of exercise outside of school because they spend so much time on electronic devices. Sedentary students need to participate in team sports. Requiring exercise also rewards students who are naturally athletic, so this is another consideration for mandatory PE.

1. Which of the following is a fact that supports the author's argument that PE should be mandatory in schools?

   A. Students spend too much time on electronic devices.
   B. Regular physical activity improves cardiovascular health.
   C. Sedentary students need to participate in team sports.
   D. It rewards athletic students.

2. Which of the following statements indicates a stereotype?

   A. Students who spend time on electronic devices are not physically active.
   B. Physical activity helps students develop stronger bodies and reduces illnesses.
   C. Students should learn to participate in team sports.
   D. Physical activity helps promote better mental health among students.

3. Which of the following describes the author's point of view regarding PE?

   A. PE rewards students who are naturally athletic.
   B. PE does little for students who spend time on electronic devices.
   C. PE requires participation in team sports.
   D. PE should be mandatory in schools.

4. Which of the following describes the tone of this passage?

   A. Pessimistic
   B. Optimistic
   C. Informative
   D. Irritated

5. In three to five sentences, describe and defend your opinion on mandatory PE in schools.

Notes:

_____

_____

_____

_____

_____

_____

_____

_____

_____

_____

_____

_____

_____

_____

_____

_____

_____

_____

_____

_____

_____

_____

_____

_____

Notes:

CHAPTER

Recognize the structure of texts in various formats

This objective includes, but is not limited to, the following examples of knowledge, skills, and abilities.

- Know the modes (e.g., persuasive, expository, narrative).
- Identify compare and contrast.
- State cause and effect.
- Recognize problem/solution.

Reading and writing is a continual puzzle-building game that can fit in different ways for diverse purposes. As a reader, you must be able to recognize various modes and types of texts. On the other hand, writers must use a blend of modes and types of writing to fulfill specific purposes. "Modes" are defined as classifications of rhetorical writing, such as persuasive, expository, and narrative.

Types of writing are the texts that fall under each mode. For example, some of the types of writing that make up expository writing are compare and contrast, procedure, and cause and effect. Some narrative structures are myths, biographies, short stories, poetry, and novels. For the TEAS, you will need to identify and evaluate these modes and the structures they employ.

The Modes of Texts

The three key modes of texts are persuasive, narrative, and informative. The persuasive or argumentative mode of writing allows the author to convince the reader to believe something about a topic. The author usually attempts to convince the reader to feel, think, or behave a certain way. In persuasive texts, the reader can find facts, details, examples, and persuasive word choice in addition to a logical order of thought development. Introductory and parenthetical phrases are common places for readers to discern the persuasive language in texts. Persuasive language must be able to portray strong opinions.

In argumentative texts, facts, details, and examples are usually organized in a logical sequence following a claim. The claim, or topic sentence, states the main focus of a paragraph and supports the main idea or thesis of the text. The reason answers why to any claim. The evidence shows—with the use of facts, details, or examples—what the claim looks like. In other words, it backs up the claim by proving it. A counterclaim is the opposition's reason against the author's claim, and a writer may anticipate and refute counterclaims. The analysis explains how the evidence is supporting the claim and wraps up the paragraph. Typically, persuasive texts follow a logical order of the weakest argument to the strongest argument.

The following table presents an example of a claim and its accompanying reasons, evidence, and analysis.

Claim	Nurses should earn a master of science in nursing (MSN) degree.
Reason	Nurses with an MSN degree gain a competitive advantage in employment in nursing.
Evidence	According to Pennsylvania University, nurses with advanced degrees are not only in higher demand but also have a higher earning potential.
Counterclaim	Advanced degrees are not worth the expense in nursing.
Refuting the counterclaim	Each level of education corresponds with higher salaries, so that the expense of an advanced degree is easily covered by salary increases.
Analysis	Earning an MSN opens the door to advanced practice nursing careers and higher salaries, so it would be well worth the time and effort.

The narrative mode of writing involves narrating or conveying a story, anecdote, or plot. Narrative writing has several purposes: Authors can entertain, inform, and challenge their readers through diverse structures. Narratives tell stories with sensory details that assist the readers in experiencing events. Whether in poetry, anecdotes, or short stories, narratives use chronological order (beginning to end or end to beginning). Yet, many authors use narrative devices that foreshadow or flash back and create images in readers' minds.

The following is a list of signal words and phrases that assist readers in following the order of events (time and sequential) in narrative writing.

formerly	originally	consequently	occasionally
previously	soon after	subsequently	ultimately
initially	to begin with	next	following

In the informative or expository mode of writing, the author informs, explains, or tells the reader how to do something. In contrast to persuasive writing, expository writing is not trying to convey an opinion or stance on a topic. The primary purpose of the expository mode of writing is to convey information. Informative writing uses a variety of structures to inform or persuade the reader, such as procedural writing, compare and contrast, cause and effect, and problem and solution.

Procedural Writing

In procedural writing, writers convey an established process. A procedure involves specific step-by-step or how-to instructions. For example, think about the steps involved in making chocolate chip cookies. To begin with, you gather ingredients and then preheat the oven. Next, you complete each step of the recipe in order and place the dough in the oven as directed. To complete the procedure, you take the cookies out and let them cool a bit before enjoying them. The following table lists words commonly found in procedural writing.

These words help the reader to identify the sequence of instructions.

first	next	then	in closing
to begin with	accordingly	last	to finish

Compare and Contrast

One structure used by writers to convey their ideas is to compare and contrast ideas about a topic. When you compare components of writing, you are finding similarities. When you contrast components of writing, you are identifying differences.

The following is a list of words and phrases used in writing that help readers identify comparing and contrasting.

Words That Signal Comparing	Words That Signal Contrasting
also, both	yet, but
in the same way	on the other hand
similarly	however
in like manner	on the contrary

Cause and Effect

Another way a text can be structured is by describing a cause and its effect. A cause is the reason that something occurs later. The effect is what occurred as a result specific conditions or causes. For example, when you step out of your car onto an icy driveway, you could fall. The cause, an icy driveway, would produce the effect of a fall. In another example, if you train for a 5K race by running regularly, you will likely complete the race and may even run a personal best time. The training would be the cause of the effect of completing the race. Writers use cause-and-effect structure when they explain the results of events or actions.

The following table contains signal words that can appear in texts that describe causes and their effects.

Words That Signal Cause	Words That Signal Effect	Cause-and-Effect Phrases
because	therefore	if . . . then . . .
since	consequently	as a result of
as	hence	as a consequence
due to	so	the sequence of

Problem and Solution

Persuasive texts or essays often use a problem-and-solution structure. This structure can include the following: an introduction naming a problem or issue, a description of the problem, a plausible solution to the problem, and a closing that challenges the reader to take action. The format can change, but these features structure a problem-and-solution essay.

The following table includes signal words and phrases that are often found in problem-and-solution essays.

| the problem | so that | for this reason | if . . . then . . . |
| because | this led to | a solution | one reason for |

CHAPTER 9 PRACTICE PROBLEMS

Read the following passage. Then answer the questions that follow.

The Centers for Disease Control and Prevention (CDC) defines secondhand smoke as smoke from burning tobacco products such as cigarettes or smoke that has been breathed out by people who are using tobacco products. Until recently, the chemicals in secondhand smoke had not been analyzed. Gradually, research on these chemicals was completed. The CDC now estimates that there are hundreds of chemicals that are toxic to human health contained in secondhand smoke and that there is no safe level of exposure to secondhand smoke. Consequently, people exposed to secondhand smoke are subject to health problems and chronic disease. Children exposed to secondhand smoke are more likely to have ear infections as well as asthma. On the other hand, adults exposed to secondhand smoke are more likely to suffer from heart disease, lung cancer, and stroke.

1. Which of the following is the primary mode of this passage?

    A. Persuasive
    B. Descriptive
    C. Narrative
    D. Expository

2. Which of the following terms signals a result in the text?

    A. Consequently
    B. Gradually
    C. Now
    D. Until recently

3. Which of the following signal words or phrases indicates a comparison?

    A. More likely
    B. Gradually
    C. On the other hand
    D. As well as

4. Which of the following structures is used in the passage?

    A. Compare and contrast
    B. Cause and effect
    C. Problem and solution
    D. Persuasion and argument

5. Secondhand smoke is a health problem faced by many people. In five to seven sentences, describe the problem and suggest a solution.

Notes:

_____

_____

_____

_____

_____

_____

_____

_____

_____

_____

_____

_____

_____

_____

_____

_____

_____

_____

_____

_____

_____

_____

_____

Notes:

CHAPTER

10 Interpret the meaning of words and phrases using context

 This objective includes, but is not limited to, the following examples of knowledge, skills, and abilities.

- Identify the correct definition of a word.
- Distinguish between figurative and connotative meanings.
- Recognize the cumulative effect of specific word choice on meaning.
- Identify a source to find vocabulary definitions.

Reading comprehension is a challenging practice made even more difficult by the multiple meanings of words. To be a successful reader, you must identify correct definitions, discern between diverse meanings, and distinguish between figurative and connotative word meaning. The TEAS will test your ability to skillfully employ these strategies and to evaluate the impact of an author's use of vocabulary in text.

Identifying Correct Definitions

Comprehending text is easier said than done. It involves multiple skills, one of which is identifying a correct definition of a word. One way to discern the meaning of an unknown word is to consider the meaning of the parts of a word. Word meaning can also be inferred by the use of a word in a sentence or context. The context is the text preceding or following a specific word. Several types of context clues provide hints to the meaning of the specific word.

 When confronted with an unknown term, first use root words and affixes to determine word meaning. Consider the word, fracture. The root is the base of the word (fract) and has the suffix (–ure). In this instance, *fract* means "to break" and the suffix, *–ure*, means "the act or process of." So, the meaning of fracture is the act or process of breaking.

If the word parts do not illuminate word meaning, use the context. Sometimes the context of a sentence provides the definition of a word. Consider the sentence: *Becoming a CPA, or a certified public accountant, requires passing a series of exams.* In this example, the definition of CPA is provided following the term.

Another type of context clue is the use of an example or illustration. Find the example in the following sentence: *The neonatal intensive care unit (NICU), where medical professionals care for premature or critically ill infants, requires staff with special certifications.* Here the reader can understand that the NICU is an area of a hospital specifically designated for the care of infants.

Signal phrases in a sentence can also help to illuminate word meaning. Notice the introductory phrase in the following sentence: *Unlike many other careers, meteorologists are required to understand statistical probabilities.* In this example, the introductory phrase provides a clue about the meaning of the term "meteorologist." A meteorologist engages in a career that involves advanced mathematics. Other parts of the text might point to the idea that meteorologists study weather. Use the entire text as the context of a word to determine its meaning.

Figurative and Connotative Meanings

Many authors employ creative ways to state ideas and make unfamiliar settings and objects more accessible to the reader. If a reader becomes aware of common figurative devices, then the text will be more manageable and comprehensible.

Figurative Device	Definition	Example
Metaphor	Comparison between unlike things without using "like" or "as"	Maria's phone was a dinosaur.
Simile	Comparison between unlike things using "like" or "as"	The hurdler cleared the barriers as gracefully as a gazelle.
Personification	Giving human attributes to something nonhuman	The gurney groaned under the weight of the injured wrestler.

The Effect of Word Choice

Comprehension of a text can depend on a reader's ability to infer the meaning of the word by reading between the author's lines. In addition to assisting comprehension, authors can influence the emotional effect on a reader. A reader's experiences will determine the positive and negative connotations of a word. Ultimately, the tone (author's feeling toward the subject) affects the mood (the reader's feeling elicited from the text).

For example, each of the following words is similar, yet experience and use result in diverse meanings.

Word	Definition	Connotation
old	advanced in age	feeble, needing care
mature	fully developed	experienced, competent

Sources for Definitions

After using roots and affixes, context, and connotations to determine word meaning, readers can confirm definitions by using a dictionary, thesaurus, encyclopedia, or other source.

Book	Online Source
Dictionary	https://www.dictionary.com/ http://visualdictionaryonline.com/
Thesaurus	https://www.thesaurus.com/ https://www.visualthesaurus.com/

CHAPTER 10 PRACTICE PROBLEMS

Read the following passage. Then answer the questions that follow.

> Theodore Roosevelt, the 26th president of the United States, took a trip late in 1913 following his defeat for a third term as president in 1912. He traveled to Brazil and joined an expedition. The team trekked through uncharted tributary of the Amazon River, the River of Doubt. The overland trip required passing through the rugged Brazilian wilderness, which proved to be a formidable opponent. The jungle's thick vegetation acted like a massive green wall blocking the team's progress. Once Roosevelt and his team arrived at the River of Doubt, they faced more extreme risks in the water and on its banks: alligators, piranhas, venomous snakes, mosquitoes, stinging insects, and even an army of ants that ate the team's food. Despite the harsh elements encountered during the adventure, and the lingering ailments afterward, Roosevelt still referred to the trip as one of the greatest he had completed.

1. Based on context in the passage, which of the following is the meaning of the word "trekked"?

    A. Defeated
    B. Carried
    C. Studied
    D. Hiked

2. Which of the following phrases provide a context clue to the meaning of the word "formidable"?

    A. Overland trip
    B. Rugged wilderness
    C. Uncharted tributary
    D. Harsh elements

3. The writer states that "The jungle's thick vegetation acted like a massive green wall blocking the team's progress." Which of the following figurative devices is used in the sentence?

    A. Personification
    B. Metaphor
    C. Simile
    D. Connotation

4. The writer refers to the wilderness as a "formidable opponent." Which of the following figurative devices is used in the sentence?

    A. Personification
    B. Connotation
    C. Denotation
    D. Simile

5. Reread the passage. Choose three words used to describe the jungle and explain their effect on the reader.

Notes:

_____

_____

_____

_____

_____

_____

_____

_____

_____

_____

_____

_____

_____

_____

_____

_____

_____

_____

_____

_____

_____

CHAPTER

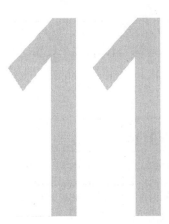

Determine the denotative meaning of words

 This objective includes, but is not limited to, the following examples of knowledge, skills, and abilities.

- Identify the correct definition of a word.
- Identify a source to find vocabulary definitions

Determining the meanings of words is one of the first and most basic skills included in learning to read and comprehending a text. Words have two levels of meaning: denotative and connotative. The denotative meaning of a word is its dictionary definition. The connotative meaning of a word is more complex and is a combination of the word's definition and its suggested meaning based on context and emotions or associations evoked by a word. For the purposes of this TEAS task, you will focus on the denotative meaning of words and strategies for locating denotative word meanings.

Identifying Definitions

Perhaps the easiest and most traditional way to find a word's meaning is to look up the word in a dictionary. There are several reliable and well-known dictionaries; *Merriam-Webster Dictionary* and *Oxford English Dictionary* are two you have probably seen in libraries, classrooms, and offices. These dictionaries are usually large books that require you to know little about a word prior to finding its meaning.

It is helpful to know how a word is spelled or at least know the first several letters of the word. This will not be a problem if you are looking up a word found in a text. However, if you have only heard the word and have not seen it in a printed text, you might have to guess how it is spelled. Once you know the first several letters of a word, you should be able to locate it in the dictionary using guide words. Guide words appear at the top of each page of a dictionary and show readers the first and last words that appear on that page. You will need to search for the two guide words that would come before and after the word you are looking up. For example, to find the word "prescribe," a page with the guide words "pneumonia" and "prayer" would not include the word, but a page with guide words "precious" and "proton" would.

Most dictionaries include a standard set of information intended to help a reader understand its meaning. Dictionaries usually include a word's part of speech, which refers to how the word functions within a sentence. Noun, verb, adjective, and adverb are common parts of speech. They are often abbreviated in dictionaries in the following ways:

Noun	n.
Verb	v.
Adjective	adj.
Adverb	adv.

Identifying Sources for Definitions

If a word has multiple meanings, dictionaries will include a numbered list of meanings, usually followed by sentences that demonstrate the word being used with each meaning. Some dictionaries even include a word's origin, which can help readers make associations or connections with other words they might know.

Finding denotative word meanings has become easier as a result of technological advances. With a smartphone, tablet, or computer, simply type a word into an online search tool and quickly retrieve denotative word meanings. Both the *Merriam-Webster Dictionary* and the *Oxford English Dictionary* offer online resources. Many of the basic principles followed in printed dictionaries also apply to online sources. Word meanings found online still typically include a part of speech and several possible definitions with examples to provide readers some context.

CHAPTER 11 PRACTICE PROBLEMS

Read the following passage. Then answer the questions that follow.

Strength training involves the entire neuromuscular system. Electrical impulses from the brain send messages to the muscles via motor units. Each motor unit is comprised of a nerve cell and the muscle fiber bundles that contract in response to signals from that nerve cell. Extra strength training for a powerlifting competition requires neuromuscular adaptations. Lifters train their muscles to work faster and work together more efficiently. Training the motor units to work faster is called "rate coding." Training muscles to work simultaneously is called "motor unit synchronization." These adaptations result in stronger and faster nerve impulses. In turn, muscles react with greater force and can manage heavier weights.

1. When looking up the definition of "powerlifting" in a printed dictionary, which of the following sets of guide words could appear at the top of a page?

   A. Practicable and Pyrex
   B. Psychoanalysis and public speaking
   C. Poseidon and poverty
   D. Powdery and pox

2. Which of the following part of speech would be included with a dictionary entry for the word, "neuromuscular"?

   A. Noun or n.
   B. Verb or v.
   C. Adjective or adj.
   D. Adverb or adv.

3. Which of the following phrases helps to define the term "motor units"?

   A. Nerve cell and muscle fiber bundles
   B. Neuromuscular adaptations
   C. Electrical impulses
   D. Rate coding

4. Which of the following phrases helps to define "neuromuscular adaptations"?

   A. Muscle fiber bundles tell them to contract
   B. Motor units work faster and simultaneously
   C. Stronger and faster nerve impulses
   D. Muscles react with greater force

5. Using a dictionary or encyclopedia, research "rate coding" and "motor unit synchronization." Define each term, and then explain these two procedures work together to train motor units.

Notes:

CHAPTER

12 Evaluate the author's purpose in a given text

 This objective includes, but is not limited to, the following examples of knowledge, skills, and abilities.

- Draw inferences about an author's purpose or message.
- Distinguish between fact and opinion.
- Distinguish between informational/expository, persuasive, and narrative/entertaining.
- Recognize tone within context.
- Summarize and compare information within a text.

Part of being an astute reader is determining the purpose of a piece of text. Determining an author's purpose, or the reason a particular piece of text was written, can help you focus on the most important details of a text. This is especially important if a text is lengthy or complex. As you read, it is important to ask yourself whether the author is trying to persuade, inform, or entertain you. It is also important to remember that one text can have more than one purpose. In preparing for the TEAS, practice determining the author's purpose for all texts you encounter.

Drawing Inferences

Knowing a writer's purpose (also called "authorial intent") can be an important component of comprehension. If you want to understand a text deeply, it is helpful to know the circumstances under which it was produced.

When trying to determine authorial intent, it is helpful to ask yourself a series of questions as you read. Some especially helpful questions include the following:

- Where does the text appear?
- What is the structure of the text?
- What is the author's tone?

Distinguishing Between Fact and Opinion

Is the text a novel, an excerpt from a novel, or a short story from an anthology? Does the text appear in a travel magazine plastered with images and advertisements for vendors associated with the area a writer is highlighting? Is the text a magazine or television advertisement? Where text appears can help you determine authorial intent.

If the text is in a newspaper, for example, the author might have intended to inform a community about issues pertinent to a specific geographical area. Novels, short stories, and poems are generally created to entertain an audience. Advertisements are created to persuade a group of people to make a purchase or act on a specific request.

Readers, however, must be careful not to assign a single purpose to any specific source. For example, although some news sources exist to inform readers, others were created to cater to a specific audience or set of beliefs. Likewise, many nonfiction texts that seek to inform readers can also be entertaining to read.

Distinguishing Between Text Structures

Structure can help you determine an author's intent. Some basic rules you can consider when examining the structure of a text follow.

Although informational or expository texts can take many forms, they often include section headings that might appear in bold or underlined type. Informational texts also often include bulleted or numbered lists, short phrases that might not be complete sentences, and images with captions, maps, and diagrams. Instructions for assembly are an example of informational text. Course textbooks are another form of informational text. Both of these are used to inform readers about a specific topic.

Some persuasive texts are easy to recognize. Writers of advertisements seek to sell a service, product, or idea to a specific audience. Newspapers often include editorials that express specific opinions intended to persuade readers about a topic of local interest. However, some persuasive texts can be disguised. For example, Upton Sinclair wrote the novel, *The Jungle*, which is widely read by many high school students today. But the fact that it is a work of fiction should not distract readers. Sinclair wrote it to inform a specific publication's audience about harsh working conditions inflicted on immigrants to the United States. *The Jungle* resulted in a public uproar about those poor working conditions and the lack of sanitation in the US meat-packing industry in the early 1900s.

Narrative structures appear in stories or poetry, which often serve to entertain an audience. Narrative texts generally include a plot and one or more characters trying to overcome an obstacle or solve a problem.

Recognizing Author's Tone

Sometimes, an author's purpose can be determined by examining specific words used in a piece of writing. Authors who intend to simply inform readers tend to use straightforward, neutral language that lacks emotional correlation (words that can be defined as exclusively happy or exclusively angry). On the other hand, authors who intend to persuade readers might use emotionally charged language coupled with images to evoke a specific emotion in readers.

 For example, an advertisement for a premium photo-printing service might ask potential customers, "How much are your memories worth?" These words, placed beneath an image of a grandparent smiling over a newborn child, might suggest that readers should not trust a local discount store to print their photos but instead should use the advertiser's services. Paying attention to an author's words can help you determine the intended message.

Summarizing and Comparing Information

A summary is a brief statement of the main ideas of a text. Creating a summary of a text involves four basic steps:

1. Identifying the topic.
2. Identifying the central idea about the topic.
3. Identifying the key details about the central idea.
4. Expressing and central idea and key details in your own words.

While reviewing a text, compare information by looking for what is alike and what is different. Look for the author's purpose or purposes and common themes. Create a chart to list details in the text and then create a Venn diagram to compare and contrast those details.

CHAPTER 12 PRACTICE PROBLEMS

Read the following passage. Then answer the questions that follow.

A local hospital published the following announcement for mandatory nurse in-service training.

To: All Nursing Staff

From: Dr. Lynette Smith, MSN, Head of Professional Development

Re: Mandatory In-Service Training

Topic: Transitional Care

All staff is required to attend in-service training regarding transitional care. This involves effective procedures for moving patients from inpatient care to a new facility and discharging patients to go home.

In this training, you will learn in greater detail how to fulfill these five standards encompassed within transitions of care:

1. Identifying at-risk patients who may transition poorly.

2. Conducting a thorough assessment for transition of those patients identified as at risk.

3. Compiling a complete and accurate medication list for each patient.

4. Developing a care management plan that is dynamic and ongoing.

5. Transferring all transitions of care information to the appropriate new caregivers or care providers.

1. Which of the following is the primary purpose of this announcement?
   A. To provide a way for nursing staff to sign up for training
   B. To inform nursing staff about an in-service training
   C To require nursing staff to memorize the five standards
   D To inform nursing staff they may miss a shift to attend training

2   Which of the following is the mode of this announcement?

   A.   Persuasive
   B.   Narrative
   C.   Argumentative
   D.   Informational

3.   Which of the following best describes the tone of this announcement?

   A.   Sincere
   B.   Relaxed
   C.   Informative
   D.   Urgent

4.   Which of the following statements expresses a fact?

   A.   Nurses are required to attend in-service on how to manage transitions of care.
   B.   Nurses must memorize the five standards involved in transitions of care.
   C.   Nurses must take time off to attend the transitions of care training.
   D.   Nurses are required to create one type of transitional care management plan.

5.   Summarize the main points of the in-service announcement.

Notes:

_____

_____

_____

_____

_____

_____

_____

_____

_____

_____

_____

_____

_____

_____

_____

_____

_____

_____

_____

_____

_____

_____

Notes:

CHAPTER

13 Evaluate the author's point of view in a given text

 This objective includes, but is not limited to, the following examples of knowledge, skills, and abilities.

- Recognize and evaluate the text source (author, publication, organization).
- Recognize different perspectives in text.
- Gather, organize, and interpret information.
- Compare texts from different sources and opinions.
- Evaluate the relevancy and accuracy of information.

Developing the ability to determine an author's point of view can serve a reader well in gaining a deep understanding of a text. Depending on the purpose of a text, an author's perspective (also known as an author's point of view) can be made clear, or it can remain intentionally hidden. For example, an editorial in a newspaper is intended to convey an author's perspective on a particular issue or topic. However, a news story written to inform a community about a serious recent tragedy is not supposed to include the writer's personal opinion about the event; the writer is simply meant to report the occurrence truthfully.

For this TEAS task, you will need to recognize and evaluate an author's point of view by thinking about who the author is, what organization(s) or group(s) he or she might be associated with, the type of publication in which a piece of writing appears, whether information the writer shares appears to be fact or opinion, and how a piece of writing fits within a larger context.

Evaluating a Source

As you develop reading skills, it is important to identify the kinds of sources being read and discern the need for more information to develop a true and full understanding about a topic. For example, if reading a biography of George Washington in which a writer casts the first president as an arrogant, cruel, and harsh person, you might read another biography written by a different author.

Recognizing Perspectives

Although some of the information included in a different book is bound to be the same, there will likely be additional information about another event in Washington's life or a different take on an event covered in the first book that presents Washington as a kind and compassionate man rather than a cruel one. Seeing these differences in interpretations of a single man might cause you to look into who the authors are, their educational backgrounds, how they developed an interest in Washington, and so on. Examining works by different authors about a single topic and comparing them can help you determine and better understand an author's point of view.

Gathering and Interpreting Information

Sometimes researching background information about authors can help you to determine the point of view they might have, regardless if it is clear within a piece of writing. For example, in researching the benefits of following a particular diet, such as the keto diet, you might stumble on a blog that appears to be a source of useful, factual, and scientific information. However, when you click on the "About" tab at the top of the page and read about the blog's author, you discover that the author is the founder of a company that sells products and memberships related to the keto diet and lifestyle. Therefore, the author's ultimate purpose is likely to grow the business and entice the general public to follow the keto diet and participate in the keto lifestyle community. This is not to say that the information included on the blog is untrue; much of it might be factual. However, you should be aware of the writer's probable purpose and seek out other sources of information to ensure that you have the most accurate information possible.

Comparing Texts

In this example, the fact that the writer was using a blog is also important to note. Blogs are widely used for a variety of purposes. Anyone can start a blog, and the information placed on one is generally not reviewed or verified to ensure accuracy. If you locate information on a blog, verify its accuracy by comparing it to other sources, especially those that have been reviewed by experts to ensure accuracy, such as peer-reviewed journals.

Evaluating Relevancy and Accuracy

Relevance of information can also be an effective way to determine a writer's point of view. Political speeches illustrate this point nicely. In a political debate, for example, two candidates asked a variety of questions focused on diverse topics may consistently frame their answers on overarching themes. One candidate might mention the environment in each answer, and another candidate might mention the burden of student loans. Although parts of their answers address the moderator's questions, the politicians each repeatedly steer their answers back to topics they most want to discuss with voters. Analyzing the relevance or irrelevance of authors' (or speakers') information can be an effective way to determine point of view.

CHAPTER 13 PRACTICE PROBLEMS

Read the following passage. Then answer the questions that follow.

A nurse educator at a long-term care facility is preparing a lesson on preventing falls. She wants to include information, examples, and hands-on exercises addressing why falls happen and how to prevent them. She is considering the following three sources of information.

1. A website features articles and videos from a medical facility. Renowned professionals provide insight on numerous topics. Their credentials and bios are included.

2. A website sponsored by a nurse-staffing organization provides qualified nurses for travel assignments. The site includes stories from nurses. It also includes lists of services provided, qualifications for nursing staff, and related resources.

3. A blog by a popular nurse influencer has a substantial following. She shares stories about her experiences in the nursing profession. She also writes promotional posts for various advertisers of products and services relevant to nursing.

1. Which of the following sources appears to be the most reliable?
   A. Blog by a nurse influencer
   B. Website by a nurse staffing organization
   C. Website from a medical facility
   D. Both answers B and C

2. Which of the following features would support the reliability of a source?
   A. A medical facility website featuring its staff's insight is most authoritative.
   B. Both websites feature relevant insight from medical staff and travel nurses.
   C. A nursing staff website features nurses' stories who gain experience in multiple settings.
   D. A nursing blog with a nurse influencer's stories is captivating and based on experience.

3. Which of the following is a reason the credentials of an author are important to know when evaluating a source?
   A. To understand their personal experience
   B. To substantiate their expertise
   C. To support an opinion about the author
   D. To understand their views on policy

4. Which of the following is a reason to evaluate the credibility of sources on falls prevention?
   A. To use only hospital-approved references
   B. To locate an alternate perspective
   C. To follow safety protocol and practice
   D. To establish relevancy and accuracy

5. Identify at least two reasons why a nurse who is also an influence blogger would not be the most appropriate source for this lesson.

Notes:

CHAPTER

14

Use text features

 This objective includes, but is not limited to, the following examples of knowledge, skills, and abilities.

- Find headings and subheadings.
- Identify features (e.g., key, legend, bold, italic, footnote, glossary, index, table of contents).
- Use navigational tools in media (e.g., search query, search engine)

Text features are parts of a text that are designed to stand out from a larger text for a specific reason. Some examples of text features include bold print, italics, and footnotes. Text features can be used for a number of purposes, such as to orient the reader, provide additional information or background knowledge, assist a reader with quickly locating information, and provide a clear organizational structure. Good readers recognize text features and are able to use them effectively to better comprehend what they read. To do well with questions in this TEAS task, you should be able to locate headings and subheadings, identify various text features, and determine appropriate key words for searching a text or set of texts.

Review the following example with various text features.

> ## SUMMER 2020 STAFF BARBEQUE
>
> The hospital event planner is looking forward to organizing a wonderful 2020 staff barbeque this summer. This year's picnic will include both indoor and outdoor games and activities, as well as a catered smorgasbord of delicious barbeque favorites.
>
> ### Eligibility
>
> All medical staff and their families are invited to attend the barbeque. There will be games and activities suitable for all ages. The barbeque menu will also include something for everyone, even those with food allergies.
>
> ### Location and Time
>
> The barbeque will be at the city park's south end. The time will be from 1 pm to 5 pm in an effort to accommodate the greatest number of staff.

Headings and Subheadings

Headings and subheadings are some of the most common text features authors use to help readers understand how a text is organized.

In the preceding example, "Summer 2020 Staff Barbeque" is the heading. "Eligibility" and "Location and Time" are subheadings. Notice that the heading appears in bold type and is larger than the subheadings and the explanatory text. The subheadings also appear in bold type, but they are set in a smaller font size. The subheadings and their explanations are indented to the right of the heading, as well. Indentation is another text feature that helps to organize and clarify text for readers.

Identifying Features

Some text features are easily identified by where they appear on a page. Sidebars, footnotes, and map legends are some examples of these types of text features. Sidebars are often used in history textbooks. The main text in the book might focus on a world leader's work and major accomplishments associated with a particular social or political movement. A sidebar can include a photograph or image of leaders, along with an additional detail or two about their personal life.

 FOR EXAMPLE:

Sidebars like this one can offer readers additional information about a text that might not be provided in the main text.

Underlined and Italicized Print

Some other common text features are underlined and italicized print. These text features can be a bit more confusing to interpret because there are many reasons why text might be italicized or underlined. Likewise, formal style guides used by writers, reporters, and scholars use different sets of rules for italic and underlined print.

It is sometimes up to a reader to infer why a portion of text appears different from the text around it. There are, however, some standard uses for text features. Italics, for example, are used for titles of works (e.g., books), foreign words or phrases, and for emphasis.

A simple rule of thumb is that writers often use text features to draw attention to specific portions of text for specific reasons. Here are some simple questions you can ask yourself if you notice that part of a text has a different appearance than the text around it.

- Is the text a title?
- Is the text a quotation that the author is using to help prove a point, introduce an idea, or make a statement?
- Is the text introducing a different section that will cover a new topic or idea?
- Is the text feature being used for aesthetic reasons only?
- Does the text feature help to organize information?
- Does the text feature have something to do with the type of text? (A script, for example, might include boldface type to indicate characters' names and italics to indicate actions of characters.)

Footnotes

Footnotes are often used in informational texts to offer readers more in-depth information about a topic. Texts that use footnotes usually use numbers in superscript, or small numbers set slightly above the line of text. Here is an example:

Dr. Benjamin F. Wells will be the special speaker at the graduation ceremony.[4]

The example indicates that at the bottom of this page, readers can find additional information about this statement next to the number 4.

Legends

Map legends are a text feature invaluable to readers wanting to understand information included on a map. Legends often translate symbols included on a map to reduce clutter and make the map easier to read. For example, many maps indicate the population of towns and cities by assigning different styles of "dots" depending on the population range of a location.

The legend, usually placed somewhere on the edge of the map, indicates which style of dot is assigned to each population range. Large urban centers with populations greater than 1 million people might be marked with a large black star with a circle around it, whereas small towns might be marked with a tiny black dot. Rather than be left to guess about what each symbol means, readers can look to the legend for help with interpretation.

CHAPTER 14 PRACTICE PROBLEMS

Read the following passage. Then answer the questions that follow.

While reviewing the upcoming semester's course list, you see a course that grabs your attention, so you review it in the course catalog.

COURSE 623 *Continuity of Care and Nurse Navigation.* (3 cr)

This course teaches procedures for ensuring appropriate community resources are established for necessary follow-up care.

This course is offered in the Willis Memorial building on campus. See the following map for its location.

Prerequisites

Enrollment in RN-to-BSN program

Minimum of five years of clinical experience

Preferred: Certification in area of specialized practice

Student Comments

"This was the best decision I ever made for my career! Taking this course rounded out my career trajectory and allowed me to eventually become a nurse navigator. I highly recommend this course to anyone who wants to be a patient advocate and to serve as a conduit for clinical resources."[1]

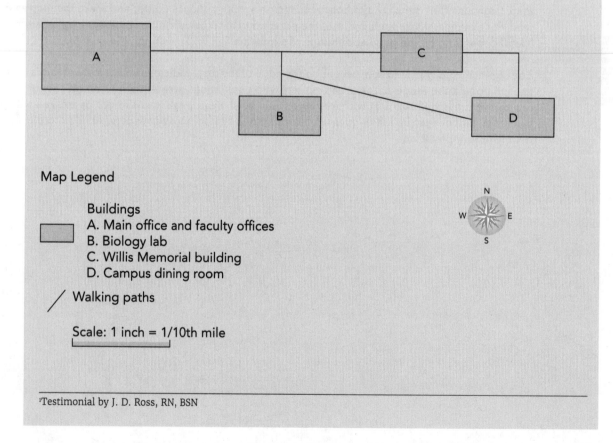

Map Legend

Buildings
A. Main office and faculty offices
B. Biology lab
C. Willis Memorial building
D. Campus dining room

Walking paths

Scale: 1 inch = 1/10th mile

[1]Testimonial by J. D. Ross, RN, BSN

1. In the preceding passage, which text feature highlights the course title?

   A. Bold font
   B. Sidebar
   C. Quotation
   D. Italics

2. Which information is included in a sidebar?

   A. Campus map
   B. Prerequisites
   C. Course description
   D. Footnote

3. What is the meaning of the superscript "1" after the quotation in the passage?

   A. It identifies the number of a footnote related to the quotation.
   B. It means that is the first quotation used in the course catalog.
   C. It signifies the importance of that quotation.
   D. It marks an in-text citation for a reference.

4. What is in the footnote?

   A. Map legend
   B. Prerequisites
   C. Testimonial by J. D. Ross, RN, BSN
   D. Course credits (cr)

5. Identify five features described in the map legend and describe their purpose.

Notes:

CHAPTER

15 Identify primary sources in various media

 This objective includes, but is not limited to, the following examples of knowledge, skills, and abilities.

- Identify primary sources.
- Recognize primary source materials (e.g., Internet, video, text, audio, artifact, print media, photograph, autobiography, document, memoir, oral history).
- Locate information in a primary source.

Primary sources exist in all types of media. The term "primary-source documents" refers to written materials, artifacts, recordings, images, and other media that have not been altered from their original state. They are created by individuals within a specific context. This TEAS task requires you to distinguish between primary sources and other types of documents and to be able to locate information within those documents.

Primary Sources

Primary sources provide immediate, firsthand evidence about a person, event, object, or work of art. When trying to determine whether something is a primary source, it can be helpful to think of how the author is related to the events they describe. If the author was a participant in or attended the event described, the document is likely a primary-source document.

Published documents are primary sources if they come from the time period discussed or were produced by a participant or eyewitness. Newspaper articles written by reporters at an event are primary sources because they are written by eyewitnesses. However, articles about historical events are secondary sources because the author was not a participant in the events discussed. Another type of primary source is original research. A dissertation titled, "Identifying Barriers to Academic Success" by Dr. Arthur Bains is an example. This is a primary source because the author is reporting a study he conducted.

Other primary-source documents include e-mails, blogs, journals, letters, editorials, and interviews. Creative writing and other artwork are primary sources. Original photography and audio and video recordings are considered primary sources because they document events as they occur. Artifacts, such as ancient tools or ancient artwork, are also considered primary sources. Remember, primary-source documents and objects are created during the time period they describe.

Secondary Sources

A secondary source describes, analyzes, or combines ideas from primary sources. They are removed from the event or time period described. Secondary sources are written or produced after events and can comment on them with hindsight. Like primary sources, secondary materials can be written documents or other media such as recordings and documentaries. Secondary sources can also organize primary source information in print or online encyclopedias and textbooks. The textbook itself is a secondary source, but items like quotes from interviews or photographs from a time period within the textbook remain primary sources. If you are asked to find a primary source in a document, look for eyewitness accounts and photographs or drawings from the event or time period.

A tertiary source will use both primary and secondary sources to discuss a topic. Research papers use encyclopedias and primary sources like interviews from eyewitnesses to describe a topic are tertiary sources.

Locating Information

Primary-source documents can be used to gain valuable information about a specific time or place. How can a reader locate information in a primary source? Primary sources can be read or viewed with a specific purpose. With that purpose in mind, readers can scan the source for key words and images that relate to the purpose. For example, a history student may be writing about the history of the participation of women in the 1968 Olympic games. The student may want to look at primary-source data on the total number of Olympians and then zoom in on how many of those Olympians were female. The student may also want to look at primary-source photographs and video recordings that document the participation of women and may also access newspaper articles from 1968 about the games, scanning them for information about women participants. Reading with a purpose helps readers locate information in documents and other media.

CHAPTER 15 PRACTICE PROBLEMS

1. A nursing student is researching treatments for dry skin. Which of the following is a primary source that the student could use to locate information about skin treatments?

    A. Medical textbook
    B. Medical encyclopedia
    C. Research done by doctors at the Centers for Disease Control and Prevention
    D. A journal article describing treatments studied by several doctors

2. Which of the following is a secondary source about baseball?

    A. A documentary about the history of baseball
    B. A telegram sent by baseball legend Babe Ruth
    C. The autobiography of pitcher Dwight Gooden
    D. The novel *The Art of Fielding* by Chad Harbach

    In 1863, Abraham Lincoln wrote a speech called "The Gettysburg Address." Read the following excerpt from this speech and answer the following two questions.

    Four score and seven years ago our fathers brought forth, upon this continent, a new nation, conceived in liberty, and dedicated to the proposition that "all men are created equal"

    Now we are engaged in a great civil war, testing whether that nation, or any nation so conceived, and so dedicated, can long endure. We are met on a great battle field of that war. We have come to dedicate a portion of it, as a final resting place for those who died here, that the nation might live. This we may, in all propriety do. But, in a larger sense, we can not dedicate—we cannot consecrate—we cannot hallow, this ground— The brave men, living and dead, who struggled here, have hallowed it, far above our poor power to add or detract. The world will little note, nor long remember what we say here; while it can never forget what they did here.

3. Which of the following describes one of the key beliefs of the founders of the United States?

    A. All men can own land.
    B. All men are created equal.
    C. All men must serve as soldiers.
    D. All men must run for office.

4. Which of the following describes why Lincoln is giving this speech in Gettysburg?

    A. To gain support for his reelection
    B. To describe why the United States was founded
    C. To explain why the Civil War started
    D. To dedicate land for the burial of soldiers

5. Conduct an online search for three primary-source documents about the development of the measles, mumps, and rubella (MMR) vaccine. Describe why the three sources you located are considered primary sources.

Notes:

CHAPTER

16

Use evidence from text to make predictions and inferences, and draw conclusions about a piece of writing

 This objective includes, but is not limited to, the following examples of knowledge, skills, and abilities.

- Synthesize information from the text to form a prediction, make an inference, and form a conclusion.
- Cite evidence from the text to support a prediction, inference, or conclusion.

Often, writers leave out certain details about a story or topic, and it is up to readers to put together details from a text to draw conclusions about the author's intended meaning. Readers draw conclusions by making reasonable inferences and predictions based on details they find in a text. Being able to cite specific evidence explaining how you came to a conclusion will help you to gain credibility as a reader and can be a benefit to others wanting to better understand a writer's work. For this TEAS task, you will need to be able to successfully identify evidence from a text to support predictions, inferences, and conclusions.

Synthesizing Information

Synthesizing information means to gather details and then discern their similarities and differences. A synthesis combines these details to form new ideas that can support a prediction, inference, or conclusion about a text. For example, fiction writers sometimes provide vague details about a character or situation as a narrative strategy or to build a sense of mystery within a text. In these instances, writers expect readers to ask questions, form hypotheses, and draw on potentially important details to predict characters' actions, plot twists, and story resolutions. One literary technique for fiction that authors use to help readers predict is foreshadowing.

Predictions

Suppose an author begins a story with the sentence, "If I had known I would end up in the hospital, I never would have gone to the gym that day." This opening line alone captures readers' attention and creates a situation in which readers are inferring and predicting what might have happened to the narrator. Did this person get into an accident on the way to the gym? Did this person do something at the gym that was too difficult, such as try to lift weights that were too heavy? Readers can make reasonable predictions about what might have happened based on details introduced in this opening line.

Inferences

An inference is similar to prediction. A prediction uses details from a text to make a judgment about what will happen next. An inference uses details and a reader's background knowledge to draw a logical conclusion about a text.

Read the following passage to make inferences about the characters and events presented.

The young woman stood alone in the corner looking down at the gym floor. She wanted to participate in a deadlift competition but was not sure if she was strong enough to lift weights significantly beyond her normal limits. Little did she know that her decision to go for it would change her life for years to come.

Because the passage ends with the idea that her decision to compete would "change her life," readers might predict that the woman will be injured or be successful. Readers can also infer ideas about the character. Because the woman "stood in alone the corner looking down," a reader can infer that she was feeling unsure or nervous in this competitive situation. She was also alone, suggesting that she did not approach others for advice before making her decision. By studying details in a passage, readers can draw logical conclusions that are not directly stated in a text.

Citing Evidence

Good readers can cite evidence to support their ideas about informational pieces of writing. Sometimes, the structure of a text can assist readers in making predictions about what an author will include. If the text includes a numbered list, a reader might predict that the author will be giving instructions in a sequence or providing a list of items in order of their importance. A title is a text feature that can also help readers make predictions about what might be included.

One thing that readers often must infer in all types of texts is word meanings. When readers come across an unfamiliar word, they might make an educated guess about its meaning before consulting a dictionary. Often, words that surround an unknown word can provide readers clues about the meaning of a word.

Whether writers intend their readers to predict, infer, and draw conclusions, it is likely that every text at some point will require a reader to do these things. In a sense, all readers are experimenters, trying out words, exploring meanings, and predicting events and outcomes.

CHAPTER 16 PRACTICE PROBLEMS

Read the passage carefully and answer the questions that follow.

Nikita's mother loves to tell anyone who will listen that she had to enroll her daughter in gymnastics to keep her safe. She would often find baby Nikita precariously perched on the highest limb of a tree or attempting double flips from the top of her bureau onto her bed. The gym was Nikita's haven growing up, but now that haven was a sheer rockface in the Sierra Nevada Mountains. Nikita clung to miniscule fissures in the rock as her climbing partner Ivan watched from below. His muscles tensed as he watched her, ready to belay her ropes to catch even the tiniest slip or fall. Nikita looked down and made eye contact with Ivan. She detached her ropes and let them fall.

1. Which of the following is a prediction based on the last line of the passage?
   A. Nikita will panic because she lost her ropes accidently.
   B. Nikita will attempt a freestyle climb without ropes.
   C. Ivan will run for help because Nikita has lost her ropes.
   D. Ivan will climb up and help Nikita reattach her ropes.

2. Which of the following is an inference that could be made about Nikita?
   A. Nikita is afraid of heights.
   B. Nikita is athletic and adventurous.
   C. Nikita is a professional climber.
   D. Nikita has traveled to many mountains.

3. Which of the following synthesizes information about Nikita's childhood and her present situation?
   A. Nikita is drawn to the outdoors and risk taking.
   B. Nikita's mother discouraged her climbing.
   C. Nikita has a deep love of geology.
   D. Nikita wanted to become an Olympic gymnast.

4. Which of the following definitions can be inferred for the meaning of "belay" in the passage?
   A. To let go of
   B. To fasten on a cleat
   C. To exert tension on
   D. To loosen

5. Read the back cover of a biography on an online website. Make a prediction about the events in the biography based on details from the back cover.

Notes:

CHAPTER

17

Compare and contrast themes from print and other sources

 This objective includes, but is not limited to, the following examples of knowledge, skills, and abilities.

- List similarities and differences across themes.
- Recognize similar themes across cultures.
- Compare and contrast a theme from one author or topic.
- Compare and contrast themes across genres.

A theme is a broad concept often thought of as a universal concern that an author addresses through a given medium. The theme of a work is different from its subject. Although the subject of a story might be living in Alaska, the primary theme of the work could be that resilience can overcome challenges, like those faced living in the wilderness. The theme of resilience will inform a reader's understanding of the story and its characters. This TEAS task requires several skills: finding similarities and differences across themes, recognizing similar themes across different cultures, comparing and contrasting the way in which a single author uses a theme, comparing and contrasting different themes related to a topic, and comparing and contrasting how a theme appears across different genres.

Similarities and Differences Across Themes

Themes are present in both short and long works of fiction and nonfiction, as well as with nonprint sources such as films and radio broadcasts. Sometimes themes are obvious because a work has a specific purpose or aim, such as to convince a person or group of people about a point of view on a topic. However, themes can be less obvious and require a reader to pull together different parts of a text to recognize them. When reading a story, watching a film, or looking at an artwork, ask yourself: What are the big ideas that the artist is engaging with? How are those concepts addressed?

Novels can engage readers by exploring a number of themes. This explains why two teachers can teach the same novel with a different emphasis. One teacher of historical fiction about pioneering nurses such as Clara Barton and Florence Nightingale might focus on the theme of the benefits of hard work and their contributions to the field of nursing. Another teacher might focus on the theme of courage and how they struggled for equal opportunities for women in the medical field.

Similar Themes Across Cultures and Genres

Some common themes across classic works of literature often studied in the United States are power, motherhood, freedom, and privilege. Much can be learned from the themes present within the works of literature in a particular culture, geographic area, or even time period. Recurring themes of oppression within the literature of a time period or culture would likely indicate an oppressive regime or social structure. Presence of a single theme across genres and authors can often signal a historically significant event or attitude among a group of people.

Although a theme can sometimes be treated in a similar manner by different authors, authors often take different perspectives on a single theme. For example, the subject of compassion is present in many works of fiction and nonfiction, but different authors have different themes or ideas about compassion to share with their readers. It is important to recognize that authors can treat the same theme differently within works of fiction or nonfiction. A story about compassion during war will be different from an informational article on compassionate care in nursing.

Often, genre will impact how a theme is addressed. A poem exploring the theme of compassion would describe caring for others in a much different way than a play does. Both texts deal with the universal theme of compassion, but one deals with it through imagery and meter, and the other explores this idea through having characters speak for themselves and express their compassion through words and actions onstage.

Films are a wonderful medium in which to note powerful themes, and filmmakers choose to display and comment on themes in many ways. For example, a director might choose to highlight the powerlessness of a certain group of people by using camera angles that look down on a group rather than a head-on or from below. Camera angles showing a subject from below can depict characters as more powerful or important than those around them. Scenes that show a subject as a small part of the screen in comparison with a vast landscape can also depict a theme of powerlessness.

Once you become adept at finding themes in all artistic genres, you will more easily be able to evaluate one author's or artist's treatment of a theme in relation to another. Likewise, you can begin to look at themes as social commentary and analyze them in relation to cultural or historic movements that might have influenced an artist.

CHAPTER 17 PRACTICE PROBLEMS

Read the following poem and passage. Then answer the questions that follow.

> Our lives, discolored with our present woes,
> May still grow white and shine with happier hours.
> So the pure limped stream, when foul with stains
> Of rushing torrents and descending rains,
> Works itself clear, and as it runs refines,
> till by degrees the floating mirror shines;
> Reflects each flower that on the border grows,
> And a new heaven in its fair bosom shows.

By Joseph Addison, c 1700

The fire crackled in the hearth as Hilda pulled the blanket closer to her for warmth. It had been a long day in the fields, with little to eat afterwards. The overseer had been especially harsh that day, with horrifying threats if anyone paused for breath. Hilda looked toward the small opening in the wall and saw the full moon shining through the only a ragged piece of oilcloth. When the moon waned and waxed just once more, it would be time to run. It would be time to head North.

1. Which of the following is a common theme in the poem and the passage?

   A. Racism poisons people's lives.
   B. Hope sustains people through difficulties.
   C. Hard work brings success.
   D. Nature can be harsh but beautiful.

2. Which of the following is one difference between the poem and passage?

   A. Only the poem uses imagery.
   B. Only the passage describes a character.
   C. Only the poem describes nature.
   D. Only the passage describes an event.

3. Which of the following describes how the writer develops the theme in the poem?

   A. The writer uses an extended metaphor.
   B. The writer uses hyperbole.
   C. The writer narrates a story with characters.
   D. The writer has characters speak for themselves.

4. Which of the following best defines the word "theme"?

   A. The topic of a creative work
   B. The tone of a creative work
   C. A universal concept explored in a creative work
   D. A universal character explored in a creative work

5. Read the passage again. Describe two themes the writer is exploring in the story. Provide evidence that supports each theme.

Notes:

_____

_____

_____

_____

_____

_____

_____

_____

_____

_____

_____

_____

_____

_____

_____

_____

_____

_____

_____

_____

CHAPTER

18 Evaluate an argument and its specific claims

 This objective includes, but is not limited to, the following examples of knowledge, skills, and abilities.

- Identify the argument.
- Identify supporting evidence.
- Examine information that supports the argument.
- Evaluate the relevance and sufficiency of the evidence.

The word "argument" can be a synonym for the word "conflict," but in writing it often means something a bit different. An author's argument is essentially a point that an author believes or seems to believe is true. The argument is what an author is claiming about a debatable issue. The author will then provide reasons for the claim and evidence that supports those reasons. To do well with this TEAS task, you will need to be able to identify an author's argument and supporting evidence and examine the information that supports the argument to determine its relevance and sufficiency.

Identifying the Argument

Identifying a writer's argument involves reading a text completely to determine the claim being made by the entire text. First, identify the topic or issue being discussed. One topic could be dairy products. Second, ask yourself if the author has stated an opinion on the topic. An informative article about dairy products would describe the different types, nutritional values, and sources. But an argumentative or persuasive text will make a claim about dairy products, such as "dairy products are damaging to human health." Third, check that the details in the text provide information about the claim you have identified. If the information supports the claim, you have identified the argument.

Supporting Evidence

It is not enough, however, for a writer to simply state an argument or make a claim. A writer should also have clear reasons and credible evidence to support why the argument is true or valid. Reasons are often stated following an argument, but some authors might purposely place their main argument at the end of a piece after they have stated all the reasons readers should agree with their perspective. Evidence can be directly or indirectly related to the claim, but it will definitely provide readers reasons to agree with the author.

Some evidence is better than others. Evidence drawn from sources that are known to be reputable and based on sound research will likely be more reliable and help to support an argument better than evidence drawn from sources that are not. When evaluating sources, ask yourself who the author(s) is(are), whether the source is peer reviewed, how new the source is, and whether that makes a difference to the argument it is being used to support.

Evaluating Evidence

Remember to examine evidence to determine its reliability. Consider whether the writer is using primary or secondary sources. If a writer cites a primary source, review the evidence to ensure that it is correct and credible. Review data in context from wherever it originated. If a writer cites a secondary or tertiary source, look it up and read it for yourself. Decide whether the writer has interpreted the source correctly in their argument.

Some authors may use evidence that is somewhat unrelated to the argument. This might be accidental, sometimes presenting unrelated evidence is a strategy. When you are evaluating the validity of an argument and its evidence, think about how closely the evidence aligns with the argument being presented. If the evidence is inconsequential or out of alignment with the argument, perhaps the author does not have enough support for the presented position.

Recognizing an author's argument and corresponding evidence is important. Readers who can distinguish between strong and weak arguments and evidence will be ultimately better informed.

CHAPTER 18 PRACTICE PROBLEMS

Read the following passage. Then answer the questions that follow.

Milk is a part of diets around the world, and milk from cows, goats, and even camels is used as a beverage and to make dairy products such as yogurt, skyr, butter, and cheese. People believe that milk is healthy because it is a natural product, but recent research suggests that drinking milk is harmful to human health. Ingesting milk has been linked to heart disease and cancer. Several studies have shown a high positive correlation between milk consumption and mortality rates from heart disease. Most large studies indicate that high dairy consumption increases the risk of prostate cancer. Proponents of milk argue that the nutrients provided by milk are important to health. Although milk does contain these components, these macromolecules can also be found in foods that do not promote disease.

1. Which of the following is the primary argument of the passage?

    A. Milk is a part of diets around the world.
    B. Milk is healthy because it is a natural product.
    C. Ingesting milk has been linked to heart disease.
    D. Drinking milk is harmful to human health.

2. Which of the following is a reason that supports the argument?

    A. There is a correlation between milk consumption and mortality.
    B. High dairy consumption increases the risk of prostate cancer.
    C. The nutrients provided by milk are important to health.
    D. Ingesting milk has been linked to heart disease and cancer.

3. Which of the following is evidence that supports the argument?

    A. Milk can be used to make yogurt and skyr.
    B. High dairy consumption increases the risk of prostate cancer.
    C. High dairy consumption increase nutrients in the diet.
    D. Milk contains macromolecules that can also be found in other foods.

4. Which of the following is a counterargument in the passage?

    A. Milk is a natural product.
    B. Milk can be obtained from cows, goats, and camels.
    C. The nutrients in milk can be found in other foods.
    D. The nutrients provided by milk are important to human health.

5. Many schools require students to wear a school uniform. Write a short argument about whether you agree with this policy. Include a claim, a reason, and supporting evidence.

Notes:

CHAPTER

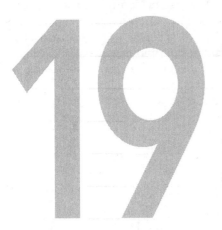

READING

Evaluate and integrate data from multiple sources in various formats, including media

 This objective includes, but is not limited to, the following examples of knowledge, skills, and abilities.

- Select relevant data.
- Examine various data sources.
- Organize data from various sources.
- Combine data from various sources into one document.
- Synthesize data from texts, charts, or graphs.

People read information about topics that interest them on a regular basis, often in newspapers, magazines, professional journals, blogs, and—of course—books. Sometimes these sources include charts, graphs, and diagrams that help to explain an idea shared in a text. If multiple sources of information are not already included in a particular text, it is often a good idea to locate additional sources that could provide more information about a topic.

Doing so will ensure that you develop a more complete understanding of an issue, which will leave you better equipped to converse with others or write more meaningfully on the topic. Most documents produced in postsecondary coursework and by professionals require the author to integrate knowledge from multiple sources. This TEAS task will test your ability to synthesize, organize, and analyze data from multiple sources.

Relevant Data

Whatever the topic, it is wise to seek multiple relevant data sources so that an understanding can be based on multiple perspectives. For example, consider researching risk factors for arthritis and calcium-deficient illnesses.

You could begin with an initial question: What data is most relevant to determining risk factors? You could look at multiple studies of these diseases and consider data on diet and exercise routines and other related health information. You could also consider qualitative data such as case studies and patient histories. It is important to select relevant data from many sources to make a reasoned judgment on what factors put people at risk for these diseases.

Various Data Sources

This initial question and round of data gathering will likely lead you to ask another question: What additional sources of information could help you? You might know some additional sources of information already, depending on how knowledgeable you are about the topic. However, if you have trouble thinking of additional sources of information, library media specialists can be excellent resources. Sometimes also known as "information specialists," they can assist with finding information relevant to a wealth of questions and topics. For the purposes of our example, you might be interested in finding information about negative impacts of traditional blood pressure medications on clients who have various health afflictions, some of which your client might have.

Organizing Data

Once you have determined the information you need and located several sources to provide that information, the next step is to organize the information in a logical manner. One way to do this is by using a coding system that makes sense to you. For the purposes of our example, you might mark articles or participant data related to the required daily allowance of calcium intake with the letters "RDA," and the milligram dosage with the letters "mg." You might also indicate participants who already have arthritis with the letters "RA" for rheumatoid arthritis or "OA" for osteoarthritis (or both, if applicable). Marking information can help physically sort it into physical or electronic folders so you can come back to it when you need it.

There are many technology tools that can help organize information in meaningful ways. These tools can help people organize articles, data, and notes into electronic files and folders. Using technology to help organize information can save money by eliminating printing costs and time sorting through pages of information to locate what is most relevant.

Synthesizing Data

After organizing the information, ask yourself, how does all of this fit together and what does it mean? This stage is often called "synthesis" because you have taken information from many sources, pulled it apart and thought about it, and now you must put it all back together in a meaningful way. For the purposes of our example, your recommendation will be supported by data you have gathered about the participant in the clinical trial and outside sources that provide guidance on best practices related to this particular instance.

Gathering, organizing, analyzing, evaluating, and synthesizing information from multiple sources is an invaluable skill in many professions. Developing the ability to use multiple sources to make decisions and respond to situations helps to ensure more sound and thoughtful actions.

CHAPTER 19 PRACTICE PROBLEMS

Read the passage and review the graph. Then answer the questions that follow.

Nurse practitioners were concerned about the growing rate of expectant mothers who do not take prenatal supplements. Expectant mothers reported that they believed that taking medication when they had no symptoms made no sense. Some believed the supplements could harm the fetus. Expectant mothers also reported that the supplements were difficult to swallow and had an aftertaste. To investigate ways to increase patient knowledge of prenatal supplements, the nurse practitioners designed a controlled study. The control group received normal individual instruction at the hospital. The treatment group received community instruction at local clinics with other expectant mothers. Expectant mothers in both groups were given a pretest and posttest on their knowledge of supplements. Results are shown in the following graph.

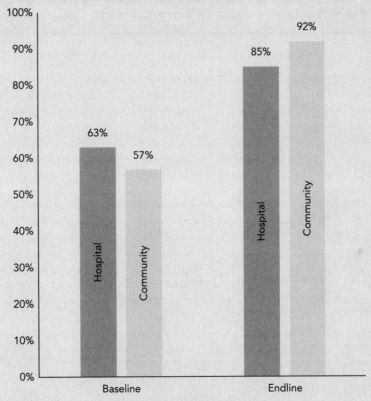

1. Which of the following best describes the results of the study?

    A. Hospital instruction was more effective than community instruction.
    B. Both types of instruction were equally effective.
    C. Community instruction was more effective than hospital instruction.
    D. Neither type of instruction increased patient knowledge.

2. Which of the following was the treatment in this experiment?

    A. Community instruction
    B. Hospital instruction
    C. Use of prenatal vitamins
    D. Use of a placebo

3. Which of the following describes the improvement in knowledge associated with hospital education?

   A. 63 percentage points
   B. 85 percentage points
   C. 35 percentage points
   D. 22 percentage points

4. Which of the following is a conclusion based on the passage and the graph?

   A. There is no difference in knowledge gains based on the way information is delivered.
   B. Community instruction can increase patient knowledge more than individual consultation.
   C. Nurse practitioners can increase patient compliance with their medication.
   D. Hospital instruction is not effective in increasing patient knowledge.

5. Reread the passage and graph. What additional data could be collected to provide more evidence about whether the community intervention helped expectant mothers learn more about prenatal supplements?

Notes:

Notes:

_____

_____

_____

_____

_____

_____

_____

_____

_____

_____

_____

_____

_____

_____

_____

_____

_____

_____

_____

_____

_____

_____

_____

_____

_____

_____

Key Terms

aesthetic. Guiding principles of a piece of work.

anecdote. A short story that illustrates a concept but is not the main idea.

anthology. A published collection of related works.

argument. A set of reasons to make a case for an idea.

argumentative. A contentious tone.

assumption. Supposition of an unstated idea.

audience. The intended consumers of information.

authorial intent. The reason an author creates a text.

bias. Tendency toward a preconceived idea.

blog. A website that is usually informal and independently run.

caption. Description of a figure or graphic.

chart. A type of diagram that graphically represents data.

chronological. In order by time.

claim. A statement that something is true.

classified. A print advertisement selling or soliciting something.

comprehension. Ability to understand.

conclusion. A deduction made by a reader about ideas in a passage based on key points and terms.

connotation. An implied meaning of a word or idea.

context. Nearby text that influences understanding.

delineate. Describe precisely.

denotation. An explicitly stated meaning of a word or idea.

diagram. A symbolic representation of information.

edit. Correct errors in a piece of writing.

evidence. Proof to support an idea.

exclamatory. With strong emotion.

explicit. Clearly stated.

fact. Statement that can be proven.

fact-checking. Verifying facts and statements in text.

figurative. By a figure of speech, usually a metaphor.

footnote. Comment at the bottom of a page that refers to something within the text.

foreshadowing. An author's hints of events to come.

forum. An online message board.

genre. A group of related writings or other media.

graph. A type of diagram that displays data mathematically.

graphic. A diagram, graph, illustration, or other piece of artwork.

guide words. Words in a dictionary that help readers locate words.

heading. A title.

identify. Distinguish a particular idea.

imply. Indicate an idea subtly without specifically stating it.

inference. An idea about a topic that is not directly stated but is based on evidence and reasoning.

information specialist. A library employee who helps patrons find information.

irrelevant. Not applicable to the idea.

key points. Ideas that support the main idea about a topic.

legend. Map feature that explains symbols and other elements.

library media specialist. A library employee who helps patrons find media sources.

logic. The framework of reasoning used to understand ideas.

main idea. The central point the author is making about the topic of a text.

memorandum. A written informal note usually used for business purposes.

modes. Forms of writing.

opinion. Statement that cannot be proven.

parts of speech. Basic types of words in English.

peer-reviewed journal. Published writings that have been analyzed by experts in the field.

persuasive. Intending to make the reader believe an idea.

point of view. Perspective.

prediction. A reader's guess of events to come.

primary source. A firsthand document or source created at the time in question.

procedure. Process for writing, editing, and revision.

professional journal. Published periodical texts that represent a specific industry.

publication. Printing or distribution of text.

query. A question.

reason. A basis or fact to support an idea.

relevant. Connected to the idea being discussed.

rephrase. To explain an idea in different words.

representation. How something is expressed.

research based. Reliant on ideas backed by study.

revision. Rewriting a piece of text.

rhetoric. The use of elements of language.

rhetorical. Used for effect only, not meaning.

scale. Ratio of distance expressed to actual measurement.

search engine. Website to locate information online.

search term. Words used to find information via a search engine.

secondary source. Secondhand account of events.

sequence. Logical order in writing.

sequential. Following a set order.

social commentary. Use of rhetoric to make statements about current culture.

social structure. The system and relationships between groups of society.

stereotype. Simplified categorization of an idea or person based on convention.

structures. Ways of logically organizing ideas.

style guide. Set of conventions and standards for a type of writing.

subheading. A title of a subdivision of information with a larger text.

superscript. Text that is smaller and above the surrounding text.

support. Lend credibility to an idea.

tertiary source. A compilation of primary and secondary sources.

theme. A foundational concept engaged with by a piece of art.

tone. The author's voice and attitude toward the topic.

topic. Subject of a text.

valid. Proven as true.

word origin. How a word came to its current use and meaning.

Practice Problem Answers

Chapter 1

1. Option B is correct. It indicates that the entire passage will describe a case of sepsis, including its cause, symptoms, and treatment. Option A indicates only that welding does have occupational hazards. Option C is only about part of the passage. Option D is not covered in this passage.

2. Option C is correct. The description of the symptoms and treatment of sepsis is the central idea of the passage. Option A is only about welding, which is a detail of the passage. Option B is a detail about two ER trips. Option D is a detail that is one part of the passage.

3. Option C is correct. Shortness of breath is one warning sign or symptom of sepsis. Option A is a condition that may or may not lead to sepsis. Option B is the opposite, as sepsis can cause faster-than-normal heart rate. Option D is the opposite, as sepsis can cause a drop in blood pressure.

4. Option A is correct. The infection was the cause of sepsis. Option B was only the material that caused a burn. Option C was one of the warning signs of sepsis. Option D was the result of the hot metal.

5. Rationale: A summary of the passage and rephrasing of key ideas could include the following.

   • Sepsis can occur due to an infection.
   • Sepsis can result in a fever and faster-than-normal heart rate.
   • Sepsis can cause a drop in blood pressure.

Chapter 2

1. Option B is correct. Clues such as "next start date for the program" and "complete cardiopulmonary resuscitation (CPR) and basic life support (BLS) training" reveal when Danielle could apply to the residency program. Option A is incorrect because that is the step before the residency program. Option C is incorrect because that is unrelated to the ability to apply to the program. Option D is incorrect because choosing a specialty would happen upon applying for the program.

2. Option A is correct because this phrase provides a sequence context for the actions that Danielle takes immediately after completing high school.

Option B simply explains Danielle's motivation for wanting to become a nurse. Options C and D do not provide any information that would reasonably allow the reader to assemble the events in the passage.

3. Option C is correct because four semesters are equivalent to two years. The other options are incorrect because each year is equivalent to two semesters.

4. Option B is correct. Nurses in the neonatal intensive care unit (NICU) are responsible for the care of the tiniest patients, the premature newborn infants, as well as critically ill infants. The others options are incorrect because they are not the patient population cared for in the NICU.

5. One possible conclusion to be drawn from the passage is that "transition to practice" means nursing students would work with nurses and gain experience while learning about nursing. This is implied by the phrase "gain professional experience and develop real hands-on nursing skills."

Chapter 3

1. Option C is correct. The topic of this passage is about the importance of exercise in maintaining a healthy heart. Option A conveys the analogy about the heart being like the engine in a car. Option B is related to the heart, but it is not the main topic. Option D is something that can potentially be avoided by regular exercise, but it is not the main topic.

2. Option B is correct. The main topic is about how to keep the heart healthy through regular exercise, and this option describes an effective exercise routine. Options A, C, and D relate to main topic but do not summarize it.

3. Option D is correct. It covers the types of exercises that can contribute to heart health.

   Options A, B, and C address details covered in the passage but are not summaries of the main topic.

4. Option A is correct. It addresses how exercise can promote heart health. Option B is not a supporting detail. Options C and D are potential benefits of exercise but not supporting details.

5. The supporting detail should be about how exercise helps improve blood circulation. None of the other options given are supporting details.

Chapter 4

1. Option B is correct. The passage is about the correct procedure for inserting an IV catheter.

   Options A, B, and D are parts of the procedure but not the procedure itself.

2. Option D is correct. Steps in a procedure include procedural signal words to demonstrate how they are related. Options A and C are true about what is conveyed in the passage but do not explain how the steps are related. Option B merely mentions a cautionary note but is not an explanation for how the steps are related.

3. Option A is correct. Order terms signify the relationship among steps. Options B, C, and D are directional terms that explain how to carry out the steps.

4. Option C is correct. One step can occur while another is occurring. In the case of this passage, "While using a soothing tone, encourage the patient to not watch the procedure." Options A and B describes individual steps occurring at specific times. Option D describes a step at the end of a procedure.

5. Suitable answers could include any of the following or related ones in the passage:

   Explain the IV catheter insertion procedure.

   Determine if the patient has needle phobia.

   Encourage the patient to not watch the procedure.

   Follow infection control protocol.

   Look for a suitable vein.

   Carefully use your fingers to locate a suitable vein.

Chapter 5

1. Option D is correct. The memo addresses the importance of following proper handwashing procedures. Options A, B, and D are addressed in the memo but are not the main point.

2. Option B is correct. Proper handwashing procedure is to wash hands for at least 30 seconds. Options A and D are not included in the rules for proper handwashing. Option C may occur, but the rule is at least 30 seconds.

3. Option C is correct. The NICU is the neonatal intensive care unit. Options A, B, and D are not among the patients cared for in the NICU

4. Option B is correct. A public announcement would address how to handle an emergency drill.

   Option A addresses procedural steps. Option C addresses directions for completing a task. Option D could be part of an online advertisement about taking a HIPAA class.

5. Option D is correct. An online classified advertisement would include a call to action. Option A would be included in a memo. Option B would be included in a procedural explanation. Option C would be included in a public announcement.

Chapter 6

1. Option B is correct. According to the BLS, between now and 2028, nursing careers are projected to grow at a rate of 12%, or from 3 million to 3.4 million nursing positions. Options A, B, and D are not included in this figure, according to the BLS.

2. Option D is correct. The bachelor of science in nursing (BSN) is the preferred degree to compete for jobs with other healthcare professionals. Option A is the associate degree in nursing and is considered a beginner degree. Option B is not a degree but is the exam nurses must pass to qualify for nursing licenses. Option C is a master of science in nursing (MSN), an advanced degree for those nurses wishing to pursue higher-ranking positions, such as nurse practitioner.

3. Option C is correct. Those patients who are aging and no longer able to care for themselves typically require nursing care in residential care facilities. Options A, B, and D include patients who require care in different types of facilities than residential.

4. Option B is correct. The National Council Licensure Examination (NCLEX)-RN is the exam nurses must pass to qualify for their nursing licenses. Options A, C, and D are fictional variations for the acronym NCLEX.

5. Option A is correct. Each nurse must apply for a nursing license from his or her own state's nursing board. Options B, C, and D are not licensing agencies

Chapter 7

1. Option B is correct. When something occurs prior to something else, that indicates a sequence of steps or events. Options A, B, and D are chronological signal words, indicating a time factor for steps or events to occur.

2. Option A is correct. Chronological signal words indicate a time factor, such as a length of time since something else occurred. Options B, C, and D are words indicating sequential order.

3. Option C is correct. Tim is thinking ahead that if he follows one prescribed plan, it could change his future plans. Options A, B, and D describe events that are sequential.

4. Option D is correct. Many nursing students choose to begin with the associate degree in nursing (ADN) and then progress to the bachelor of science in nursing (BSN) followed by the master of science in nursing (MSN) to become a nurse practitioner. Options A, B, and C are not the correct sequence of degrees to follow to become a nurse practitioner.

5. Option B is correct. The registered nurse (RN) to bachelor of science in nursing (BSN) path is considered the bridge program for nurses who only have a nursing diploma or associate degree in nursing (ADN). Options A, C, and D are not part of the bridge program.

Chapter 8

1. Option B is correct. Physical education does promote a healthier lifestyle. Options A, C, and D are opinions of the author.

2. Option A is correct. It is a stereotype to believe all students spend too much time on electronic devices. Options B and D are factual statements. Option C is an opinion.

3. Option D is correct. The author believes PE should be mandatory. Options A and C are opinions, and option B was not a conclusion made by the author.

4. Option C is correct. Overall, the author presented information about the benefits of PE. The author does not present this information with optimism about gaining mandatory PE or pessimism that mandatory PE will ever occur. The author uses no words to indicate that there is irritation regarding the topic.

5. PE should not be mandatory in schools. First, requiring PE would mean that students lose a class period where they could take an advanced academic class. Next, PE is upsetting for many students. Many students feel compared to others and bullying can occur when a student is teased during athletic activities. Last, mandatory PE does not improve health. Exercise for a single class period does not result in the sustained exercise that improves fitness.

Chapter 9

1. Option C is correct. The mode of this passage is expository to inform the audience about the causes and effects of secondhand smoke. It does not present an opinion about secondhand smoke to persuade the audience. It does not describe a setting or event or narrate events.

2. Option A is correct. The term "consequently" signals a consequence or a result. "Gradually" indicates how time passed during an activity. "Now" and "until recently" also indicate time and not a result of something.

3. Option D is correct. The phrase "as well as" indicates something similar to what was stated previously. The phrases "more likely" and "on the other hand" indicate contrast. "Gradually" is a term that indicates time.

4. Option B is correct. The article describes secondhand smoke as the cause of many health problems. The effects are conditions such as ear infections, asthma, and heart disease. Although secondhand smoke is a problem, the writer does not propose a solution. Secondhand smoke is not compared to another issue. The writer is not presenting an opinion about secondhand smoke to persuade the reader. The writer is presenting facts.

5. Secondhand smoke is a problem for many people because they are exposed to this smoke in their homes and public places. Secondhand smoke is dangerous at all levels, but repeated exposure is especially harmful and can cause chronic diseases. One solution to this problem is to pass laws banning smoking in public places. Another solution is education. Governments and health facilities need to advertise the health consequences of breathing secondhand smoke.

Chapter 10

1. Option D is correct. The overall mood conveys the determination of Roosevelt and his team to complete the expedition. Options A, B, and C may have occurred at different points but not in the overall mood or tone.

2. Option B is correct. The rugged wilderness proved to be formidable, daunting, or challenging. Option A describes the type of trip the team took to get to the river. Option C describes the type of river it was. Option D describes the type of conditions they faced.

3. Option C is correct. A simile uses the word "like" to compare two unlike things. Options A and B were not used in this line. Option D, "connotation," means a suggestion or implication of a word's meaning, but it is not accurate here.

4. Option A is correct. Personification attributes human qualities to nonhuman entities. Option B is a suggestion or implication of a word's meaning, whereas option C is the actual meaning. Option D, a simile, uses "like" to compare unlike things.

5. Learner answers will vary. Three terms that describe the jungle are rugged, harsh, and formidable. Rugged creates the idea of an uneven terrain that is difficult to cross. Harsh creates the feeling that the jungle will have terrible conditions and can cause harm. Formidable conjures the feeling of a strong enemy that is difficult to defeat. All of these terms create the effect that the jungle is a frightening place.

Chapter 11

1. Option D is correct. Alphabetically, "powerlifting" comes after "powdery" and before "pox." In options A and B, "powerlifting" comes before both "practicable" and "Pyrex," and "psychoanalysis" and "public speaking." In option C, "powerlifting" comes after both "Poseidon" and "poverty."

2. Option C is correct. "Cardiovascular" is an adjective used in this passage to describe health. Options A, B, and D are not adjectives and are not the correct parts of speech to describe health.

3. Option A is correct. Motor units are composed of nerve cells and muscle fiber bundles. Options B, C, and D are related but are not correct definitions of the term.

4. Option B is correct. Neuromuscular adaptations involve having motor units work faster and simultaneously. Options A, C, and D are events that occur during and as results of adaptations.

5. Learner responses will vary based on what sources learners find. They should cover how rate coding addresses making motor units work faster and how motor unit synchronization makes motor units work together simultaneously. Together, they cause nerve impulses to be stronger and faster and increase muscle development and capacity.

Chapter 12

1. Option B is correct. The announcement is primarily to provide information about the in-service training. Option A is part of the task for nurses to complete, but it is not the primary purpose. Although option C may be desirable, it is not the primary purpose. Option D is not correct because staff will need to alternate times they participate in the training so some staff remain on duty.

2. Option D is correct. The announcement conveys information. Options A, B, and C are not the modes of the announcement.

3. Option C is correct. The author of the announcement conveys an authoritative tone. Options A, B, and D are not expressed in the tone of the announcement.

4. Option A is correct. Nurses need to know how to manage transitions of care. Option B may be helpful, but it is not required. Option C was not stated as a necessity, and Option D will be included in the training.

5. Learner responses will vary but should include the audience for the announcement, the topic of the training, the definition of transitions of care, and a paraphrased version of the five standards.

Chapter 13

1. Option C is correct. The website by the staff of a medical facility would be the most reliable. Options A and B are not as reliable. Option D is incorrect because it includes one answer that is not as reliable.

2. Option A is correct. Insight from medical professionals would be most reliable and authoritative. Option B is incorrect because the nursing staff website does not necessarily include insight about the prevention of falls. Options C and D do not necessarily include insight about preventing falls.

3. Option B is correct. For an important topic like preventing patients from falling and sustaining injuries, authority and expertise would be essential. Although options A, C, and D all have some merit, they are not as important.

4. Option D is correct. Information on the topic of preventing falls should be both relevant and accurate. Options A and C may have some basis for consideration, but they are not the most important reasons. Option B would likely not be a desirable choice if it does not align with sound practice.

5. Learner responses will vary. Suitable answers for why a blog would not be a reliable source for information on preventing falls include that the blog relates personal experiences and opinions and not researched procedures. The reader would also need to consider that social-media influence and loyalty to advertisers and sponsors may bias the blogger's information on the topic of fall prevention.

Chapter 14

1. Option D is correct. The course title, *Continuity of Care and Nurse Navigation*, is italicized. Options A and B are text features in the sidebar, and Option C is a text feature of a quotation from a graduate.

2. Option B is correct. Prerequisites for the course are included in the sidebar. Options A, C, and D are included in other parts of the course catalog page.

3. Option A is correct. A superscript number after a line indicates there is a corresponding footnote. Options B, C, and D are unrelated to the footnote.

4. Option C is correct. The superscript identifies the footnote as a testimonial by J. D. Ross, RN, BSN. Options A, B, and D are not included in footnotes.

5. Learner responses will vary but should include that the descriptions of the buildings and the walking paths are important to locating these on campus. The scale should be mentioned as important to understanding the distances across campus. The compass rose should be described as important to understanding the direction in which to move to travel to a desired location from a given starting point.

Chapter 15

1. Option C is correct. A research study is a primary source. Textbooks and encyclopedias are secondary sources that compile medical information. Option D would be secondary sources.

2. Option A is correct. A documentary about the history of baseball will combine a variety of primary and secondary sources to tell about the past of this sport. A telegram is a primary source because it is written by the sender. An autobiography is a primary source because it is written about a person by that person. A novel and other creative writing are primary sources written by a person about their own ideas.

3. Option B is correct. One of the key beliefs of the founders is that "all men are created equal." The speech is about consecrating land and not owning land. The speech is about the death of soldiers and not serving as soldiers. The speech does not refer to running for office.

4. Option D is correct. Lincoln is giving this speech in Gettysburg to dedicate land for the burial of soldiers. He makes no mention of reelection. He does describe why the United States was founded, but this is in the introduction and is not the purpose of the speech. Lincoln discusses the Civil War but not why it started.

5. Answers will vary. Students may cite a variety of primary sources about the MMR vaccine, such as photographs of the developer of the vaccine Maurice Hillman. There are also photographs of procedures that helped to develop the vaccine, such as workers making openings in chicken eggs in preparation for a measles vaccine. There

are also publications on the research conducted to verify the efficacy of the vaccine by Hillman and the Merck company. Newspaper articles from 1971 about the vaccine could also be cited as primary sources. Students should explain that any source they cite was done by an eyewitness or participant or produced at the time of the vaccine development.

Chapter 16

1. Option B is correct. Because Nikita detached the ropes deliberately, the reader can predict she may freestyle climb. Nikita will likely not panic because she deliberately detached her ropes. Ivan will not run for help or climb up because there is no evidence to predict that Nikita needs assistance.

2. Option B is correct. Because she has loved to climb all her life, the reader can infer that Nikita is athletic and adventurous. It is unlikely that Nikita is afraid of heights because she loves to climb. There are no details in the passage that suggest that Nikita is a professional climber or has traveled to many mountains.

3. Option A is correct. The reader can synthesize information on Nikita climbing trees as a baby and her current rock climbing to conclude that Nikita is drawn to the outdoors and risk-taking. Nikita's mother encouraged her climbing by placing her in gymnastics. The passage does not discuss whether Nikita has a deep love of geology or wanted to become an Olympic gymnast.

4. Option C is correct. A climbing partner belays or puts tension on a rope to keep the climber from falling. Letting go of the rope or loosening it would not help the climber. There is no evidence that Ivan has a cleat to fasten the rope to.

5. Answers will vary. One example of a biography is *Frida, a Biography of Frida Kahlo* by Hayden Herrera. The back of the book states that it is about the life of Frida Kahlo, an important Mexican painter. She was born in Mexico City and was injured in a devastating tram accident. She was involved in international exhibitions and politics. She had many relationships that influenced her and her work. From this information it can be predicted that the biography will discuss how her injury affected her life and paintings.

Chapter 17

1. Option B is correct. Both the poem and passage discuss hope. The poem says that hope will help a person through their woes, and in the passage, we see the character Hilda surviving harsh labor by hoping for freedom. Racism and hard work are only discussed in the passage. Nature is described in both passages but not described as harsh.

2. Option B is correct. Only the passage describes a character. Both genres use imagery, describe nature, and describe an event.

3. Option A is correct. The writer develops the theme in the poem through the extended metaphor of a stream slowly clearing representing our lives following woe. Eventually the woe will be over. The writer does not use hyperbole or exaggeration. The writer does not narrate a story or have characters speak for themselves.

4. Option C is correct because a theme is a universal concept explored in a creative work. It is not a topic; it is what the writer is saying about the topic. It is not a tone or feeling related to an artistic work, or an exploration of a universal character in a work, although stock characters are often used in creative works.

5. Answers will vary. Two possible themes the writer is exploring in the story are resilience in the face of cruelty and the will to survive. Resilience is illustrated by Hilda's ability to keep working despite the overseer's cruelty and the will to survive is seen in her plans for escape.

Chapter 18

1. Option D is correct. The writer is arguing that drinking milk is harmful to human health. The writer provides background by saying that milk is a part of diets around the world and that people believe that milk is healthy because it is a natural product. The fact that ingesting milk has been linked to heart disease is evidence that supports the claim.

2. Option D is correct because one reason for the claim that milk is unhealthy is that ingesting milk has been linked to heart disease and cancer. The correlation between milk consumption and mortality and increases the risk of prostate cancer are evidence for the reason. The fact that nutrients provided by milk are important to health is a counterargument.

3. Option B is correct. Research that shows high dairy consumption increases the risk of prostate cancer is evidence that dairy products increase heart disease and cancer rates. That milk can be used to make yogurt and skyr and contains macromolecules that can also be found in other foods is background information about milk. The fact that high dairy consumption increase nutrients in the diet is part of the counterargument.

4. Option D is correct. The counterargument is the opposite of the claim. The opposite of the claim that milk is unhealthy is that the nutrients provided by milk are important to human health. That milk is a natural product and can be obtained from cows, goats, and camels is background information. That nutrients in milk can be found in other foods is a rebuttal to the counterargument.

5. Answers will vary. One claim is that schools should require students to wear a school uniform. One reason for this is that it will save families money on clothing. For example, the average teenager will need 7 to 10 outfits to wear to school. With a school uniform, this is cut down to 2 to 3 outfits because the student is wearing the same outfit daily.

Chapter 19

1. Option C is correct. Looking at the graph, community instruction was more effective than hospital instruction. This is shown by the larger increase in the percentage points from pretest to posttest. Community instruction increase knowledge by 35 points, whereas hospital instruction increased patient knowledge by 22 points. Both types of instruction increased knowledge, but community instruction increased it by 6 points more.

2. Option A is correct. Community instruction was the treatment in this experiment because it was a new way of presenting knowledge to patients devised by the nurse practitioners to increase patient understanding of supplements. Hospital instruction was the control because it was the normal instruction patients received. This enabled the nurses to discern whether the new method was better than the old method. This study did not test medications or a placebo.

3. Option D is correct. To calculate the improvement in knowledge associated with hospital education, subtract the pretest score (63) from the posttest score (85), and a difference of 22 percentage points is found. This is the measure of the average improvement in knowledge. Sixty-three percentage points is the average pretest score of hospital instruction participants, and 85 percentage points the average pretest score of hospital instruction participants. Thirty-five percentage points is the average improvement in knowledge associated with community instruction.

4. Option B is correct. Community instruction can increase patient knowledge more than individual consultation. This is shown when considering the increases in knowledge produced by each type of instruction. Community instruction increase knowledge by 35 points, and hospital instruction increased knowledge by 22 points. So, community instruction was more effective by 13 points. So, in this study, the method of instruction did matter. The study did not address compliance with taking the supplements, only knowledge of the supplements.

5. Answers will vary. One type of additional data that could be collected to provide more evidence would be to interview participants about what they learned. Qualitative studies like this can reveal how patient knowledge differed between groups and what participants felt about the two types of instruction. Patient emotional reactions can enhance or interfere with retention of knowledge.

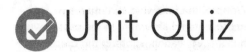 # Unit Quiz

The next six questions are based on this passage.

The Apprentice

Luigi, following his friend Mario, dashed over the cobbled street in the November rain. He'd left his village in the southeast and traveled north to the renowned city of Rome. After several months, the urban environment was becoming second nature. Above all, Luigi adored art—sculpture, frescos, and mosaics—and Rome contained innumerable artistic treasures. Great masters toiled endlessly, drawing, chiseling, grinding pigments, and mixing paints.

Luigi had apprenticed himself to sculptor and painter Marco de Luca. His body ached from intense, grueling work and endless days, but Luigi derived satisfaction from the uniqueness of creation. However, his greatest desire was to encounter the master of all masters, the young Michelangelo Buonarroti. Luigi and his fellow apprentice, Mario, deemed Michelangelo's work to be superior; the **Pietà** was their favorite sculpture.

One afternoon, while chiseling milky-white marble, Mario whispered, "After we're done with work today, follow me on an errand for Master Marco; you'll be surprised."

Luigi had eyed his companion curiously, while still concentrating carefully on the hard, white stone. After plodding through the drizzle with a satchel of assorted pigments, Mario and Luigi entered a large door, navigated a series of hallways, and eventually found themselves in a chapel. Scaffolding obscured considerable sections of the ceiling, but evidently a great masterwork was in progress: Flowing figures in soft blues, glowing golds, and raucous reds emerged from behind the scaffold.

"I've brought your requested pigments, sir," squeaked Mario, his knees shaking.

A pale, elongated face outlined with ebony hair appeared over the scaffolding, contrasting with the luminous figures above it.

"Thanks to you and Master Marco, this segment will be completed today!" the man exclaimed. "But painting is secondary for me these days—I prefer sculpture. Surely you've seen my **Pietà**?"

Speechless, Luigi gazed upward at Michelangelo Buonarroti, master of all masters.

1. Which of the following statements best summarizes the passage?
   A. Luigi and his friend Mario find themselves running an errand in the rain.
   B. After working long hours, Luigi and Mario, newcomers to Rome, enjoy their time off.
   C. Luigi goes to Rome to work, and his friend Mario helps him meet someone he admires.
   D. Mario and Luigi are friends and coworkers who enjoy meeting famous artists.

2. Which of the following is a logical conclusion that can be drawn from the passage?
   A. Mario is interested only painting.
   B. Luigi came to Rome to study art.
   C. Marco de Luca is from Luigi's hometown.
   D. Luigi is from a large city.

3. Which of the following is a supporting detail for the idea that "a great masterwork was in progress"?
   A. "Flowing figures in soft blues, glowing golds, and raucous reds emerged from behind the scaffold."
   B. "Scaffolding obscured considerable sections of the ceiling"
   C. "After plodding through the drizzle with a satchel of assorted pigments"
   D. "A pale, elongated face outlined with ebony hair appeared over the scaffolding"

4. Which of the following best describes what happened immediately after Mario asks Luigi to follow him on an errand?
   A. Luigi leaves his home to go to Rome.
   B. Mario and Luigi meet Michelangelo.
   C. Luigi and Mario find their way to the chapel.
   D. Luigi and Mario carry a satchel of pigments through the rain.

5. The passage states that "Scaffolding obscured considerable sections of the ceiling." Which of the following is the most accurate interpretation of this phrase?
   A. The scaffolding had removed parts of the paintings on the ceiling.
   B. Parts of the paintings were hidden from view behind the scaffolding.
   C. The scaffolding had been built to cover parts of the ceiling.
   D. Sections of the ceiling were missing entirely.

6. Which of the following excerpts from the passage is an opinion?

    A. "Luigi had apprenticed himself to sculptor"
    B. "Mario and Luigi entered a large door"
    C. "Luigi dashed over the cobbled street"
    D. "Mario deemed Michelangelo's work to be superior"

The next two questions are based on this passage.

Do Uniforms Matter?

School uniforms are an invaluable means for educational administrators. They prevent problems within student populations by promoting order and discipline. They help students learn the importance of adhering to regulations and recognizing that deviation from expectations produces consequences. Dressing appropriately for school helps young people learn that life requires different styles of attire, depending on the situation. Uniforms also promote standardization. They limit the promotion of ideas or values that are inappropriate in schools, such as students showing allegiance to a gang or like groups or wearing clothing that others may find offensive. Dr. Karen P. Braun of Southern University, an adolescent behavioral expert, believes that students who wear uniforms are more accepting of their same-age peers.

7. Which of the following statements would strengthen the argument in the passage?

    A. A study that shows students who wear uniforms do better academically
    B. A quote from an expert about the need for young people to be individuals
    C. A report on the costliness of buying and maintaining school uniforms
    D. A series of photographs of students in school uniforms

8. Which of the following is a primary source that could be used to provide opposition to the argument in the passage?

    A. The study "Uniforms and Peer Acceptance" by Dr. Karen P. Braun
    B. An interview with a school principal who wrote an editorial called "The Harm of Uniforms"
    C. A newspaper article that cites several cases about the usefulness of uniforms
    D. A catalog that includes different designs and fabrics for school uniforms

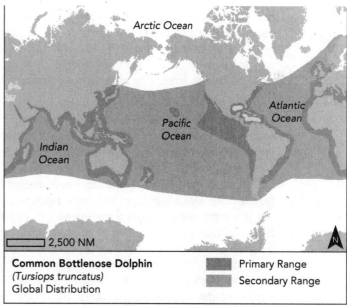

2,500 NM

Common Bottlenose Dolphin
(Tursiops truncatus)
Global Distribution

    Primary Range
    Secondary Range

9. Based on the map, which ocean contains the northernmost secondary range of the common bottlenose dolphin?

    A. Arctic
    B. Atlantic
    C. Pacific
    D. Indian

10. Which of the following is the meaning of "inquisitive" as used in the sentence?

    Maya's inquisitive nature led her to answer her own questions as a research scientist.

    A. Logical
    B. Methodical
    C. Curious
    D. Careful

The next six questions are based on this passage.

The Tragedy of the RMS Titanic

Preparation is the key to success and being prepared for an emergency can mean the difference between life and death. Lack of preparation was one of the key factors in the tragedy of the *Titanic* in which more than one thousand people perished in the cold waters of the Atlantic.

The tragedy began when the *Titanic* hit an iceberg off the coast of Newfoundland in the North Atlantic at approximately 11:40 p.m. on April 14, 1912. The ship eventually sank in the early hours of April 15. But the profound loss of life of approximately 1,500 people could have been greatly reduced—or even avoided—had there been sufficient planning for the possibility that the ship could sink and was not, in fact, unsinkable. There were only 20 lifeboats available, and they could only hold 1,178 people, but 2,240 were on board. Additionally, during the panic of the tragedy, boats were launched when they were only half-full of passengers. Therefore, too few lifeboats, combined with too few passengers on each lifeboat, resulted in the staggering loss of life.

There was also a difference in the survival of passengers depending on gender, age, and class. The law of the sea dictates that women and children should board the lifeboats first. It wasn't only women and children who were more likely to survive, though; the type of ticket that a passenger had made a difference, too. It is estimated that passengers who were traveling first class were 44% more likely to survive than other passengers. Because of the tragedy of the *Titanic*, ships today are required to adhere to rigorous safety protocols. These include meeting requirements for the number of lifeboats, having clear directions in cases of emergency, and conducting emergency practice drills before sailing. Because of the *Titanic*, sailing is much safer today.

11. Which of the following provides the best summary of the passage?

    A. Men who were first-class passengers and women were the most likely to survive the sinking of the *Titanic*.
    B. The cold waters of the Atlantic is why passengers and crew who did not reach a lifeboat ultimately perished.
    C. The loss of life on the *Titanic* could have been reduced had there been more lifeboats and had they been filled to capacity.
    D. Because of the law of the sea, more women and children survived the sinking of the *Titanic*.

12. Which of the following can you infer about the number of people who survived the sinking of the *Titanic*?

    A. No crew members or passengers survived.
    B. Most passengers and crew did not survive.
    C. Most members of the crew survived.
    D. Most passengers and crew survived.

13. According to the passage, which of the following describes why ships are safer today?

    A. Ships have more crew to maintain safety.
    B. Ships have to follow rigorous safety procedures.
    C. Ships must allow women and children to board lifeboats first.
    D. Ships have to be built with equipment for breaking icebergs.

14. Which of the following events in the passage occurred first?

    A. The *Titanic* hit an iceberg.
    B. Only a few hours after it hit an iceberg, the *Titanic* sunk.
    C. Women and children boarded onto lifeboats.
    D. Ships began to follow rigorous standards, including lifeboat requirements.

15. Which of the following best describes the structure of the passage?

    A. Compare and contrast
    B. Problem and solution
    C. Chronological order
    D. Cause and effect

16. Which of the following is the purpose of this selection?
    A. Entertain readers with a narrative about events regarding the *Titanic*
    B. Inform readers about why the loss of life was so high on the *Titanic*
    C. Persuade readers that the design of the *Titanic* caused the ship to sink
    D. Describe to readers the design of lifeboats on the Titanic in detail

The next two questions are based on this passage.

Using a product created by Alltech Enterprises will always give users a better experience. For example, the Alltech Desktop Computer is user friendly and less likely to crash and contract viruses than other laptops currently on the market. In addition, when a customer takes the leap of faith and buys multiple Alltech products, such as the Alltech Superphone and Supertablet, there will be a variety of pleasant surprises. The Calendar application on both Alltech's Desktop and Supertablet will sync with its Superphone. Customers can also see texts on all three products simultaneously. Overall, having Alltech products will make a customer's life better and easier.

17. Which of the following statements is a fact cited in the passage?
    A. Alltech products make a customer's life easier with a variety of features.
    B. The calendar on an Alltech Superphone can sync with the calendar on an Alltech Supertablet.
    C. Using a product created by Alltech always gives users a better experience.
    D. The Alltech Desktop Computer is more user friendly than other laptops.

18. Which of the following is the author's argument in the passage?
    A. Having Alltech products will make users life better and easier.
    B. Alltech Desktop Computers are less likely to crash.
    C. Alltech products are less likely to contract viruses.
    D. Buying multiple Alltech products results in pleasant surprises.

	Price per ounce	Replacement Needed
Soap A	$0.10	3 months
Soap B	$0.11	3 months
Soap C	$0.10	4 months
Soap D	$0.12	4 months

19. A frugal couple is looking to save money and are considering the cost of their hand soap. They are considering four different soap products. Each soap bottle contains 6 ounces. The chart shows the cost per ounce and how often the soap would need to be replaced. Which of the following options cost the least over 4 months?
    A. Soap A
    B. Soap B
    C. Soap C
    D. Soap D

20. Which of the following is a primary source that is best to use when writing an article about the effort to convert a vacant lot into a community garden?
    A. An interview with local expert gardeners involved in the project
    B. An interview with local business owners who work near the vacant lot
    C. An article in the local newspaper about the effort to create a community garden
    D. A video clip on the local news reporting on a potential community garden

Directions: Soil Incorporation Composting

To make compost, try soil incorporation, a relatively simple method for composting small amounts of organic waste. Start by digging a hole at least 12 inches deep in your yard. Collect the leftovers you want to compost, such as coffee grounds and vegetables. (Do not include oily or fatty scraps, such as meat because they can lure hungry animals.) Next, chop up the scraps and mix them into some of the soil you removed; the soil will speed up the decomposition process. Fill the hole about 4 inches deep with the mixture of scraps and soil, and cover it up with at least 8 inches of soil. The buried food wastes will decompose in 1 month to 1 year, depending on the size of the hole, becoming nutrient-rich compost in the process.

21. Which of the following is the final step in the process of soil incorporation composting?

   A. Chop up food scraps and mix them with soil for faster decomposition.
   B. Place a mixture of food wastes and soil at the bottom of a hole at least 12 inches deep.
   C. Cover the mixture of food wastes and soil with 8 or more inches of soil.
   D. Wait for the buried food wastes to decompose over time, creating rich compost.

Directions: Registering Online for a 5K Run

1. On the home page of the official website for the 5K race, click on the Register or Sign Up link. Fill in all the fields. You may be asked to provide your birthdate and sex (for placement in competitive running groups) and emergency contact information.

2. Click on Agree to Terms to read the waiver. Verify that you understand the race legalities by clicking the Agree box. Then click Continue.

3. Follow the rest of the steps until you get to the Final Checkout page.

4. Review all the information entered.

5. Click on Check Out or Cart and enter your credit card information to pay the entry fee. You may be given the option of buying a race T-shirt. Click Confirm Payment.

22. According to the directions, when should you click the Agree box on the Agree to Terms link?

   A. After you have entered your credit card information on the Final Checkout page and read the waiver.
   B. After you have filled out all the fields in the Register section and read the waiver.
   C. Before you have filled out all the fields in the Register section or read the waiver.
   D. Before you have provided your birthdate and sex in the Register section.

The next two questions are based on this passage.

Timeline: *The History of Sugar*

c. 8000 BCE Sugarcane first cultivated in New Guinea

c. 350 CE First crystal form of sugar made in India

c. 1000 Arabs improve manufacturing process of sugar and add sugar to many foods

c. 1096–1150 Crusaders returning from the Middle East introduce sugar to Europe

1480–1540 Portuguese explorers bring sugar to the New World

1550–1770 Thousands of sugar mills are built in the Americas and the Caribbean; millions of African and American Indian slaves are forced to harvest sugarcane

1951–present Technology increases sugar yields, but health concerns about sugar consumption lead to the development of new artificial and natural sweeteners

23. According to the timeline, which of the following events likely led to Europeans' desire for sugar?

   A. Crusaders bringing sugar back from the Middle East
   B. The cultivation of sugarcane in New Guinea
   C. Development of the first crystal form of sugar in India
   D. Arab people adding sugar to sweeten foods

24. According to the timeline, what significant negative effect did sugar production have on world history?

   A. It caused the European Crusaders to travel to the Middle East.
   B. It caused the Portuguese to introduce sugar to the Americas and Caribbean.
   C. It led to the enormous growth of slavery in the Americas and Caribbean.
   D. It led to the development of artificial sweeteners to replace sugar.

The next two questions are based on this passage.

Leafy seadragons are related to seahorses, but they look more like tiny dragons than tiny horses—that is, if dragons could sprout leaves! Found in the ocean off southern Australia, leafy seadragons can grow to 14 inches. They have a long snout, which is similar to seahorses. The leaf-like appendages sprouting all over their bodies do not help them swim, but these protrusions serve an important function. They look like strands of kelp or seaweed and can change color. Leafy seadragons cannot swim fast with their tiny pectoral and dorsal fins, and because their bony bodies are fragile, elaborate camouflage is essential for survival. Leafy seadragons have not only been threatened by pollution and climate change but also by people capturing them for use in home aquariums. As a result, they are now a protected species.

25. According to the passage, what important function do the leafy seadragons' appendages serve?

    A. They enable the leafy seadragons to swim in deep water.
    B. They serve as protective camouflage for the leafy seadragons.
    C. They protect the leafy seadragons from pollution and climate change.
    D. They help the leafy seadragons quickly swim away from predators.

26. What is the primary purpose of this text?

    A. To entertain readers with a story about leafy seadragons
    B. To persuade readers that leafy seadragons are worth saving
    C. To inform readers about leafy seadragons
    D. To explain that leafy seadragons are not seahorses

The next two questions are based on this passage.

Annie Oakley (1860–1926) was one of several women of the "Wild West" known for her exceptional talent at wielding shotguns. She traveled with Buffalo Bill's Wild West Show for 16 years, starting in 1885. Because of her talents with a shotgun, the Lakota Sioux leader, Sitting Bull, gave her the nickname "Little Sure Shot." Oakley toured not only the United States but also England and many parts of Europe. She was the first female "international sensation" from the United States. More than that, Oakley was also a strong advocate for women and children. She encouraged and taught women to handle guns for self-protection. When World War I broke out, Oakley offered to create and train an all-female regiment of excellent shooters; however, the government never responded to her offer.

27. Which of the following statements best expresses the point of view in this passage?

    A. Annie Oakley had an exceptional ability with shotguns and was as adept with a gun as any man.
    B. Annie Oakley was a colorful Wild West figure who was worthy of becoming a legend.
    C. Annie Oakley accomplished things that no other woman of her time and, few today, could accomplish.
    D. Annie Oakley was more than just an international star; she also tried to improve the lives of women.

28. Which of the following details from the passage supports the inference that Annie Oakley was not always taken seriously?

    A. Sitting Bull gave her the nickname "Little Sure Shot."
    B. The government ignored her idea of training female sharpshooters.
    C. She traveled in Europe and became the first female international star from the United States.
    D. Sixteen years of her career were spent traveling with Buffalo Bill's Wild West Show.

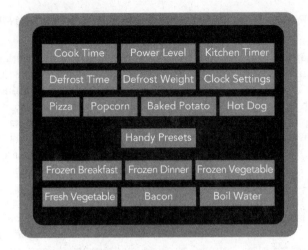

This diagram represents the touchpad control of a microwave oven.

29. Which of the following buttons on the touchpad should be pressed to cook a 12-oz package of frozen peas?

    A. Defrost Weight
    B. Frozen Vegetable
    C. Defrost Time
    D. Power Level

Literature and Life

Index

30. According to the index, which of the following pages would contain information on static and dynamic characters?

    A. Pages 25 to 27
    B. Pages 25 and 26
    C. Pages 20 to 22
    D. Pages 20, 26, and 27

Directions for returning a package:

1. Print your return shipping label.

2. Print a duplicate label to include inside the package.

3. If the shipping label is blank, fill out any required information.

4. Label the package. Place the second label inside the package; this will be helpful if the label on the box is lost or damaged. Securely seal the package.

5. Take the package to a pack-and-ship store, or to a US post office, UPS station, or other shipping location.

6. Pay for the return postage, unless your return is free.

7. Retain your receipt. This is proof of the shipment and contains useful information.

8. Track the shipment online to ensure it arrives at its destination.

31. According to the passage, which of the following steps should be completed after retaining the receipt for proof of shipment?

    A. Securely seal the package.
    B. Track your shipment online.
    C. Place a duplicate shipping label inside the package.
    D. Take the package to a US post office.

Directions for replacing a window

1. Measure for replacement glass, deducting 1/8 inch from both width and height.

2. Purchase replacement glass.

3. Carefully remove glass and any remaining adhesive. Brush the frame free of any dust or particles of adhesive.

4. Place a layer of adhesive around the frame. Place glass over adhesive, press gently, and add a second layer of adhesive around the edge of the glass.

5. Make sure the adhesive does not extend beyond the frame. Allow adhesive to dry before painting or washing the window.

32. Which of the following should be done after placing the glass in the window?

    A. Clear the window frame of debris.
    B. Deduct 1/8 inch from the width and height.
    C. Measure the replacement glass.
    D. Add a second layer of adhesive.

The next two questions are based on this passage.

Historians are defined as interpreters of the past; that is, they are more than chroniclers, who simply tell what happened in the past. History is much more difficult than that. Historians carefully use primary sources—materials that originate in the period being studied—to write an understanding of the past. Naturally, this assumes that there is not one static version of what has happened. Rather the past is subject to interpretation and does not conform to an objective truth. In writing their subjective accounts, historians acknowledge that their version may differ from that of other historians.

33. Which of the following best paraphrases the topic sentence of this passage?

  A. The work of historians is subjective.
  B. "Historian" and "chronicler" are synonymous.
  C. Historians will agree on any given subject.
  D. Historians look for one version of the past.

34. Which of the following details support the main idea of the passage?

  A. "Historians carefully use primary sources—materials that originate in the period being studied."
  B. "They are more than chroniclers, who simply tell what happened in the past."
  C. "Historians acknowledge that their version may differ from that of other historians."
  D. "History is much more difficult than that."

The next two questions are based on this passage.

To the residents of the South Washington Condominiums:

During the week of November 3 through 12, hallways on all odd-numbered floors will be painted. This means that we will need access to your apartments to paint the frames of front doors. All residents should make sure the manager has their current contact details for notification approximately half and hour before work begins near their apartment. The schedule for painting even-numbered floors has not yet been determined. Thank you for your cooperation.

35. Which of the following is true according to this memo?

  A. Residents on the third floor should vacate their apartments between November 3 and 12.
  B. Fourth-floor residents should make sure their contact information is up to date.
  C. There are no plans to paint the hallways on the second floor.
  D. Residents will need to leave their apartments while their hallway is being painted.

36. Which of the following is implied but not stated by this memo?

  A. The sixth-floor hallways will be painted after the third-floor hallways.
  B. Odd-numbered floors will be painted between November 3 and 12.
  C. Residents must remain available during the entire period of the project.
  D. Only some of the hallways will be painted in November.

The next two questions are based on this passage.

Although the majority of those residing in the United States can vote, significant portions of the population are excluded from voting. For example, many people convicted of a crime are not allowed to vote, even if they never served time in jail. In some cases, people who have served their sentences may regain the right to vote, but this is not the case in all states. Being born in a foreign country does not necessarily disbar people from voting, but they must be, or become, a US citizen to vote. Becoming a citizen is a long and, sometimes, arduous process. In addition, minors—those younger than age 18—cannot vote. A person must be 18 years of age before the date of an election, although some believe the voting age should be lowered to 16. Citizens who are 17 years old can register to vote if they will turn 18 before the date of the election. Another requirement for voting is a valid US Postal Service street address. This requirement has caused many people to be disenfranchised because their street addresses are not recognized by some electoral boards.

37. Which of the following best describes the structure of the passage?

  A. Problem and solution
  B. Procedural text
  C. Cause and effect
  D. Compare and contrast

38. If this were the opening paragraph of an online article, which of the following conclusions could be drawn about the purpose?

   A. Elections should have fewer amounts of voters.
   B. The voting age should be lowered to 16 years of age.
   C. Governments should take steps to enfranchise more voters.
   D. Disenfranchised voters do not deserve the right to vote.

1. Construction of a recombinant DNA molecule

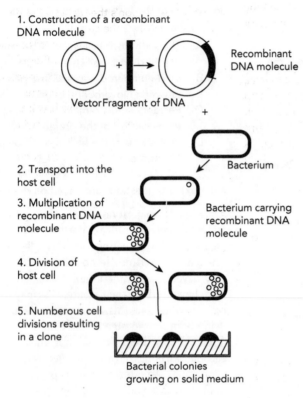

Recombinant DNA molecule

Vector Fragment of DNA

Bacterium

2. Transport into the host cell

3. Multiplication of recombinant DNA molecule

Bacterium carrying recombinant DNA molecule

4. Division of host cell

5. Numberous cell divisions resulting in a clone

Bacterial colonies growing on solid medium

39. Which of the following are the essential components of a recombinant DNA molecule?

   A. A vector and a DNA fragment
   B. A recombined DNA template
   C. A host cell
   D. Cell division

40. Which of the following describes the role of the bacterium in this process?

   A. The bacterium carries the fragment of DNA that contains new information.
   B. The bacterium provides the vector for recombination.
   C. The bacterium is the newly created DNA molecule.
   D. The bacterium is the host for the recombination process.

The next three questions are based on this passage.

All along Seymour Avenue, the blinding white that had been yesterday's snowfall had turned to a mass of dingy gray. The pollution index had skyrocketed, resulting in overcast skies with a brown, hazy glow. Incandescent lights flicked inside the windows of the cold, repetitive apartment blocks. The smells of fried fish, burning rubber, and gasoline-powered generators mingled with the sounds of factory workers drifting out for the late shift. A lone, wizened woman, her pale hair drawn up in a fierce bun, struck at a stoop with a broom, attempting to eradicate the traces of the stray, mangy dog who'd spent the night there.

41. Based on the context, which of the following is the meaning of the word "eradicate" in the passage?

   A. Gather up
   B. Crush
   C. Remove
   D. Wash clean

42. Which of the following statements best describes the point of view in the passage?

   A. There is little hope for the future here.
   B. Pollution is bad for the environment.
   C. Factory workers are not to be trusted.
   D. Cities are full of interesting people.

43. Which of the following statements most likely describes the woman in the passage?

   A. She enjoys living in the neighborhood.
   B. She has a husband who works at the factory.
   C. She likes to keep her apartment tidy and clean.
   D. She is angry at the dog who'd slept on her stoop.

The next two questions are based on this passage.

Women's Suffrage and a Little-Known Warrior

In 1848 the first women's rights convention, in Seneca Falls, New York, allied strong-minded, resolute women to fight for suffrage—the right to vote. After the Civil War, Congress ratified the Fourteenth and Fifteenth Amendments, which bestowed rights—including suffrage—on males who had been enslaved and continued to exclude women from this significant privilege. In 1872 suffragists intensified their battle, challenging the status quo with lawsuits and by voting illegally. In 1890, women achieved a landmark decision:

The state of Wyoming granted women suffrage. After acquiring support from important politicians, women finally accomplished their objective with the ratification of the Nineteenth Amendment in July 1920. The decisive vote was cast by Harry Burn of Tennessee—who voted "aye" at the urging of his mother, Febb Burn.

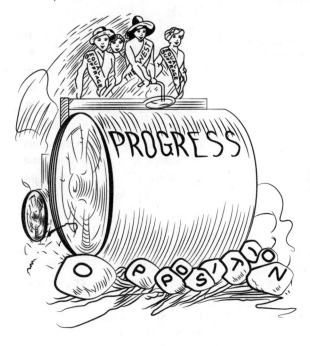

44. Which of the following is a common theme in the passage and cartoon?

   A. Change will always crush those who are against it.
   B. Women are a powerful force for change.
   C. Politicians can help people achieve their dreams.
   D. Accomplishments come to those who try hard.

45. Which of the following best describes how the themes in the cartoon and passage are different?

   A. The cartoon's themes and the passage's themes are the same.
   B. The passage has a theme of how men stood in the way of women's suffrage, but the cartoon shows how men helped.
   C. The passage displays a theme that sometimes it is okay to break the law, and the cartoon shows that following the rules leads to progress.
   D. The theme of the passage is that women's suffrage made slow progress, but the cartoon shows opposition to women's progress being crushed quickly.

The next two questions are based on this passage.

A customer who owns an equestrian training business outlines the following criteria when shopping for a preowned automobile. Her vehicle needs to include a preinstalled with a trailer hitch, and her preference is for a recent model—2017 or later. Another must-have is a powerful eight-cylinder piston engine, and the potential buyer appreciates music, so a high-end eight-speaker sound system is essential. Being ecologically minded, her requirements include achieving at least 17 miles per gallon on long-range highway travel. Finally, the automobile should have fewer than 10,000 miles on the odometer. Which of the following would be appropriate for this customer?

Vehicle A

Mileage

10,500

Year

2017

Engine

4 cylinder

Amenities

Moon roof, trailer hitch

Miles per gallon (mpg)

14 mpg local; 17 mpg highway

Vehicle B

Mileage

8,750

Year

2018

Engine

8 cylinder

Amenities

High-performance tires, 8-speaker sound system, heated seats, trailer hitch

Miles per gallon (mpg)

15 mpg local; 20 mpg highway

Vehicle C

Mileage

7,000

Year

2019

Engine

Eight cylinder

Amenities

Heated seats, back-up camera, 6-speaker sound system

Miles per gallon (mpg)

18 mpg local; 21 mpg highway

Vehicle D

Mileage

12,200

Year

2015

Engine

8 cylinder

Amenities

Leather interior, trailer hitch

Miles per gallon (mpg)

15 mpg local; 18 mpg highway

46. Which of the following vehicles would be appropriate for this customer?

   A. Vehicle A
   B. Vehicle B
   C. Vehicle C
   D. Vehicle D

47. Which of the following is the meaning of "cumulative" as used in the sentence?
The popularity of the new Fidget Widget has increased dramatically over the past 3 years, with cumulative sales topping more than 15 million units.

   A. Carefully calculated
   B. Randomly figured
   C. Reduced in number
   D. Summed values of

Unit Quiz Answers

1. Option C is correct. This summary sentence identifies major points in the plot of the passage. Option A only addresses one aspect of the plot. It does not state that they meet a famous artist. Option B misses the main point of the plot: that they met Michelangelo. Option D makes an inference that cannot be drawn from the passage.

2. Option B is correct. This conclusion can be drawn because Luigi loves all kinds of art and is apprenticed to a painter and sculptor. Option A is not logical because Mario is apprenticed to a man who is both a painter and sculptor. Nothing in the passage suggests that Option C is correct because Luigi does not seem to have a previous connection to Marco. The passage states that Rome's urban nature was becoming more familiar, which suggests that Luigi is from a small town, rather than from a large city.

3. Option A is correct. This detail describes the artist's work using vivid imagery, suggesting that he is a master. Options B and C does not provide evidence to the reader that the artists work is great. Option D describes the artists, but not the work itself.

4. Option D is correct. According to the passage, Luigi goes to Rome, where he meets Mario. One day Mario asks Luigi to join him on an errand, and they carry a satchel of pigments in the rain on their way to give them to Michelangelo.

5. Option B is correct. The word "obscured" provides a context clue that indicates that the scaffolding hid parts of the paintings. Option A misinterprets the meaning of "obscured"; the word does not mean "removed." Option C misses that point that scaffolding is temporary. The ceiling was not deliberately hidden by it. Option D reflects an incorrect understanding of the word "obscured"; it does not mean "removed".

6. Option D is correct. This is an opinion because it is what Mario believes about Michelangelo, and it is not a fact that can be verified. All of the other choices are events that can be checked; they are not feelings or ideas about a topic that can vary.

7. Option A is correct because it supports the idea that uniforms promote order and discipline. Option B provides a foil to the idea that standardization is important. Option C is an argument against uniforms because of the financial burdens they may place on some families. Option D, although it might illustrate what the uniforms look like, does not contribute to the overall argument.

8. Option B is correct. The principal has direct experience of school uniforms and has written about the harm they caused, and this refutes the argument of the passage that uniforms are beneficial. Option A is a primary source, but it supports the argument. Option C is a secondary source because it interprets primary sources, the cases. Option D is a secondary source that does not present an argument about uniforms.

9. Option B is correct. The light blue range extends the furthest north in the Atlantic Ocean off the coast of Europe. The Arctic Ocean does not include any range of the dolphin. The Pacific and Indian Oceans contain substantial portions of the secondary range, but they do not extend as far north as the range in the Atlantic.

10. Option C is correct. An inquisitive person asks questions and has natural curiosity. Being logical, methodical, and careful are all possible characteristics of a scientist, but these terms are not associated with asking questions.

11. Option C is correct. This summary sentence offers the most complete summary of the passage. Option A is correct, but it does not encompass the passage as a whole. Option B is partially true because the Atlantic was cold, but it was not the only reason people died; additionally, this information was not contained in the passage. Option D is partially true because women and children were more likely to survive, but not all of them did, and it does not encompass the passage as a whole.

READING

12. Option B is correct. Of the 2,240 passengers and crew on board, approximately 1,500 lost their lives. Therefore, most passengers did not survive. Option A is incorrect because the passage noted that some people survived, and option D is incorrect because only 740 of 2,240 survived. Option C is incorrect because the passage does not mention how many of the crew survived.

13. Option B is correct. The passage states that "ships today are required to adhere to rigorous safety protocols." Protocols mean procedures. The passage does not refer to requiring more crew, equipment for breaking icebergs, or who must board lifeboats first.

14. Option A is correct because this occurred first at at 11:40 p.m. on April 14, 1912. Women and children then boarded the lifeboats. The *Titanic* sank several hours later. After it sank, ships began following rigorous standards, including requirements for the number of lifeboats.

15. Option D is correct. The causes of the loss of life during the sinking of the *Titanic* are described. The passage also discusses how the lack of safety procedures on the *Titanic* influenced safety protocols today. The passage does not compare or contrast events, and only a portion of the passage concentrates on a sequence of events. It does not focus on the problem of ship safety but, rather, focuses on the causes of the sinking and their effects.

16. Option B is correct. It serves to inform readers about the reasons that more than a thousand passengers perished on the *Titanic*. The author's purpose is not to entertain the reader because it does not focus on events or characters. The passage does not focus on the design of the *Titanic*, except for the detail of the lack of lifeboats. It does state that first-class passengers were more likely to survive the sinking, but this is a detail and not the overall purpose.

17. Option B is correct. This is information that can be verified and can be proven to be true or false. The ideas that Alltech products can make a customer's life easier, provide a better experience, or that the Alltech Desktop Computer is more user friendly are opinions with which people can disagree.

18. Option A is correct. The author is trying to convince the reader that having Alltech products will make life better and easier. The other options are reasons that support this argument, such as Alltech products are less likely to crash, contract viruses, and result in pleasant surprises.

19. Option C is correct. Soaps A and C are the same price per ounce, but Soap C lasts longer. Soap B is more expensive than A or C and does not last as long as C. Soap D is the most expensive; even though it lasts as long as Soap C, it costs more.

20. Option A is correct. An interview with local expert gardeners would provide insight on the effort. The gardeners would be considered a primary source because they are directly involved in the event. Local business owners are a primary source, but the article is focusing on creating the garden, so business owners may not have information about that. Options C and D are considered secondary sources because they are not direct participants in the event but are reports on the event.

21. Option C is correct because according to the directions the last step in soil incorporation composting is covering the matter to be decomposed with a thick layer of soil. Option D, decomposition resulting in nutrient-rich compost, is not a final step of the directions but, rather, an outcome of the actions taken.

22. Option B is correct because the Agree to Terms link appears after the Register section, and the registrant must read the waiver before clicking the Agree box. Option A is incorrect because a registrant cannot even access the Final Checkout page without first clicking the Agree box.

23. Option A is correct because the timeline says that the Crusaders introduced sugar to Europe, meaning that the Europeans did not even know of sugar until that time. Option D, Arabs adding sugar to food, only indirectly led to the European desire for sugar because the Crusaders would have likely first become alerted to the existence of sugar by tasting it in Middle Eastern foods.

24. Option C is correct. Historians say that sugar cultivation in the New World led to the Age of Slavery. Harvesting sugarcane was difficult and dangerous work, and with thousands of sugar mills to staff, Europeans pressed millions of Africans and American Indians into service, which resulted in countless deaths. Options B and D are incorrect; even though it could be argued that the introduction of sugar to the New World led to many problems or that artificial sweeteners have often had adverse health effects, by far the worst impact of the sugar trade was the growth of the institution of slavery and the abuse and degradation of countless Africans and American Indians over two centuries. Option A is false.

25. Option B is correct because the passage clearly states that the leafy appendages are not used for swimming, which makes Options A and D incorrect. The phrase "an elaborate camouflage is essential" directly refers back to the statement that, "They [the leafy appendages] look like strands of kelp or seaweed and can change color," which follows the assertion that "these protrusions serve an important function." Students should infer that the important function, based on the description of what the leafy appendages do, is to provide camouflage. Option C is not supported by information in the passage.

26. Option C is correct. The passage is a brief informative piece describing a sea creature that may be unfamiliar to students. Option A is incorrect because the passage is not a narrative, and although the endangered status of the leafy seadragon is mentioned, it is not the main point, and there is no argument about protecting the species. Option D is incorrect. Even though comparisons are made to the more familiar seahorse, this is done to help readers better visualize and understand the leafy seadragon; the passage is not a comparison and contrast between the species.

27. Option D is correct. By mentioning Oakley's advocacy of, and work with, women, and prefacing it with "More than that," the author shows a positive valuation of Oakley's contributions to society beyond her status as a celebrity and entertainer. The anecdote about the government's failure to acknowledge Oakley's idea to help in the war effort shows that the author feels Oakley was never fully appreciated for her championing of women. Option A is true but is only one aspect of Oakley's greatness, and Option C is not supported by the passage. Option B is possibly true but, like Option A, is only a small part of what the author thinks of Oakley.

28. Option B is correct. Oakley's idea to train women to be sharpshooters in the war was ahead of its time and courageous on many levels. The government's failure to respond was more than a lack of imagination on its part but a patronizing response that as much said that Oakley's idea was not worthy of consideration (and, likely, that women were incapable of accomplishing such a thing). Options C and D point to the fact that, for most of her life, Oakley was seen as only an entertainer, but these options do not have anything to do with her not being taken seriously. At first glance, Option A might seem like an example of Oakley not being taken seriously because "Little Sure Shot" could seem like a patronizing nickname, but the author makes it clear that the nickname derived from a sense of admiration and not mockery.

29. Option B is correct. On seeing the word "frozen," students might first think of defrosting (Option C), and on seeing "12-oz package" they might think of weight (Option A), but the diagram shows that this microwave model has presets that allow for, among other things, the cooking of frozen vegetables. Thus, to be efficient, the first control a user would touch would be Frozen Vegetable.

30. Option A is correct. Static characters are treated on page 25 and dynamic characters on pages 26 to 27, so to get information about both types, a reader would have to read that three-page span. Option B, pages 25 and 26, would leave out part of the information on dynamic characters.

31. Option B is correct because the label needs to be printed out before the package can be labeled. The label can be placed inside the package first but that can be done after the package is labeled.

32. Option D is correct because the other three choices need to be done before the glass is placed in the window. The second layer of adhesive needs to be applied *after* the replacement glass is placed in the window.

33. Option A is correct. The thesis of this passage is that the work of historians is essentially subjective, reflecting their personal interpretation of the materials used.

34. Option C is correct because the passage claims that historians write more subjectively, and chroniclers merely record the past.

35. Option B is correct because *all* residents have been asked to update their information. Options A and D are incorrect because no one needs to leave their apartment during painting. Option C is not correct because it is implied that the even-numbered floors will be painted at later date.

36. Option A is correct because it can be inferred that the even-numbered floors will be painted after the odd-numbered floors. B and D are stated in the passage, and Option C is neither stated nor implied.

37. Option C is correct. The structure of this passage is cause and effect. It contains key words and phrases such as "has caused." Option A is incorrect because the passage may discuss some problems, it does not offer solutions. Option B is incorrect because a procedure is not discussed, and Option D is incorrect because nothing is compared or contrasted. People don't have to register to vote at 17 years of age (Option B), and if they are born in a foreign country (Option D), they may become a citizen and earn the right to vote. If they are younger than 18 years of age, they cannot lose the right to vote because they never had that right.

38. Option C is correct because the passage uses words and phrases with negative connotations, such as "disenfranchise," hinting at the purpose. Options A, B, and D are logical conclusions that can be drawn from this passage.

39. Option A is correct. These are the only two essential building blocks of a recombinant DNA molecule. Option B is the result of recombination. Options C and D are necessary for the process of recombination but are not the components of a recombinant DNA molecule.

40. Option D is correct. See step 2 "Transport into the host cell." The other options are incorrect because the new DNA molecule carries the new information (Option A), the vector is a DNA molecule (Option B), and the bacterium is not a molecule (Option C).

41. Option C is correct. A broom is used to remove dirt and debris.

42. Option A is correct. The overall tone of the passage is depressed, which the author uses to express lack of hope. Pollution is mentioned, but Option B is not correct because it does not capture the whole paragraph. Option C is not correct because there is nothing in the passage to imply this point of view. Option D assumes that the setting is in a city, but the focus is not on the people who live there.

43. Option D is supported by the words "fierce" and "struck," words that indicate anger. Option A is incorrect because there is nothing to suggest that the neighborhood is nice to live in or that she enjoys living there. The passage does not imply that the woman is married. Although she uses a broom, which might suggest Option C, there is no indication that she keeps a clean house.

44. Option B is correct because both passage and cartoon portray women as leading progress in society. Option A applies to the cartoon only and states an absolute. Option C is illustrated in the passage, but it is not in the cartoon. Option D is best illustrated by the passage only.

45. Option D is correct. The passage tells the story of how it took decades for women's suffrage to finally be law. Option A is incorrect because, although there are some themes that are similar, there are still key differences. Option B is incorrect because the cartoon does not show men helping. Option C is incorrect because the cartoon does not show a theme of following the rules leading to change.

46. Option B is correct because it is the only option that meets all the customer's criteria. The correct answer is revealed through a process of elimination. Option A has too many miles, the wrong engine, and no sound system is mentioned. Option C does not have a trailer hitch or eight-speaker sound system. Option D has too many miles, is too old of a model, and does not mention a sound system.

47. Option C is correct. Cumulative refers to the values added up over time.

Mathematics

The following 15 chapters cover the tasks from the ATI TEAS test plan for the Mathematics unit. These are focused on assessment of basic mathematical skills and are organized into two sections:

- Number and algebra
- Measurement and data

Each chapter in this unit introduces knowledge, skills, and abilities relevant to the Mathematics task and provides an overview of some essential topics, along with specific examples to highlight important concepts. Practice questions at the end of each chapter will allow you to test your knowledge of select concepts. In addition, there are key terms included at the end of each section and a practice Mathematics quiz at the end of the unit. This unit quiz includes the same number of questions as the Mathematics unit on the ATI TEAS and matches the test plan task allocations (shown below). The quiz will give you a good idea of the number and types of sources you will encounter and the questions that will accompany those sources. Keep in mind that these chapters are a great starting point and guide to your studies, but they are not an exhaustive review of all concepts that might be tested in the Mathematics unit of the ATI TEAS. You should use other sources (textbooks, online resources, etc.) for additional study and practice in areas that you haven't mastered.

Items pertaining to numbers and algebra cover fractions, decimals, percentages, rational and irrational numbers, and the operations of adding, subtracting, multiplying, and dividing. Also included in this section are items related to translating phrases and sentences into expressions, equations, and inequalities. The measurement and data section includes items related to interpreting and evaluating information in tables, charts, and graphs using statistics, as well as explaining the relationship between variables and calculating geometric quantities.

There are 32 scored Mathematics items on the TEAS. These are divided as shown below. In addition, there will be four unscored pretest items that can be in any of these categories.

Section	Number of scored items on the ATI TEAS
Number and algebra	23
Measurement and data	9

CHAPTER

20 Convert among non-negative fractions, decimals, and percentages

 This objective includes, but is not limited to, the following examples of knowledge, skills, and abilities.

- Know the relationship between the numerator and denominator in a fraction.
- Demonstrate knowledge of place value within decimals.
- Define percent as a number out of 100.

Numbers can be written in many ways, including fractions, decimals, and percentages. For this task on the TEAS, you'll need to understand each of these forms and the process of converting from one form to another. You should practice converting from one number quantity to another until you've mastered the processes. There are plenty of exercises available on the Internet for more practice converting fractions, decimals, and percentages. The following overview will provide the base of knowledge you'll need to succeed at this task.

Fractions

A fraction is a numerical quantity that represents a part of a whole. Fractions can be written in the form a/b or $\frac{a}{b}$, where a and b are integers. The bottom integer is called the denominator. It represents the whole quantity. The top integer is called the numerator. It represents the part of the whole number that the fraction represents. So, if you have 1/3 of a cup of flour, you've divided the 1 cup into 3 parts, and you only have 1 out of the three parts filled with flour. You can divide the numerator by the denominator to determine a decimal value for the fraction.

 Let's look at an example of converting a fraction to a decimal.

5/8 or $\frac{5}{8}$ is five-eighths, or five parts (portion) out of eight parts (the whole thing).

To convert $\frac{5}{8}$ to a decimal, divide numerator 5 by denominator 8 ("5" into calculator first, then "/," then "8").

$5 \div 8 = 0.6250$

Decimals

Another form of number quantity is decimal form. Numbers in decimal form have place values, some of which are illustrated by the following chart.

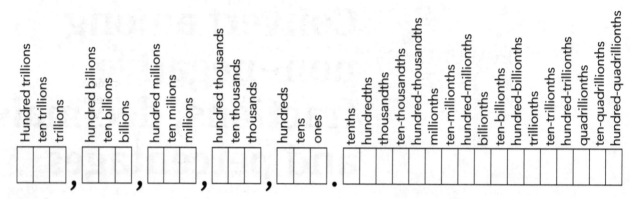

 The chart shows two examples of decimal numbers and how they are read.

Number	In Words
2,134.14	two thousand one hundred thirty-four and fourteen hundredths
0.00036	thirty-six hundred-thousandths

The decimal part of any number can be read ending with the decimal place of the last nonzero digit. In the case of 0.00036, the 6 is the last nonzero decimal digit. Because the 6 is in the hundred-thousandths place, this is how it is expressed.

Converting Decimals to Fractions

To convert from decimal to fraction form, there are two scenarios to consider: a value greater than 1 and a value less than 1. If a decimal value is less than 1—for example, 0.48—simply use 48 as the numerator and the place value of the last decimal digit as the denominator. In this case, the denominator would be hundredths. The decimal 0.48 would be written as $\frac{48}{100}$ and read "forty-eight hundredths." If the decimal was 0.048, it would be written as $\frac{48}{1000}$ and read "forty-eight thousandths."

If a decimal value is greater than 1, there are more steps involved. Let's convert the decimal 3.24 to a fraction.

1. Move the decimal to the right until you have a whole number (in this case, 324). This whole number becomes the numerator.

2. Keep track of how many decimal places you moved the decimal. Your denominator becomes a 1 followed by the number of zeros that matches the number of places the decimal moved. Changing 3.24 to 324 implies that the decimal moved to the right two places. The denominator becomes a 1 followed two zeros (100).

3. The fraction representation of 324 is thus $\frac{324}{100}$. You can also try to simplify, or reduce, fractions if possible.

Let's use these steps in another example.

1. If the decimal was 4.064, move the decimal to the right until you have a whole number: 4,064. This whole number becomes the numerator.
2. You've moved the decimal 3 places. The denominator becomes a 1 followed by 3 zeros (1,000).
3. The fraction representation of 4.064 is thus $\frac{4064}{1000}$.

Percentages

A percentage is a third form of number quantity. A percentage, or percent, means "per 100." It is showing the value of a number in terms of 100. If a product is 100% whole wheat, it means that all of the item is made of whole wheat. If it is 50% whole wheat, only half of the item contains whole-wheat grains. One

percent can be interpreted as one one-hundredth $\frac{1}{100}$ of something.

 The following chart shows some example percentages, how these convert to fractions, and their decimal equivalents. To change a percent to a fraction, simply put the percent over 100. To convert a percentage to a decimal, write the number over a denominator of 100 and then divide by 100. Remove the percent symbol.

Percent	Fraction	Decimal
35%	$\frac{35}{100}$	0.35
28.4%	$\frac{28.4}{100}$	0.284
55%	$\frac{55}{100}$	0.55
100%	$\frac{100}{100}$	1
0.09%	$\frac{0.09}{100}$	0.0009

Converting Decimals and Fractions to Percentages

A decimal can be converted to a percent by multiplying it by 100 and adding a percent sign. For example, 0.78 can be multiplied by 100 to give 78; then add the percent symbol. So 0.78 equals 78%.

To convert a fraction to a percent, one strategy is to convert to decimal form first. Then convert the decimal to a percent. For example, ¼ is 1 divided by 4, which is 0.25. This is 25/100, or 25%.

CHAPTER 20 PRACTICE PROBLEMS

1. Convert each decimal to a percent.

   A. 3.25
   B. 0.215

   Convert each percent to a decimal.

   C. 62.9%
   D. 145%.

   Convert each decimal to a fraction.

   E. 0.265
   F. 1.39

   Convert each fraction to a decimal.

   G. $\dfrac{26}{10}$

   H. $\dfrac{16}{25}$

2. Which of the following percentages is equivalent to $\dfrac{17}{10}$?

   A. 0.17%
   B. 1.7%
   C. 17%
   D. 170%

3. Which of the following fractions is equivalent to 56.4%?

   A. $\dfrac{564}{1000}$

   B. $\dfrac{564}{100}$

   C. $\dfrac{564}{10}$

   D. 564

4. Which of the following decimals is equivalent to 3.75%?

   A. 3.75
   B. 0.375
   C. 0.0375
   D. 0.00375

5. Which of the following decimals is equivalent to $\dfrac{16}{50}$?

   A. 0.32
   B. 0.68
   C. 1.47
   D. 3.125

Notes:

_____

_____

_____

_____

_____

_____

_____

_____

_____

_____

_____

_____

_____

_____

_____

_____

_____

_____

_____

_____

_____

_____

Notes:

CHAPTER

21

Perform arithmetic operations with rational numbers

 This objective includes, but is not limited to, the following examples of knowledge, skills, and abilities.

• Complete computations with integers using the four basic operations.
• Complete computations with decimals using the four basic operations.
• Complete computations with fractions and mixed numbers using the four basic operations.
• Complete computations involving the order of operations, excluding complex fractions.

Completing basic computations by hand can at times be quicker than using a calculator. Additionally, calculators do not always complete the mathematical order of operations in ways you assume they will. For this TEAS task, you need to be competent at doing arithmetic calculations by hand. You will apply the order of operations—including addition, subtraction, multiplication, and division—and be expected to do so using integers, decimals, fractions, and mixed numbers. Practice makes perfect, so it might be helpful to search the Internet for additional practice problems.

Order of Operations

Knowing the order of operations is crucial to success on this task. One mnemonic device for the mathematical order of operations is PEMDAS, which stands for parentheses, exponents, multiplication and division, addition and subtraction. There are some exceptions to PEMDAS, but these will not appear on the TEAS. Exponents will also not appear on the TEAS. You will need to use parentheses, multiplication and division, and addition and subtraction in the correct order. To successfully execute these operations, you must follow these rules in order.

1. First, perform any calculations inside parentheses.
2. Next, perform all multiplication and division, completing the operations as they occur from left to right.
3. Finally, perform all addition and subtraction, completing the operations as they occur from left to right.

Computations with Integers

The following are three basic computations with rationales.

Ex. 1:

$3 + 5 \times 9 = 3 + \mathbf{5 \times 9}$	Multiply first.
$= 3 + \mathbf{45}$	Then add.
$= 48$	

Ex. 2:

$24 \div 3 - 5 = \mathbf{24 \div 3} - 5$	Divide first.
$= \mathbf{8 - 5}$	Then subtract.
$= 3$	

Ex. 3:

$(18 - 7) \times 4 = \mathbf{18 - 7} \times 4$	Perform operations in parentheses first.
$= \mathbf{11 \times 4}$	Then multiply.
$= \mathbf{44}$	

Multiple-Step Problems

The following are several examples involving multiple steps.

Ex. 4: $5 + 7 \times (4 + 8) \div 6 - 9$

Solution:

Step 1:	$5 + 7 \times \mathbf{(4 + 8)} \div 6 - 9 = 5 + 7 \times \mathbf{12} \div 6 - 9$	Parentheses
Step 2:	$5 + \mathbf{7 \times 12} \div 6 - 9 = 5 + \mathbf{84} \div 6 - 9$	Multiplication
Step 3:	$5 + \mathbf{84 \div 6} - 9 = 5 + \mathbf{14} - 9$	Division
Step 4:	$\mathbf{5 + 14} - 9 = \mathbf{19} - 9$	Addition
Step 5:	$19 - 9 = 10$	Subtraction

Ex. 5: $8 - 4 \div (5 - 3) \times 3 + 11$

Solution:

Step 1:	$8 - 4 \div \mathbf{(5 - 3)} \times 3 + 11 = 8 - 4 \div \mathbf{2} \times 3 + 11$	Parentheses
Step 2:	$8 - \mathbf{4 \div 2} \times 3 + 11 = 8 - \mathbf{2} \times 3 + 11$	Division
Step 3:	$8 - \mathbf{2 \times 3} + 11 = 8 - \mathbf{6} + 11$	Multiplication
Step 4:	$\mathbf{8 - 6} + 11 = \mathbf{2} + 11$	Subtraction
Step 5:	$2 + 11 = 13$	Addition

In the last two examples, you will notice that multiplication and division were evaluated from left to right according to rule 2. Similarly, addition and subtraction were evaluated from left to right, according to rule 3.

Operations Within Parentheses

When two or more operations occur inside a set of parentheses, these operations should be evaluated according to rules 2 and 3. This means multiplication and division from left to right are completed first. Then addition and subtraction from left to right follow. This is done in the following example.

Ex. 6: $225 \div (3 + 2 \times 11) - 4$

Solution:

Step 1:	$225 \div (3 + \mathbf{2 \times 11}) - 4 = 225 \div (3 + \mathbf{22}) - 4$	Multiplication inside parentheses
Step 2:	$225 \div (\mathbf{3 + 22}) - 4 = 225 \div \mathbf{25} - 4$	Addition inside parentheses
Step 3:	$\mathbf{225 \div 25} - 4 = 9 - 4$	Division
Step 4:	$9 - 4 = 5$	Subtraction

Computations with Fractions

When a problem includes a fraction bar, this means we must divide the numerator by the denominator. Think of a fraction bar as a grouping symbol like parentheses. However, we must perform all calculations above and below the fraction bar BEFORE dividing. Let's look at an example.

Ex. 7: $\dfrac{47 - 5}{5 + 9}$

Solution:

This problem includes a fraction bar, so divide the numerator by the denominator. Perform all calculations above and below the fraction bar BEFORE dividing. Thus:	$\dfrac{47 - 5}{5 + 9} = \dfrac{(47 - 5)}{(5 + 9)}$
Evaluating this expression, we get:	$\dfrac{(47 - 5)}{(5 + 9)} = \dfrac{42}{14} = 3$

Extensions of the preceding example include decimals, fractions, and mixed numbers. With decimals, all processes are identical. With fractions, you might need to find a common denominator or convert fractions to decimals. With mixed numbers, you might need to convert to a fraction first. To help prepare for the TEAS, search the Internet for order of operations practice and work on your mastery of these types of problems.

CHAPTER 21 PRACTICE PROBLEMS

1. Solve the following problems:

   $6 + 8 \times (12 \times 9)$

   $(14 - 5) \div (7 - 4)$

   $7 \times 4 + 8 \div 4 - 3 \times 6$

   $\dfrac{50 - 2 \times 7}{6 + 4 \times 3}$

2. Which of the following is the correct value of $3 + 2 \times 6 - 4$?

   A. 32
   B. 10
   C. 11
   D. 26

3. Which of the following is the correct value of the following expression?

   $$\dfrac{15 + 2 \times 5}{11 - 24 \div 4}$$

   A. 21
   B. 5
   C. ≈ 9.9
   D. ≈ 5.9

4. Which of the following is the correct value of the following expression?

   $$50 - (8 \times 3) + \dfrac{9 + 6}{3}$$

   A. 31
   B. 35
   C. 131
   D. 135

5. Which of the following is the correct value of the following expression?

   $$17 + \dfrac{18 - 2 \times 3}{6}$$

   A. 14
   B. 19
   C. 25
   D. 34

Notes:

Notes:

CHAPTER

22

Compare and order rational numbers

 This objective includes, but is not limited to, the following examples of knowledge, skills, and abilities.

- Demonstrate knowledge of the meaning of rational numbers.
- Know the terms and symbols for "greater than," "less than," and "equal to."
- Order three or more quantities (least to greatest, greatest to least).
- Compare two quantities using symbols.
- Know place value with decimals.
- Rewrite numbers to have a common denominator.

Rational numbers are those that we see and use every day, decimals and fractions included.

Defining Rational Numbers

What makes rational numbers unique is that those fractions can be written as either terminating or repeating decimals. For instance, ½ can be written as 0.5. This is a terminating decimal. One-third is a repeating decimal because it is equivalent to $0.\overline{3}$. Whole numbers such as 4 can be written as rational numbers such as $\frac{12}{3}$ or $\frac{16}{4}$, but we usually see it in its simplified form: 4. Integers can be written as fractions by simply writing them over 1. For example, -7, 13, and 100 can be written as $\frac{-7}{1}$, $\frac{13}{1}$, and $\frac{100}{1}$.

Conversely, irrational numbers *cannot* be written in fraction form (for example, $\sqrt{2}$ and π converted to decimals are not terminating or repeating). Other examples of irrational numbers include $\sqrt{\text{any non-perfect square number}}$ and the natural number e.

Ordering Rational Numbers

It is important to be able to put rational numbers in numeric order as well as visualize and predict situations involving ordered quantities. At times, interpreting ordered number inequality statements is useful as well (like equations, but with inequality symbols instead of equal signs). The TEAS test requires you to compare and order rational numbers. Try searching the Internet using any of the glossary terms to find additional explanations and practice problems.

It is important to note that any negative number is "smaller" than any positive number. Essentially, if a number is to the left of another number on the number line, it is smaller. All negative numbers are to the left of all positive numbers.

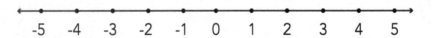

To put rational numbers in numeric order (either increasing or decreasing), it can be useful to write the numbers as decimals (unless they are already integers, like -2, -1, 0, 1, 2). Once in decimal form, you can write the numbers vertically, lining up the decimals.

 For example, the numbers 4.356, 4.635, and 0.6534 can be stacked this way.

4.356
4.635
0.6534

The next thing you do is, starting with the digit with the highest place value (in this case, the ones place), decide which is the largest (or smallest). Let's put them in decreasing order. Therefore, we need to identify and write the largest value. There are two numbers with 4 in the ones place, so we next need to compare the tenths place for these two numbers.

In this case, the largest is 4.635. 6 tenths is larger than 3 tenths. Then determine the next largest number in the same way: 4.356. And continue this process until all are in order. The decreasing and increasing lists are summarized below.

Decreasing list: 4.635, 4.356, 0.6534

Increasing list: 0.6534, 4.356, 4.635

If the numbers are not in decimal form and you're unsure how to order all of them, you can divide the fractions or fraction parts to get them in decimal form. For instance, for 3 5/6, you can divide 5 by 6 to get 0.8333, so the value becomes 3.8333. Now you can compare to other decimal form numbers.

Comparing Rational Numbers

You can use comparison symbols to compare and order rational numbers.

Symbol	Meaning
>	greater than
<	less than
≥	greater than or equal to
≤	less than or equal to

Using the decreasing list 4.635, 4.356, 0.6534, we can write 4.635 > 4.356 > 0.6534.

Using the increasing list 0.6534, 4.356, 4.635, we can write 0.6534 < 4.356 < 4.635.

We can also write inequalities like 4.356 ≤ 4.635 because 4.356 is truly less than OR equal to 4.635. Here the qualifying portion is the "or."

You can compare fractions and mixed numbers with different denominators by rewriting the numbers as equivalent fractions or mixed numbers.

To find the lowest common denominator, do the following.

1. Find the least common multiple of the denominators (also called the least common denominator).
2. Rewrite each fraction as an equivalent fraction using the lowest common multiple of the denominators.

 Example: Use the least common denominator for $\frac{2}{5}$, $\frac{1}{6}$, and $\frac{4}{15}$ to compare and order the fractions.

- List the **multiples** of each denominator:
  Multiples of **5** are 5, 10, 15, 20, 25, **30**, 35, 40, …
  Multiples of **6** are 6, 12, 18, 24, **30**, 36, 42, 48, …
  Multiples of **15** are 15, **30**, 45, 60, 75, 90, 105 …
- 30 is the lowest common multiple appearing in each list.
- Therefore, the **least common denominator** of $\frac{2}{5}$, $\frac{1}{6}$, and $\frac{4}{15}$ is **30**.

- The equivalent fractions are $\frac{2}{5} = \frac{12}{30}$, $\frac{1}{6} = \frac{5}{30}$, and $\frac{4}{15} = \frac{8}{30}$.

- Decreasing order: $\frac{2}{4}, \frac{4}{15}, \frac{1}{6}$ $\frac{12}{30}, \frac{8}{30}, \frac{5}{30}$

- Increasing order: $\frac{1}{6}, \frac{4}{15}, \frac{2}{5}$ $\frac{5}{30}, \frac{8}{30}, \frac{12}{30}$

This method works well for numbers that aren't too big. The TEAS test will stick to more manageable numbers.

CHAPTER 22 PRACTICE PROBLEMS

1. Write in increasing order: $-8, 8\frac{3}{4}, 8.43$.

2. Which of the following is a correct comparison of 9.14 and $9\frac{1}{6}$?

   A. $9.14 > 9\frac{1}{6}$

   B. $9.14 < 9\frac{1}{6}$

   C. $9.14 = 9\frac{1}{6}$

   D. $9.14 \geq 9\frac{1}{6}$

3. Which of the following lists the numbers in decreasing order: $-4, 0.4, 4\frac{1}{5}, -0.04$?

   A. $-4, 0.4, 4\frac{1}{5}, -0.04$

   B. $-0.04, -4, 0.4, 4\frac{1}{5}$

   C. $4\frac{1}{5}, 0.4, -4, -0.04$

   D. $4\frac{1}{5}, 0.4 - 0.04, -4$

4. Which of the following lists the numbers in increasing order: $\frac{3}{8}, \frac{3}{4}, \frac{11}{16}, \frac{1}{2}$?

   A. $\frac{1}{2}, \frac{3}{8}, \frac{3}{4}, \frac{11}{16}$

   B. $\frac{11}{16}, \frac{3}{8}, \frac{3}{4}, \frac{1}{2}$

   C. $\frac{3}{8}, \frac{1}{2}, \frac{11}{16}, \frac{3}{4}$

   D. $\frac{3}{4}, \frac{3}{8}, \frac{1}{2}, \frac{11}{16}$

5. Which of the following lists the numbers in decreasing order: $-1\frac{3}{5}, -1.45, -1.8, -1\frac{3}{4}$?

   A. $-1.45, -1\frac{3}{5}, -1\frac{3}{4}, -1.8$

   B. $-1.8, -1\frac{3}{4}, -1\frac{3}{5}, -1.45$

   C. $-1\frac{3}{4}, -1.45, -1\frac{3}{5}, -1.8$

   D. $-1\frac{3}{5}, -1.45, -1.8, -1\frac{3}{4}$

Notes:

Notes:

_____

_____

_____

_____

_____

_____

_____

_____

_____

_____

_____

_____

_____

_____

_____

_____

_____

_____

_____

_____

_____

_____

CHAPTER

23 Solve equations in one variable

 This objective includes, but is not limited to, the following examples of knowledge, skills, and abilities.

- Understand the meaning of a variable.
- Understand the structure of an algebraic equation.
- Demonstrate knowledge of inverse arithmetic operations.

Variables, Constants, and Coefficients

An equation is a statement that shows that two expressions are equal to each other. Algebraic equations consist of variables (usually letters that represent an unknown quantity) and constants (numbers). A term is a number, variable, or product of numbers and variables. Terms are separated by addition and subtraction signs. A coefficient is the numerical part of a variable term. A variable written without a numerical part has a coefficient of one.

To succeed at this TEAS task, you'll need to practice solving a range of equations with one variable.

 Algebraic equations with one variable can have one or more terms in that same variable.

Equation	Variable Terms	Constants	Coefficients
$x + 6 = 10$	x	6, 19	1
$4x - 7 = 2x + 11$	$4x, 2x$	−7, 11	4, 2

Inverse Operations

Inverse mathematical operations are the opposites of each other and undo each other. These include but are not limited to:

- addition and subtraction
- division and multiplication

If you want to undo multiplication by a fraction, you may undo the multiplication by division. Recall that to divide by a fraction, you need to multiply by the reciprocal of the fraction.

Solving Equations

To solve an equation means to find the value of the variable that will make the equation true (i.e., both sides of the equation have the same value).

Here are some guidelines to follow:

1. Collect all variable terms on one side of the equal sign using inverse operations.
2. Collect all constants on the other side using inverse operations.
3. Use inverse operations to get the variable alone.

 The following examples illustrate using inverse operations to solve algebraic equations with one variable. Notice when the solution is substituted into the equation to check the answer, the left side of the equation is equal to the right side.

Solve: $x + 35 = 74$. Check your answer.

$x + 35 = 74$	Original equation.
$x + 35 - 35 = 74 - 35.$	Subtract 35 from both sides. Subtraction undoes addition.
$x = 39$	Simplify.
$39 + 35 = 74$	Check your answer.
$74 = 74$	

Solve: $x - 8 = -14$. Check your answer.

$x - 8 = -14$	Original equation.
$x - 8 + 8 = -14 + 8.$	Add 8 to both sides. Addition undoes subtraction.
$x = -6$	Simplify.
$-6 - 8 = -14$	Check your answer.
$-14 = -14$	

Solve: $4x = 7$. Check your answer.

$4x = 7$	Original equation.
$\dfrac{4x}{4} = \dfrac{7}{4}$	Divide both sides by 4. Division undoes multiplication.
$x = \dfrac{7}{4}$	Simplify.

$$\frac{4}{1} \cdot \frac{7}{4} = 7 \qquad \text{Check your answer.}$$

$$\frac{28}{4} = 7$$

Solve: $\frac{4}{5}x = 20$

$$\frac{4}{5}x = 20 \qquad \text{Original equation.}$$

$$\frac{5}{4} \cdot \frac{4}{5}x = \frac{20}{1} \cdot \frac{5}{4} \qquad \text{Multiply both sides by the reciprocal of } \frac{4}{5}.$$

$$x = 25 \qquad \text{Simplify.}$$

$$\frac{4}{5} \cdot \frac{25}{1} = 20 \qquad \text{Check your answer.}$$

$$\frac{100}{5} = 20$$

Solve: $5x + 5 = 2x - 10$

$5x + 5 = 2x - 10$	Original equation.
$5x - 2x + 5 = 2x - 2x - 10$	Subtract $2x$ from both sides. Collect variable terms on one side.
$3x + 5 = -10$	Simplify.
$3x + 5 - 5 = -10 - 5$	Subtract 5 from both sides. Collect constants on other side.
$3x = -15$	Simplify.
$\dfrac{3x}{3} = \dfrac{-15}{3}$	Divide both sides by 3.
$x = -15$	Simplify.
$5(-5) + 5 = 2(-5) - 10$	Check your answer.
$-25 + 5 = -10 - 10$	
$-20 = -20$	

CHAPTER 23 PRACTICE PROBLEMS

1. $x - 17 = 48$

    Solve the equation above. Which of the following is correct?

    A. 65
    B. 55
    C. 31
    D. 21

2. Solve: $2x - 6 = -4x$

3. Solve: $6x = 19$

4. Solve: $\frac{7}{5}x = 35$

5. Given the equation $6x - 9 = 3x + 12$, which of the following is an acceptable first step toward solving the equation?

    A. Subtract 9 from both sides of the equation.
    B. Add 12 to both sides of the equation.
    C. Subtract $3x$ from both sides of the equation.
    D. Add $6x$ to both sides of the equation.

Notes:

Notes:

CHAPTER

24

Solve real-world one- or multi-step problems with rational numbers

 This objective includes, but is not limited to, the following examples of knowledge, skills, and abilities.

- Differentiate among necessary, erroneous, and extraneous information in a word problem.
- Determine the necessary operation(s) from contextual clues in a word problem.
- Perform arithmetic operations with rational numbers in a real-world context.
- Check the reasonableness of the solution to a problem.
- Solve equations in one variable in a real-world context.

Mathematics is a tool we use to observe the world around us, collect and analyze data about our world, and help answer questions and solve problems. Many simple problems can be solved with one or two steps using simple rational numbers. Being able to recognize the patterns used in these problems will make the solutions easier. Repeated practice will help this process to become automatic and prepare you for success at this TEAS task.

Problem–Solving Plan

Most problems you encounter will not include specific instructions to guide you to a solution. Following are four major ideas and more specific strategies to keep in mind when solving problems.

Understand Problem	Devise Plan	Carry Out Plan	Look Back
• Identify given information. • Determine what you need to find or show. • Determine what is happening in the problem. • Determine whether you have enough information to solve the problem.	• Guess and check. • Make an orderly list. • Eliminate possibilities. • Use direct reasoning. • Solve an equation. • Look for a pattern. • Draw a picture. • Use a model. • Work backward. • Use a formula.	• Implement your chosen plan. • If the plan does not seem to be working, try a different approach.	• Check to make sure you answered the question. • Check to see if your answer is reasonable. • Make sure all of the parts of the problem are answered.

When you are first in the phase of understanding the problem, look for situations that are modeled by the four operations: addition, subtraction, multiplication, and division. Some of the ways to think about each operation are listed in the following table.

Addition	Subtraction	Multiplication	Division
• joining • putting together	• separate • remove • distance • comparing differences	• total number in equal groups • area • scaling • comparing—multiplication (e.g., three times as much)	• how many in each group/portion • how many groups/portions

Rational Numbers in the Real World

Rational numbers are used in these problems. Rational numbers can be represented by fractions. This includes whole numbers, positives and negatives, zero, and all decimals that either terminate or repeat. Irrational numbers, such as the square root of five, will not be discussed here.

Most problems will be in a real-world context. In the real world, you will likely not have a boss that says, "Solve these 10 quadratic equations and have them on my desk by 5 o'clock." Instead, you will have to take information from several sources, analyze it, determine what the question is that you need to solve, pick out the pertinent information, choose the correct procedure, solve the problem mathematically, and check the reasonableness of the answer. This takes practice.

CHAPTER 24 PRACTICE PROBLEMS

1. Jayden wants to use square pavers that are 4 inches on each side to completely surround his flower garden. The garden is 8 feet long and 2 feet wide. How many pavers should Jayden buy?

2. A cat owner gets a vitamin prescription from his veterinarian that lists the dosage as 2.5 mL twice a day. The bottle contains 200 cc. How many days will the bottle last?

3. On Monday, the nurse determined that her patient's total fluid intake for the day was 1,800 mL. On Tuesday, the same patient's total fluid intake was 2,350 mL. If the patient's total fluid outtake over the two days was 1,775 mL, what was his net result?

4. A recipe for 1 batch of cookies calls for $\frac{3}{4}$ cup of flour. How much flour is required to bake $1\frac{5}{8}$ batches of cookies?

5. In a small community, 1,225 students take the bus to school. If there are a total of 1,955 students enrolled in the school system, approximately what percentage of students take the bus to school?

MATHEMATICS

Notes:

_____

_____

_____

_____

_____

_____

_____

_____

_____

_____

_____

_____

_____

_____

_____

_____

_____

_____

_____

_____

CHAPTER

25 Solve real–world problems involving percents

This objective includes, but is not limited to, the following examples of knowledge, skills, and abilities.

- Define percent in terms of a real-world context.
- Calculate the percent of a number in terms of a real-world context.
- Find percent of increase or decrease between two numbers in terms of a real-world context.

Percent Revisited

Percent is a form of number quantity. For this task on the TEAS, you'll need to understand what percent means in real-world contexts as well as how to work with percents within these contexts. You will have to find the percent of a number quantity as well as percent increase or decrease. You will need to utilize the problem-solving skills discussed in the previous chapter and, if needed, search the Internet for additional practice problems of these types.

Percent means "per 100," or a value's proportional equivalent compared to 100. One percent can be interpreted as one one-hundredth of something. Examples of percent expressions are 25%, 19.2%, 50%, and 0.08%.

When a percent is less than or equal to 100%, then you can say "out of" 100. For example, 75% is 75 out of 100. But if a percent is more than 100%, you need to rethink the wording. It doesn't make sense to say that 175% is 175 out of 100. 175% is 175 for each 100. For example, 175% of 20 is 35.

 Following are 100 small squares, and 50 have been shaded.

| 0 | 10 | 20 | 30 | 40 | 50 | 60 | 70 | 80 | 90 | 100 |

One way to describe the shading is to say 50% has been shaded—in other words, 50 out of 100. Likewise, 50 cents is 50% of 100 cents (or 50% of $1.00).

Other real-word percentage contexts include percent off for a sale price, annual percent interest rates at a bank, annual percent gain or loss for a company or business, percent commission for a salesperson, percent depreciation of assets, and percentages of ingredients in a mixture or recipe.

You will need to find the percent of a number to determine a part or portion.

 Example: At a major airport, 15% of all flights experienced a delay or cancellation due to weather. If there were 220 flights in all, how many flights experienced a delay or cancellation?

15% = 0.15 Rewrite 15% as a decimal.

220 × 0.15 = 33 Multiply 220 by the decimal equivalent.

There were 33 flights that experienced a delay or cancellation due to weather.

Percent Increase or Decrease

You also need to find the percent of a number to solve problems involving increase or decrease. In the next two examples, two methods are presented, but they will yield the same solution.

 Example: Kathryn purchases $60 worth of groceries and pays 8% state tax. How much is her total bill with tax?

Method 1		Method 2	
8% = 0.08	Rewrite 8% as a decimal.	100% + 8% = 108%	Add 8% to 100%.
0.08 × 60 = $4.80	Multiply the decimal equivalent by $60.	108% = 1.08	Rewrite 108% as a decimal.
60 + 4.80 = 64.80	Add.	60 × 1.08 = 64.80	Multiply the decimal by $60.

Kathryn's total grocery bill is $64.80.

 Example: James purchases a new jacket originally priced at $140.00. The store offers a 30% discount. How much does James pay for the jacket with the discount?

Method 1		Method 2	
30% = 0.30	Rewrite 30% as a decimal.	100% − 30% = 70%	Subtract 30% from 100%.
140 × 0.30 = 42	Multiply the decimal equivalent by $140.	70% = 0.70	Rewrite 70% as a decimal.
140 − 42 = 98	Subtract.	140 × 0.07 = 98	Multiply the decimal by $140.

James pays a discounted price of $98.00 for the jacket.

Given that you are solving many problems that may have an increase or decrease, remember to pay attention to the type of situation in the problem. Some situations are summarized below.

Increase	Decrease
tax, mark up, increased by, gained	discount, markdown, decreased by, depreciation, loss

CHAPTER 25 PRACTICE PROBLEMS

1. Your current salary is $55,000. Next year you will get a 4.5% increase in your salary. How much more money will you make next year?

2. Which of the following is 35% of 900 pounds?

   A. 315 pounds
   B. 595 pounds
   C. 865 pounds
   D. 1,205 pounds

3. While shopping, you find a shirt that is marked 25% off. If the regular price is $50, which of the following is the reduced price?

   A. $12.50
   B. $25.00
   C. $37.50
   D. $62.50

4. A computer tablet costs $550.00. If the sales tax is 6.5%, what is the total cost of the tablet with sales tax?

   A. $35.75
   B. $514.25
   C. $556.50
   D. $585.75

5. A car salesperson earns $900 each month plus 6% commission on her monthly car sales. If she sells $58,000 worth of cars on a given month, what is her total monthly salary?

   A. $4,380.00
   B. $3,534.00
   C. $3,480.00
   D. $3,426.00

Notes:

CHAPTER

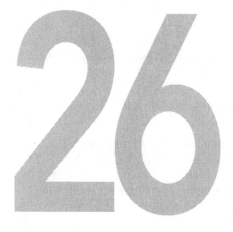

Apply estimation strategies and rounding rules to real-world problems

 This objective includes, but is not limited to, the following examples of knowledge, skills, and abilities.

- Estimate metric measurements (e.g., area, length, weight, volume).
- Know when it is appropriate to use a given estimation or rounding procedure.
- Know rounding rules (e.g., rounding to ones, tenths, hundredths; rounding fractions and mixed numbers).
- Demonstrate knowledge of estimation strategies (e.g., using a simpler problem).

Metric Measurements

While the United States still clings to standard measurements, you will work primarily with the metric system in medical studies. And for the purposes of the estimation strategies and rounding rules described by this TEAS task, you will be using metric measurements. It can be helpful to practice thinking metrically in your daily life as well, such as when you shop and drive. You will also want to practice using rounding rules and estimation strategies when solving word problems.

First, you must have knowledge of some simple approximations for common metric units. Study the following table.

Metric Unit	Household Approximation
Millimeter (mm)	The thickness of a cell phone
Centimeter (cm)	The width of a wedding ring
Meter (m)	A doorway is just over 2 m tall
Kilometer (km)	1 km equals about 2/3 of a mile
Gram (g)	The weight of a grape
Kilogram (kg)	A 10-pound bag of rabbit pellets is just over 4 kg
Degrees Celsius (°C)	Zero is freezing, 10 is not; 20 is warm, and 30 is hot!

Note that metric units do not have a period after them. Volume is measured in cubic units, such as cubic centimeters (cm^3). The exponent 3 is used for metric volume, and the abbreviation cu. is usually used for standard system units. Liquid volume is measured in liters (L) or milliliters (mL). Because carbonated beverages are sold in 2-liter bottles, this is one conversion you are probably already familiar with. One liter contains 1,000 milliliters or 1,000 cubic centimeters (1 L = 1,000 mL = 1000 cc). Helpful tip: 1 cc is the same as 1 mL.

Estimation and Rounding

Estimating and rounding are two skills that make many problems quicker and easier to solve. Good judgment should be used when deciding if estimating and rounding are appropriate. Sometimes a "ballpark" figure is reasonable. Even in a laboratory setting, where precision and accuracy are extremely important, a quick estimate can tell you whether you have the decimal point in the right place and can help determine if your mathematical procedure was correct.

Estimation strategies that you should be familiar with include front-end estimation, in which you focus on the first digits of numbers when adding or subtracting and solving a simpler problem. There are plenty of good examples of solving a simpler problem and other estimation strategies available on the Internet, so be sure to search these key words and familiarize yourself with these strategies.

The decimal place to which you need to round depends on the problem. When rounding to a decimal place, such as the tenths or the hundredths place, look only at the digit immediately to the right of the place to which you are rounding. For five or larger, round up. Less than five, drop the digits that follow. Study the following table.

Round	To This Place	And the Answer Is
73.281	Ones	73
73.281	Tens	70
73.281	Hundredths	73.28
0.6467	Thousandths	0.648
0.6467	Hundredths	0.65

When rounding fractions to the ones place, if the numerator is greater than or equal to half of the denominator, round up to the next whole number. If the numerator is less than half of the denominator, round down to the next whole number. Study the following table.

Round to the Ones Place	And the Answer Is
1/12	0
7/12	1
7 2/8	7
19 8/20	19
19/5 = 3 4/5	4

Rounding decimals and fractions to whole numbers—which are easier to calculate in your head or quickly with scratch paper—will enable you to estimate whether your detailed calculations are reasonable. One frequent error is when the digits are correct but the decimal point is placed incorrectly.

CHAPTER 26 PRACTICE PROBLEMS

1. Which of the following gives the best estimate for $\dfrac{346.8 \times 5.231}{49.6}$?

   A. $\dfrac{347 \times 5}{50}$

   B. $\dfrac{350 \times 5}{49}$

   C. $\dfrac{300 \times 5}{50}$

   D. $\dfrac{346 \times 6}{49}$

2. Round the numbers in the table to the place indicated.

Number	Round to This Place	Your Answer	Number	Round to This Place	Your Answer
34.19	Tenths		$7\frac{4}{3}$	Ones	
$\frac{6}{7}$	Ones		64.736	Tenths	
7.219	Hundredths		547	Tens	
933.74	Thousands		878	Hundreds	
2.739	Hundredths		87.357	Hundredths	
32.834	Tenths		32.95	Tenths	
37.494	Tens		483.34	Hundreds	
$\frac{23}{50}$	Ones				

3. Which metric unit best represents the length of a paper clip?

   A. Meter
   B. Millimeter
   C. Liter
   D. Milliliter

4. Which household object is best approximated by kilograms?

   A. a pet rabbit
   B. spilled water
   C. a piece of paper
   D. a tablet of ibuprofen

5. The value of $\dfrac{873.5 \times 4.72}{59.6}$ is closest to what number?

   A. 75,000
   B. 7,500
   C. 750
   D. 75

Notes:

_____

_____

_____

_____

_____

_____

_____

_____

_____

_____

_____

_____

_____

_____

_____

_____

_____

_____

_____

_____

_____

_____

Notes:

CHAPTER

27

Solve real–world problems involving proportions

 This objective includes, but is not limited to, the following examples of knowledge, skills, and abilities.

- Define proportion.
- Set up a proportion.
- Solve a proportion.
- Identify a constant of proportionality.

Proportional thinking is a valuable real-world problem-solving approach. Proportions come up in scenarios from map reading to money exchange rates. To succeed on this TEAS task, you will need to understand not only what a proportion is but also how to set one up, solve it, and identify the rate of change, also known as the constant of proportionality. The practice problems in this chapter will provide some good examples, but you might want to seek out more practice in other sources as well.

Introduction to Proportion

A proportion is a ratio in fraction form set equal to another ratio in fraction form. The numerator and denominator of each ratio are "scaled" up or down by the same factor. For instance, if one ratio is $\frac{3}{8}$, a scaled-up ratio might be $\frac{9}{24}$, because $\frac{3}{8} \times \frac{3}{3} = \frac{9}{24}$. Similarly, if one ratio is $\frac{4}{5}$, the other might be $\frac{24}{30}$ because $\frac{4}{5} \times \frac{6}{6} = \frac{24}{30}$.

Writing and Solving a Proportion

One application of proportion is using a map (a type of scale drawing). If the legend on a map reads 1 cm = 20 miles and you measure 6.4 cm between destinations, a proportion can be used to calculate how many miles (x) are represented by 6.4 cm.

$$\frac{1\,cm}{20\,miles} = \frac{6.4\,cm}{x\,miles}$$

$$\frac{1\,cm}{20\,miles} \times \frac{6.4}{6.4} = \frac{6.4\,cm}{128\,miles}$$

$$x = 128\,miles$$

If x is in the numerator of a proportion, you can multiply both sides by the corresponding denominator to obtain an expression that may be simplified to find x.

$$\frac{3}{5} = \frac{x}{9}$$

$$\frac{3}{5} \times 9 = \frac{x}{9} \times 9$$

$$\frac{3 \times 9}{5} = x, \text{ or } x = \frac{27}{5}$$

Direct Proportion and Constant of Proportionality

Two variables are directly proportional when they increase or decrease at the same rate. This rate is called the constant of proportionality. An equation can be written as $y = k \times x$, where k is the constant of proportionality.

You might also recall from studying linear equations that equations of lines can be written in the form of $y = mx + b$ (slope-intercept form). When $b = 0$ (y-intercept = 0), the equation becomes $y = mx$ (i.e., $y = k \times x$) and is directly proportional. Since m is the slope, in the case where $b = 0$, m is the constant of proportionality k.

Study the table to see what examples of directly proportional equations look like.

Directly Proportional Equations	Not Directly Proportional
$y = 4x$, $y = 8x$, $y = \frac{x}{5}$, $y = \frac{2}{3}x$	$y = 2x + 9$, $y = x - 3$, $y = \frac{4}{x}$, $y = 6$

CHAPTER 27 PRACTICE PROBLEMS

1. Micah spends 27 hours in a 3-week period practicing piano. At this rate, how many hours will he practice in 7 weeks?

2. The success rate for a salesperson is 2 out of 11 calls. At this rate, how many sales would the salesperson expect to get out of 55 calls?

   A. 5
   B. 6
   C. 10
   D. 16

3. A company found an average of 4 defective televisions for every 1,000 checked. If the company produced 95,000 televisions in 1 year, how many of them would be expected to be defective?

   A. 11
   B. 380
   C. 905
   D. 1095

4. On a map, 1 cm = 75 miles. If the distance between two cities measures 8.6 cm, what is the actual distance between the two cities?

   A. 8.7 miles
   B. 66.4 miles
   C. 82.6 miles
   D. 645 miles

5. Which of the following equations is directly proportional?

   A. $y = x - 5$

   B. $y = 3x - 5$

   C. $y = 3x$

   D. $y = 5$

MATHEMATICS

Notes:

CHAPTER

28

Solve real–world problems involving ratios and rates of change

 This objective includes, but is not limited to, the following examples of knowledge, skills, and abilities.

- Define ratio.
- Define rate of change.
- Determine rate of change in a given context.
- Formulate a ratio in a given context.
- Convert a ratio to a unit rate.

A popular question in every math class is "When are we ever going to use this?" Ratios and rates are one part of math that is used on a daily basis. How often do you ask the following?

Question	Answer
"How much does a cashier earn working?"	dollars/hour
"How fast is the train going?"	miles/hour
"Do I drink enough water?"	cups/day
"Does my smartphone data plan meet my usage needs?"	gigabytes/month
"Can I afford the mortgage payment for that house?"	(principal + interest + escrow)/month

It is the nature of our world today to think in terms of ratios and rates. Fortunately, the mathematical procedures for working with ratios and rates are quite simple. On the TEAS, you'll encounter a range of real-world problems that involve ratios and rates of change, so you'll want to understand these concepts and how to put them into practice.

Ratio

A ratio is a comparison of two numbers by division that is often represented as a fraction, which may or may not be written in lowest terms. Examples of ratios include $\frac{2}{3}$, $\frac{7}{10}$, and $\frac{7}{2}$.

Rate, Unit Rate, and Rate of Change

Ratios with units are called rates. Examples of rates include $\frac{2\ cats}{3\ dogs}$, $\frac{7\ absent}{10\ present}$, and $\frac{7\ miles}{2\ hours}$.

 A unit rate is a rate that is expressed per 1 unit. For example, for the rate $\frac{7\ miles}{2\ hours}$, the unit rate would be $\frac{3.5\ miles}{1\ hour}$ or 3.5 miles per hour. To find a unit rate, simply divide the numerator by the denominator.

Using Ratio and Rate of Change to Solve Problems

Mike manages a small crew of men at the local utility company that clears trees that fall on electric lines. They use chainsaws that require an oil-and-gasoline fuel mixture with a ratio of oil to gas of 1:50. Normally, Mike uses 12.8 fluid ounces of oil and 5 gallons of gasoline. Today is a small job, and he plans to use 1 gallon of gasoline. The normal rate is $\frac{12.8\ fl\ oz}{5\ gal}$. In order to have a 1 in the denominator, Mike divides both numerator and denominator by 5. This is the same procedure we use to reduce fractions. After dividing by 5, the rate has been reduced to approximately $\frac{2.6\ fl\ oz}{1\ gal}$. This is Mike's unit rate. All rates must also be labeled with the units in the numerator and denominator.

Because rates relate two numbers with units or variables, they can be represented on a graph. The unit rate is also called the rate of change.

Melinda keeps a chart on the money she saves each week from her weekly paycheck.

By the end of the third week, she has saved $75.00, and by the end of the eighth week, she has saved a total of $200.00. The graph of this situation is shown.

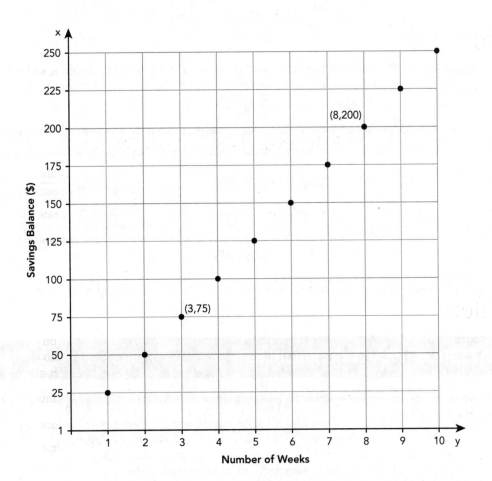

Now let's find the rate of change, or slope, of the line containing these two points. To find the rate of change, m, find the change in the y-coordinates $(y_2 - y_1)$ divided by the change in the x-coordinates $(x_2 - x_1)$. The rate of change for Melinda's weekly savings (3 weeks, \$75) and (8 weeks, 200) is found this way:

$$m = \frac{\$200 - \$75}{8\,\text{weeks} - 5\,\text{weeks}}$$

$$= \frac{\$125}{5\,\text{weeks}}$$

$$= \frac{\$25}{1\,\text{week}}$$

You do not need to draw a graph to find the rate of change between two rates. To find the rate of change, use the slope formula, $m = \frac{y_2 - y_1}{x_2 - x_1}$, where $(y_2 - y_1)$ is the difference between the y-coordinates and $(x_2 - x_1)$ is the difference between the x-coordinates.

Jackson, who is an artist, has created 256 paintings over the course of four years. He has created paintings that are either portrait (taller than wide) or landscape (wider than tall). He has 145 landscape paintings and 111 portrait paintings. We can write several ratios from this information.

Portrait to landscape: $\dfrac{111}{145}$

Landscape to portrait: $\dfrac{145}{111}$

Portrait to total: $\dfrac{111}{256}$

Landscape to total: $\frac{145}{256}$

Ellen works at a bakery. She pulls out the recipe and discovers that the number of cups is unreadable for a cake recipe. Her boss tells her that yesterday, the bakers used a total of 22 cups of cake flour to bake 6 cakes. The ratio of cups of cake flour to cakes is $\frac{22 \text{ cups}}{6 \text{ cakes}}$.

Ellen needs to know the number of cups of cake flour to make one cake, so she writes down the ratio $\frac{22 \text{ cups}}{6 \text{ cakes}}$. She calculates the unit rate, or number of cups of flour needed to make one cake by dividing the numerator and denominator by 6.

$$\frac{22 \text{ cups}}{6 \text{ cakes}} \div \frac{6}{6} = \frac{\frac{22}{6}}{1} = \frac{\frac{11}{3}}{1} = \frac{3\frac{2}{3} \text{ cups}}{1 \text{ cake}}$$

This is the same procedure we use to reduce fractions. After dividing by 6, the rate has been reduced to $\frac{3\frac{2}{3} \text{ cups}}{1 \text{ cake}}$. This is Ellen's unit rate. All unit rates must also be labeled in the numerator and denominator.

CHAPTER 28 PRACTICE PROBLEMS

1. Use unit rates to determine which is the better vacation deal: $900 for 4 nights or $1,443 for 7 nights.

   Nancy enters a fitness challenge with her friends at work. They all go walking during lunch to stay fit. Nancy decides to track her total steps over 1 month. At the end of the month, she looks back at her records and finds them incomplete. Here is what she sees.

Day	Total Steps Taken This Month at Lunch
3	1,950
7	4,550
20	13,000
22	14,300

2. Which of the following expresses the unit rate in steps per day?

   A. $\frac{3 \text{ days}}{1,950 \text{ steps}} = \frac{0.002 \text{ days}}{\text{step}}$

   B. The unit rate is $\frac{1,950 \text{ steps}}{3 \text{ days}}$.

   C. The unit rate is $\frac{650 \text{ steps}}{\text{day}}$.

   D. The unit rate is $\frac{650}{1}$.

3. A box of cereal costs $4.80 for 24 ounces. Which of the following represents the unit rate per ounce?

   A. $\dfrac{\$0.04}{oz}$

   B. $\dfrac{\$4.80}{24.\ oz}$

   C. $\dfrac{20}{1}$

   D. $\dfrac{\$0.20}{oz}$

4. Three months into a new Internet/phone/cable plan, Jason has paid a total of $360. Ten months into the plan, Jason has paid a total of $1,130. What is the rate of change for Jason's cable plan?

   A. $\dfrac{\$110.00}{month}$

   B. $\dfrac{\$113.33}{month}$

   C. $\dfrac{\$113.67}{month}$

   D. $\dfrac{\$114.00}{month}$

5. Joe has a drawer full of 28 different-colored markers. He knows he has 7 red markers and 4 black markers. Which of the following expresses the ratio of red markers to total markers?

   A. $\dfrac{1}{7}$

   B. $\dfrac{1}{4}$

   C. $\dfrac{7}{4}$

   D. $\dfrac{4}{7}$

MATHEMATICS

Notes:

CHAPTER

29

Translate phrases and sentences into expressions, equations, and inequalities

 This objective includes, but is not limited to, the following examples of knowledge, skills, and abilities.

- Define expression.
- Define equation.
- Define inequality.
- Write variables for unknowns.
- Determine the necessary operation(s) from contextual clues in a phrase or sentence.

Expressions, Equations, and Inequalities

Expressions contain numbers, variables, and/or operations. Equations relate expressions equal on another. Inequalities use comparison symbols involving greater than or less than.

Some examples are shown.

Expressions are mathematical sentences that consist of numbers, variables, and/or operations. When two expressions are set equal, it is called an equation, and when one expression is less than or greater than another, it is called an inequality.

Expressions	Equations	Inequalities
$9 - 2y$	$9 - 2y = 27$	$9 - 2y < 27x$
$-Z$	$x = 8$	$x < 8$
$-3(x - 12)$	$-3(x - 12) = 2(3x + 15)$	$-3(x - 12) \geq 2(3x + 15)$

Translation to Equations and Inequalities

One of the foundational steps of solving problems is translating written text in the problem into algebraic notation. This involves turning words and phrases into variables, numbers, operations, and a statement about equality. You will need to understand how those elements combine in expressions and equations. To be successful at this TEAS task, you will need to practice shifting between the concrete and the abstract.

Translating written language into algebra reduces the information to its most basic level. Sentence fragments become expressions, and full sentences become equations or inequalities.

You will be the author of these translations. Think of this as naming characters in your story, using variables as names to represent unknown quantities.

Xavier attends a local fair. He spends a total of $25.00, which includes $5.00 admission to the fair and 8 rides. When he returns home, his dad wants to know how much it costs for a single ride.

This is a story problem. Identify the extraneous or erroneous information. Pick a variable and tell what it represents. This is called defining the variable. Traditionally, x and y are used for variables, but it is helpful to use a letter that better represents the quantity in the context of the problem.

r = the cost of one ride

Decide what the context of the story tells you about the relationship. "... He spends a total of $25.00, which includes $5.00 admission to the fair and 8 rides."

$$8r + 5 = 25$$
$$8r + 5 - 5 = 25 - 5$$
$$8r = 20$$
$$\frac{8r}{8} = \frac{20}{8}$$
$r = 2.5$, so each ride costs $2.50.

Now let's try a more ambitious problem.

Vivian is at the supermarket and wants to spend no more than $70 on groceries. She knows that she will spend $45.00 on necessities, but wants to buy pepperoni, which costs $7.49 per pound. How much pepperoni can she buy and stay within her spending limit?

Define the variable.

p = pounds of pepperoni

Total cost of pepperoni.

$7.49p$

She will spend $45.00 on necessities.

$7.49p + 45$

Finally, make the total less than or equal to $70.

$7.49p + 45 \leq 70$

CHAPTER 29 PRACTICE PROBLEMS

1. Sue decides to collect postcards. She starts her collection with nine cards. Every week, she buys two more cards to add to her collection. Write an inequality that would allow her to find how many weeks until she has more than 35 cards.

2. James is saving money to go to a concert. From his part-time job, he is able to save $20 per week. His older brother gave him $15 to start. If W = number of weeks, which of the following expressions represents the number of weeks until James has saved at least $255?

   A. $20W + 15 = 255$
   B. $(15 + 20)W \geq 255$
   C. $20W + 15 \geq 255$
   D. $20W + 15 < 255$

3. Melissa wants to take a taxi to a restaurant. She has only $25 for a taxi ride plus some change in her purse for the driver's tip. The taxi company charges $2.00 to get in the taxi plus $1.75 per mile. If M = miles to a restaurant, which of the following expressions represents the maximum distance to a restaurant that Mary can afford?

   A. $1.75M < 25$
   B. $2.00 + 1.75M > 25$
   C. $(2.00 + 1.75)M \leq 25$
   D. $2.00 + 1.75M \leq 25$

4. Grant spent the morning driving 100 miles. He drives at an average speed of 60 miles per hour. Which of the following inequalities may be used to determine the time, T, it will take to drive at least 350 miles?

   A. $60T < 350$
   B. $100 + 60T > 350$
   C. $100 + 60T \leq 350$
   D. $100 + 60T \geq 350$

5. Which of the following inequalities models the following?

   Three more than five times a number x is greater than three times the same number, decreased by nine.

   A. $5x + 3 \geq 3x - 9$
   B. $5x + 3 > 3x - 9$
   C. $(5 + 3)x > (5 - 9)x$
   D. $5x + 3 > 9x - 3$

Notes:

CHAPTER

30 Interpret relevant information from tables, charts, and graphs

 This objective includes, but is not limited to, the following examples of knowledge, skills, and abilities.

- Demonstrate knowledge of the structure of graphical displays.
- Demonstrate knowledge of the structure of data tables.
- Interpret the labels of a graph or chart.
- Interpret the legend of a graph or chart.
- Interpret the scale of the axes of a graph.
- Identify the meaning of a point on a graph in terms of the axes of the graph.

You have probably heard the saying, "a picture is worth a thousand words." Now, imagine how much information is packed into a data table or graph. You can extrapolate all types of useful details from such data. The amount of information available in our society is multiplying at an incredible rate. Using charts, graphs, and tables helps to relay such relevant information. Charts, graphs, and tables make the presentation of data much clearer. They help readers understand the relationship between quantities, how fast they are changing, and the importance of the data. For the TEAS, you'll need to understand the various parts of these graphical displays and how to interpret information from tables, charts, and graphs.

Graphs and Tables

Most graphs you study will represent the relationship between two sets of data or parameters. These types of graphs are bivariate. Traditionally, this is shown as a Cartesian coordinate graph. When plotting a point or reading the coordinates of a point, remember to move from the origin in the horizontal direction first and then in the vertical direction. This ensures a unique point that corresponds to one pair of coordinates.

Compare the following graph with the table of points and coordinates.

Point	Coordinates
A	(4, 6)
B	(–4, 0)
C	(0, 0) the origin
D	(8, –4)
E	(0, 7)
F	(–7, –4)
G	(–4, 8)

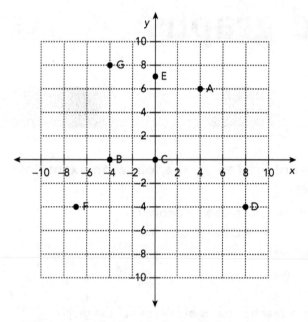

Notice points D and G. Reversing the coordinates results in two completely different points, and in this case, they are even in different quadrants.

Graphs tell a story and show the relationship between variables. The graphs you study will not be random collections of points. Consider the following graph.

The title conveys what the graph shows: the ounces of water Monique drank on a Saturday. The x-axis displays the time of day, from 8:00 a.m. until 6:00 p.m. The y-axis shows the total number of ounces drank. The scale says to multiply by 10, so 2 on the axis represents 20 ounces of water. Using a scale such as this is often saves space and makes the graph easier to read. Any point on the graph can be read as a pair of coordinates. Can you find the point for 4 p.m. when Monique had drunk 100 ounces of water? What did Monique do between 4 and 6 p.m.? Monique drank another 20 ounces of water. Do you see that by 6 p.m. Monique drank 120 ounces of water? A simple graph can contain a large amount of information.

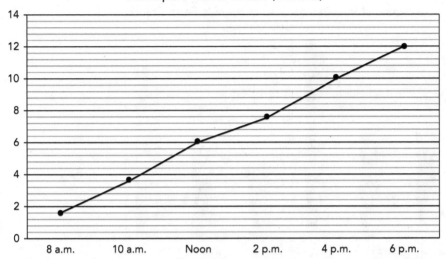

Monique's Water Intake (Ounces)

CHAPTER 30 PRACTICE PROBLEMS

The chart shows the annual costs of maintaining a car.

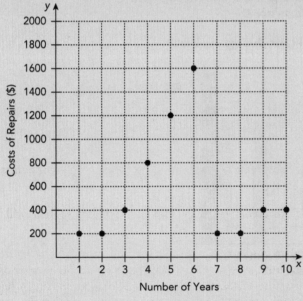

1. Which of the following observations based on this graph is correct?

   A. The cost of maintaining a car is constantly increasing each year.

   B. For the first 3 years, it costs $400 to maintain the car.

   C. The average rate of change between year 1 and year 4 is $\dfrac{\$800 - \$200}{4 \text{ years}} = \dfrac{\$600}{\text{year}}$.

   D. The average rate of change between year 1 and year 4 is $\dfrac{\$800 - \$200}{4 \text{ years} - 1 \text{ year}} = \dfrac{\$600}{3} = \$200.00$ per year.

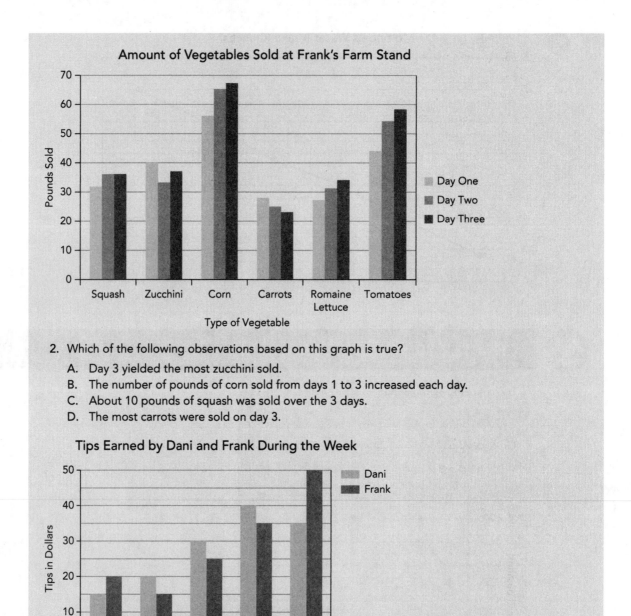

Amount of Vegetables Sold at Frank's Farm Stand

2. Which of the following observations based on this graph is true?

   A. Day 3 yielded the most zucchini sold.
   B. The number of pounds of corn sold from days 1 to 3 increased each day.
   C. About 10 pounds of squash was sold over the 3 days.
   D. The most carrots were sold on day 3.

Tips Earned by Dani and Frank During the Week

3. Use this graph to fill in the two tables and answer the questions.

Dani's tips

Night	Tips
Monday	
Tuesday	
Wednesday	
Thursday	
Friday	

Frank's tips

Night	Tips
Monday	
Tuesday	
Wednesday	
Thursday	
Friday	

On what night did Dani's daily tips decrease from the previous night?

On what night(s) did Frank earn more in tips than Dani?

What is the average rate of change for Frank from Monday to Friday?

Max's Music Machine DJ Service

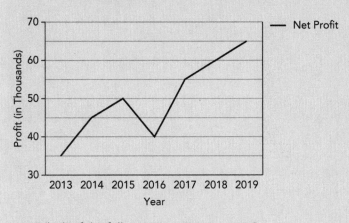

4. Which of the following statements is true?

A. Max's Music Machine's annual profits increase annually.
B. The greatest increase in profits was between 2016 and 2017.
C. Max earned $0 in 2013.
D. There were two increases of $5,000 between 2013 and 2019.

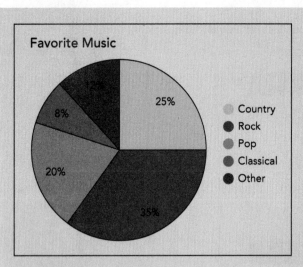

5. The given chart based on a survey of 200 people shows a favorite genre of music. Which of the following statements is true?

A. Country music is the favorite of 25 people.
B. Country music is preferred by 5 more people than pop music.
C. The most popular music is rock.
D. There were 40 people who chose neither rock nor country.

Notes:

Notes:

CHAPTER

Evaluate the information in tables, charts, and graphs using statistics

 This objective includes, but is not limited to, the following examples of knowledge, skills, and abilities.

- Calculate measures of central tendency (e.g., mean, median, mode).
- Calculate range.
- Identify the spread of a data distribution.
- Identify the shape of a data distribution.
- Identify a trend based on a graph or table of data.
- Explain a point on a graph, chart, or table in terms of a given context.
- Identify expected and unexpected values (e.g., outliers).

Statistics and data analysis are important parts of what many professionals do quantitatively. These two disciplines help us understand the world of numbers. They help us clear up areas in which there may be uncertainties. The TEAS test requires that you understand some basic concepts and carry out basic statistical calculations. The Internet is a good resource for glossary term definitions, additional explanations, and practice problems.

Mean, Median, and Mode

The mean, median, and mode are three measures of central tendency. They are used to summarize a set of data. Their definitions and examples are given in the following table.

Measure of Central Tendency	Definition	Example
Mean	The average. Add all the numbers in a set or list and divide by how many numbers there are in the set.	A number set includes: 3, 3, 3, 7, 8, 9, 9, 13. First, add 3 + 3 + 3 + 7 + 8 + 9 + 9 + 13, which equals a sum of 56. Next, divide the sum by how many numbers are in the set. There are eight numbers, so divide 56 by 8 for a mean of 7.
Median	Median is the middle number of an ordered list. If there are an odd number of terms, there is one middle number. If there is an even number of terms, there are two middle numbers, so the mean of those two numbers is the median.	For the same set of numbers as given for the mean (i.e., 3, 3, 3, 7, 8, 9, 9, 13), there are eight numbers. Because this is an even number, there are two middle numbers: 7 and 8. Next, find the mean of those two numbers to find the median for the number set. The median of this set is 7.5.
Mode	Mode is the number(s) in a list that occurs the most. If a list includes two modes, it is *bimodal*.	For the same set of numbers as given for the mean (i.e., 3, 3, 3, 7, 8, 9, 9, 13), 3 is the mode because it occurs three times.

Range

Range is a measure of spread for a data set. To find the range, subtract the minimum value from the maximum value. For the example given in the table for the mean, median, and mode, 13 − 3 = 10, so 10 is the range. Spread can be determined from a graph as well. The highest *y*-value is the maximum value, and the lowest *y*-value is the minimum value. Once these are determined, the same process to find the range is used. The spread reflects the variability of the data. Observations that cover a wide range have a large spread. Observations that are clustered near a single value have a small spread.

The shape of a data distribution can reveal valuable information. There are several common distribution patterns.

Symmetry

A symmetric distribution can be divided at the center with each half mirroring the other. Dividing below distribution at 51, both halves mirror each other.

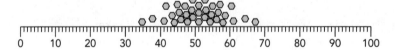

Number of Peaks

Distributions of data can have few or many peaks. A distribution with a single clear peak is called "**unimodal**," and a distribution with two clear peaks is called "**bimodal.**"

Bimodal

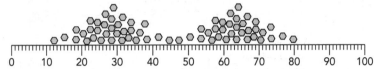

Bell-shaped, unimodal

When a symmetric distribution has a single peak at the center, it is referred to as "bellshaped." Bell-shaped, unimodal peaks are also referred to as "normal distribution."

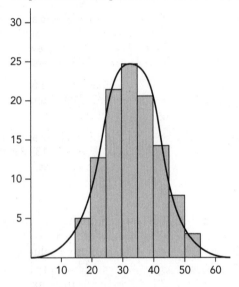

Skewness

Some graphic distributions have more observations that fall on one side of the graph compared to the other. Distributions with fewer observations on the right, toward higher values, are **skewed right.**

- **Skewed right**

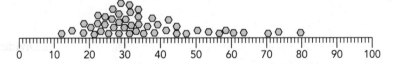

- **Skewed left**

Distributions with fewer observations on the left (toward lower values) are **skewed left.**

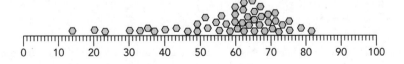

Uniform

When the observations in a data set are spread equally across the range of the distribution, this is a called a "uniform distribution." A uniform distribution has no clear peaks.

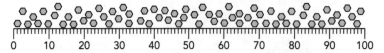

Trends in Graphs and Tables

Data sets in a graph or a table also reveal trends, or patterns, in the data. Data trends are usually easy to see in simple data tables, like the one shown here. As the value of x gets closer to 6.0 from either direction, the number of y increases.

Does the value of x affect y?	
Value of x	Number of y
1.0	50
3.5	70
6.0	100
8.5	80
11.0	60
13.5	30

Trends can be more difficult to find in complicated data tables. This is where graphs can be used. Graphs are valuable because they make trends easier to notice. The following graph clearly shows that as the value of x increases, the number of y increased, until the value is 6.0. After that, the number of y has a decreasing trend in relation to the value of x.

An individual point on a graph of a real-world situation has meaning. On this graph, the maximum point is at (6.0, 100). The meaning of this point is that there are 100 y when the x value is 6.0. Similarly, the first entry can be represented by the point (1.0, 50), indicating an x value 1.0 paired with a y count of 50.

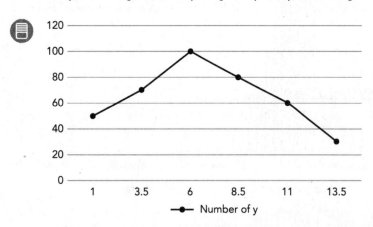

Data set models can reveal what are known as expected values and outliers. An "outlier" is an unexpected value that does not fit any trend or pattern in the data. The following graph illustrates an example of an outlier.

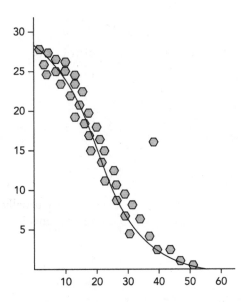

All points on the graph follow along the trend curve except the one that is way above the rest of the data. Visually, we can qualify this point as an outlier, or unexpected value. All of the other data points follow the same trend and, thus, are expected values.

CHAPTER 31 PRACTICE PROBLEMS

1. Find the mean, median, and mode of the following data set: 0, 1, 2, 2, 3, 5, 6, 7, 8, 16

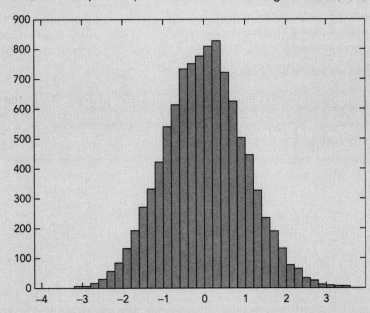

2. Which of the following best describes the distribution portrayed in the graph?

   A. Bell-shaped
   B. Normal
   C. Skewed left
   D. Skewed right

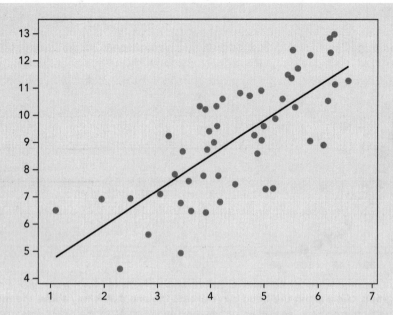

3. Which of the following describes the trend of the data portrayed in the graph?

    A. Decreasing
    B. Increasing
    C. Stable
    D. No trend

4. Which of the following statements best describes a distribution that is skewed left?

    A. The data peaks closer to lower values.
    B. The data peaks closer to higher values.
    C. The data peaks closer to middle values.
    D. There are no clear peaks.

5. Which of the following describes a decreasing trend?

    A. As one set of values decreases, the other set of values also decreases.
    B. As one set of values increases, the other set of values decreases.
    C. As one set of values increases, the other set of values remains constant.
    D. Both sets of values neither increase nor decrease.

Notes:

_____

_____

_____

_____

_____

_____

_____

_____

_____

_____

_____

_____

_____

_____

_____

_____

_____

_____

_____

_____

_____

Notes:

CHAPTER

32

Explain the relationship between two variables

This objective includes, but is not limited to, the following examples of knowledge, skills, and abilities.

- Describe how changes in one quantity affect changes to another quantity.
- Demonstrate knowledge that a variable represents a set of potential values.
- Identify positive and negative covariation.
- Identify dependent and independent variables.

The concept of a variable is one of the most powerful and important ideas in mathematics. Variables allow us to work with both known and unknown quantities. A variable represents a quantity that can truly vary. Much of your work will involve the relationship of two variables and how the change in one causes a change in the other. Being able to mathematically describe or interpret this dynamic relationship between two variables is essential for your success on this TEAS task.

Nothing happens in isolation. When you sit down to study, you increase your knowledge and decrease your free time. When you buy a new video game, your use of technology goes up and the money in your pocket goes down. When you exercise, you increase the calories you burn and decrease your weight.

Correlation

The time you spend working at a job is a constantly changing number. For every hour you work, the money you earn increases for that pay period. The time is a quantity that varies. We can represent it with a variable. Let t = the number of hours worked. In between pay periods, the money you earn varies, and it can be represented with a different variable. Let m = money earned from working. As t increases, m increases. The variables t and m are positively (or directly) related.

My monthly bills decrease, when I work. And when I work, I always pay my monthly bills. As the money I earn increases, my monthly bills decrease.

Again let m = money earned from working. Let b = balance of monthly bills. As m increases, b decreases. The variables m and b are negatively (or inversely) related.

We describe this relationship between variables as "covariance." If both variables increase, a positive covariance exists, and the variables are directly related. If one increases and the other decreases, there is a negative covariance, and the variables are inversely related.

Dependent and Independent Variables

In all of these examples, one variable depends on another variable. When the first quantity changes, the second quantity changes in response. The first quantity is called the "independent variable" and the second quantity is called the "dependent variable." Let's look at one more example.

As the temperature of a glass of water decreases the speed at which water molecules move also decreases. The temperature is the independent variable, and the molecule speed is the dependent variable.

You can transfer variables to a graph. The independent variable goes on the x-axis (horizontal axis), and the dependent variable goes on the y-axis (vertical axis). This helps you visualize the relationship between the variables. In the following example, you are traveling 100 miles in total. You can see that as your speed (independent variable) increases, your travel time (dependent variable) decreases. These two variables are inversely related.

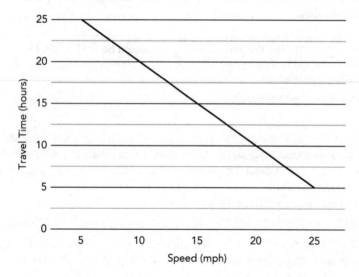

CHAPTER 32 PRACTICE PROBLEMS

From 2006 to 2012, it was found that MLB players with higher batting averages tended to score more runs. This relationship makes sense because higher batting averages suggest that the players get more hits onto the field, which in turn, allows teammates already on base to reach home plate and score a run.

1. Which of the following sentences best describes this relationship?

    A. The two parameters show positive covariance.
    B. The two variables are constants and represent fixed points in time.
    C. The batting average is the dependent variable.
    D. The two parameters are inversely related.

    The table represents the side of a square compared to its area.

Side	Area
1 inch	1 square inches
2 inches	4 square inches
3 inches	9 square inches
4 inches	16 square inches

2. For this relationship, the side of the square and the area of the square are directly related and show positive covariance. Based on this relationship, which of the following statements is true?

    A. If these two variables were graphed, the slope of the line between any two points would be negative.
    B. If these two variables were graphed, the side of the square would be the dependent variable.
    C. The points on the graph should be connected with a straight line to show that they represent variables.
    D. If these two variables were graphed, the slope of the line between any two points would be positive.

3. Determine whether each statement is true or false.

    A. Every scatterplot is an example of covariance.
    B. The more I practice the piano, the better my performance at the recital is. This is an example of positive covariance.
    C. "No pain, no gain" is an example of direct variation, positive covariance.
    D. "The more I cough, the less likely I can run at a fast pace," is an example of direct variation, negative covariance.

4. Which of the following represents a negative covariance?

    A. The more snow we get, the less likely school is open.
    B. The less you drive, the less money you spend on gasoline.
    C. The more snow we get, the more likely school will be closed.
    D. The more you drive, the more money you spend on gasoline.

MATHEMATICS

The table represents the average daily temperature in degrees Fahrenheit compared to daily sales for a small ice cream stand.

Temp.	Sales
95	$7,800
85	47,350
75	$6,750
65	$5,900
55	$5,100
45	$3,850

5 Which of the following statements is true?

  A. There is an inverse relationship between temperature and ice cream sales.
  B. There is a negative covariance.
  C. There is a positive covariance.
  D. The rate of change for any two points is always negative.

Notes:

Notes:

CHAPTER

33
Calculate geometric quantities

 This objective includes, but is not limited to, the following examples of knowledge, skills, and abilities.

• Demonstrate knowledge of area as a square measure.

• Demonstrate knowledge of circumference as the perimeter around a curved shape.

• Understand the concepts of length, area, and surface area.

• Calculate area of an irregular shape by finding the sum of the areas of sections.

• Calculate linear measures by finding the sum of the lengths of sections.

Geometric quantities, such as length and area, are part of our daily lives. It may never cross your mind, but it is a skill you experience quite often. How long is the route to the grocery store? How big is the living room that has to be vacuumed? On the TEAS, you need to be able to calculate length and area of shapes (regular and irregular) using various units.

Length is measured with a tool such as a ruler or tape measure. The table summarizes some units of length, some of which are US customary and some of which are metric.

US Customary	Metric
inches (in), feet (ft), yards (yd), miles (mi)	millimeters (mm), centimeters (cm), meters (m), kilometers (km)

Perimeter and Circumference

Both straight and curved figures possess length, or the distance of a side or around a curve. Curved figures include circles or arcs, which are incomplete circles. The "circumference," or length around a circle, may be found by using the formula $C = 2\pi r$ (π is approximately 3.14, and r is the radius of the circle). The length of an arc (part of a circle) can be found by using the formula $C = 2\pi r$ and then multiplying by the fraction $\dfrac{\text{central angle measure}}{360}$ (the fraction of the circle that the arc covers). This is illustrated in the following diagram.

$Length = \dfrac{n°}{360°} \times 2\pi r$

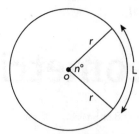

Another aspect of length is perimeter. "Perimeter" is the length around an entire shape. Perimeter is the sum of the individual lengths of the parts of the shape going around the shape once. Some shapes have all straight sides (e.g., rectangle, square, trapezoid, triangle). A somewhat more complex version might look like the following.

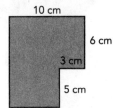

To find the perimeter, simply add the lengths of all of the sides together. To get the missing long side, add 6 cm and 5 cm. To get the missing short side, subtract 3 cm from 10 cm.

Some shapes are curved, and some have a combination of straight and curved, like the following shape.

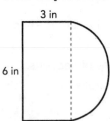

To find the perimeter of this shape, add 3 + 3 + 6 + the length of the semicircular top.

The length of the semicircle can be calculated by finding half of $C = 2\pi r$, or just πr. The radius is half of 6 in, so 3 in. Therefore, the semicircle distance is $\pi \times 3$, or approximately 9.42 in.

Thus, the entire perimeter is 3 + 3 + 6 + 9.42 = 21.42 in.

Area

Area is how much surface space something takes up. When measuring area, the units are squared. Area units include square inches (in²), square feet (ft²), square yards (yd²), square miles (mi²), and square meters (m²). Areas can cover a flat surface (such as a shipping crate) or curved surface (such as an orange). Area and surface area have one simple, yet important, difference: area is for two-dimensional space (flat), and surface area is for three-dimensional space (curved).

The following table provides basic area formulas with examples.

Shape		Formula	Example
Square	*square with side l*	$A = l \times l = l^2$	Length = 4 ft $A = 4 \times 4 = 16 \text{ ft}^2$
Rectangle	*rectangle with width w and length l*	$A = l \times w$	Length = 8 cm, width = 6 cm $A = 8 \times 6 = 48 \text{ cm}^2$
Triangle	*triangle with height h and base b*	$A = \frac{1}{2} \times b \times h$	Base = 3 m, height = 8 m $A = \frac{1}{2} \times 3 \times 8 = 12 \text{ m}^2$
Parallelogram	*parallelogram with height h and base b*	$A = h \times b$	Height = 6 cm, base = 9 cm $A = 9 \times 6 = 54 \text{ cm}^2$
Trapezoid	*trapezoid with bases b_1, b_2 and height h*	$A = \frac{1}{2} \times h \times (b_1 + b_2)$	Height = 6 ft, base 1 = 8 ft, base 2 = 5 ft $A = \frac{1}{2} \times 6 \times (8 + 5) = 39 \text{ ft}^2$
Circle	*circle with radius r*	$A = \pi \times r^2$	Radius = 5 mm $A = \pi \times 25 = 25\pi \approx 78.5 \text{ mm}^2$
Rhombus	*rhombus with diagonals d_1, d_2*	$A = \frac{1}{2} \times d_1 \times d_2$	Diagonal 1 = 4 yd, diagonal 2 = 9 yd $A = \frac{1}{2} \times 4 \times 9 = 18 \text{ yd}^2$

 For the previous example, the area of the shape can also be found by using a combination of formulas from the table.

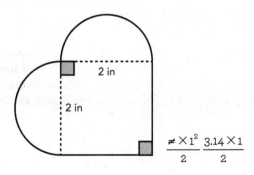

$$\frac{\pi \times 1^2}{2} \quad \frac{3.14 \times 1}{2}$$

The square area is l × l, or 2 in × 2 in, or 4 in².

For each semicircle, find the area of a circle with a 1 in radius and then divide by 2. This would be $\frac{\neq \times 1^2}{2}$ and $\frac{3.14 \times 1^2}{2}$ or approximately 1.56 in².

Then add the areas, which comes to approximately 7.14 in² for the combined area.

CHAPTER 33 PRACTICE PROBLEMS

1. Find the area of the shaded region.

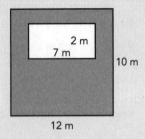

2. Which of the following is the perimeter of the following shape?

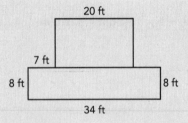

   A. 77 ft
   B. 82 ft
   C. 89 ft
   D. 108 ft

3. What is the area of the following shape?

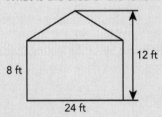

   A. 192 ft²
   B. 240 ft²
   C. 288 ft²
   D. 336 ft²

4. What is the area of the following shape?

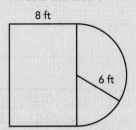

A. 114.88 ft²
B. 133.68 ft²
C. 152.52 ft²
D. 209.04 ft²

5. What is the area of the following shape?

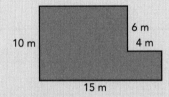

A. 170 m²
B. 150 m²
C. 116 m²
D. 90 m²

MATHEMATICS

Notes:

CHAPTER

34

Convert within and between standard and metric systems

 This objective includes, but is not limited to, the following examples of knowledge, skills, and abilities.

• Convert between units of measure (e.g., mL and L, fl oz and mL, lb and kg, mcg and mg, mg and g, tsp and L, oz and g, cm and m, Fahrenheit and Celsius).

No matter what career you pursue, you will work with numerical quantities in some form every single day. Equally important to these numbers are the units attached to those numbers. Measuring quantities accurately with the correct units is an extremely important skill to master. The health and safety of clients depend on it. You should be familiar with all of the standard and metric units used in medicine. This primarily involves length, volume, mass, and temperature. The TEAS will test your ability to convert among various values accurately, and you should be familiar with some of the most common conversions.

Metric System

The metric system was designed to make conversions easier. The units for length, volume, and mass are directly related to each other. The prefixes indicate the degree of quantity of the root, no matter what characteristic is being measured. There are many prefixes for the metric system, but those you will use on a daily basis are limited and shown in the following table.

Prefix	Meaning	Example
kilo	1,000	1 kg = 1,000 g 1 kL = 1,000 L 1 km = 1,000 m
deca	10	1 dag = 10 g 1 dal = 10 L 1 dam = 1 m
deci	$\frac{1}{10}$	1 dm = $\frac{1}{10}$ m, or equivalently, 10 dm = 1 m
centi	$\frac{1}{100}$	1 cm = $\frac{1}{100}$ me, or equivalently, 100 cm = 1 m
milli	$\frac{1}{1000}$	1 mg = $\frac{1}{1000}$ g, or equivalently, 1,000 mg = 1 g

Standard System

The following table summarizes some useful conversions within the US customary system.

Original Unit	Equivalent Unit
1 ft	12 in
1 yd	3 ft
1 mi	5280 ft
1 lb	16 oz
1 pt	2 c
1 qt	2 pt
1 gal	4 qt
1 T	2000 lb

Converting Between Standard and Metric Systems

Here is a table that is useful in converting between US customary system measurements and the metric measurements.

Original Unit	Equivalent Unit
1 gal	3.8 L
1 kg	2.2 lb
1 in	2.54 cm
1 m	3.28 ft
1 mi	1.6 km
1 oz	28.35 g
1 m	1.09 yd

To convert between units, use the unit conversion method. Start the mathematical equation with what you know and end with what you are trying to find. For example, if you needed to convert 14 pounds to kilograms, you'd set up your equation like this:

14 pounds	=	x kilograms
What we know		What we are trying to find

Here the needed conversion factor is 1 lb = 0.45 kg. Multiply what you know by the conversion factor (*hint:* write it as a fraction).

$$\frac{14 \text{ lb}}{1} \times \frac{0.45 \text{ kg}}{1 \text{ lb}}$$

The lb in the numerator and the lb in the denominator cancel out, leaving only the desired kg unit in the answer.

$$\frac{14 \text{ lb}}{1} \times \frac{0.45 \text{ kg}}{1 \text{ lb}} = 6.3 \text{ kg}$$

Multiplying by a conversion factor is nearly the same as multiplying by 1. This is because the numerator and denominator name the same quantity. Thus, the value of what we know is not changed; only its representation is changed.

As long as you can find the conversion factor, any conversion can be accomplished. One more example:

 Convert 250 g into ounces. The conversion factor is 1 oz = 28.35 g.

250g = x oz

$$\frac{250 \text{ g}}{1} \times \frac{1 \text{ oz}}{28.35 \text{ g}} \approx 8.818 \text{ oz}$$

So, for this example, 250 g = 8.818 oz.

CHAPTER 34 PRACTICE PROBLEMS

Steve is preparing dinner. He is using a cookbook his aunt sent him from Europe. The recipe calls for 10 mL vanilla extract. Steve only has a teaspoon for measuring. He finds that 1 tsp equals 4.93 mL.

1. Which of the following calculates the needed amount?

   A. $\frac{4.93 \text{ mL}}{\text{tsp}} \times 5\text{mL} = 24.65 \text{ mL}$

   B. $\frac{4.93 \text{ mL}}{\text{tsp}} = 0.986 \text{ tsp}$

   C. $\frac{4.93 \text{ mL}}{\text{tsp}} \times \frac{1 \text{ tbsp}}{14.8 \text{ mL}} = 0.333 \text{ tsp}$

   D. $\frac{5 \text{ mL}}{1} \times \frac{1 \text{ tsp}}{4.93 \text{ mL}} = 1.014 \text{ tsp}$

Patricia is in Ireland on vacation. While shopping, she sees a pretty sweater in a shop window. The price is marked €50 . Patricia had seen the same scarf in the United States for $45. The conversion rate in the bank window next to the store says €1 = $1.20. Patricia is deciding whether the sweater in the window is a good deal or if she should wait until she returns to the United States to purchase it.

2. Which of the following describes how to solve this dilemma?

   A. Divide €50 by $1.20.
   B. Divide €50 by 12.
   C. Multiply €50 by $1.20 per €.
   D. Divide €50 by $45.

3. In the following table, match the equivalent quantities. Refer to the conversions presented in this lesson. If necessary, you may consult the Internet.

Original Unit	Equivalent Unit
750 mL	12 kg
75 mL	4 cm
26.4 lb	5 in
100°C	75 cc
600 m	212°F
12.7 cm	0.75 L
40 mm	0.72 kg
720 g	0.6 km

4. Approximately how many feet are in 3 m?

   A. 0.9 ft
   B. 1.18 ft
   C. 7.62 ft
   D. 9.84 ft

5. Harry had 5 gal of gas remaining in his tank when he stopped at a gas station in Canada. He added 35 L of gas to his tank to fill the car. How much gas does Harry have?

   A. 54 L
   B. 40 L
   C. 19 L
   D. 14.2 L

Notes:

Notes:

Key Terms

addition. Calculation of a total of two or more numbers.

algebraic equation. A mathematic equation that includes one or more variables.

arc. Part of the circumference of a circle.

area. The amount of space inside a two-dimensional boundary.

axis. A reference line for measurement of coordinates.

bivariate. Containing two variables.

Cartesian coordinate. An ordered pair or ordered triple used to specify a point on a plane or space, respectively.

chart. Information in the form of a table or graph.

circumference. The length around a circle.

combine like terms. Simplifying an expression by using the distributive property.

common denominator. In a set of two or more fractions, an integer that is divisible by each denominator. That is, a multiple of all of the denominators.

constant of proportionality. The ratio between two quantities.

constant. A number that is not "attached to," or does not multiply, a variable.

contextual. Related to surrounding content.

conversion factor. The number used to multiply or divide to convert from one value to another.

conversion. Changing one value or unit of measurement to another that is equivalent.

covariance. The way two variables change together.

data trend. General tendency of numbers in a set.

decimal place value. Powers of ten by position away from the decimal point. Going left: units, tens, hundreds, etc. Going right: tenths, hundredths, thousandths, etc.

decimal. A number expressed in powers of 10.

denominator. The bottom number of a fraction.

dependent variable. A variable that depends on at least one other variable.

division. Separation of numbers into parts; the inverse of multiplication.

equation. A mathematical statement that indicates the equality of two expressions.

erroneous. Incorrect.

estimation. A rough calculation of numbers.

expected value. The most likely value of a random variable.

expression. A finite string of mathematical symbols (numbers, operations, variables) that are grouped to show a value.

extraneous. Irrelevant.

fraction. A number expressed as a numerator and denominator.

graph. A drawing that represents relationships between numbers or data.

independent variable. A variable that determines the value of another variable.

inequality symbols. Less than ($<$), greater than ($>$), less than or equal to ($\leq$), and greater than or equal to ($\geq$).

inequality. A mathematical statement with two expressions that do not have the same value.

integer. Whole numbers and their opposites: ..., -3, -2, -1, 0, 1, 2, 3, ...

inverse arithmetic operations. Mathematic operations that undo each other.

irrational number. A real number that cannot be expressed as terminating or repeating decimals.

irregular shape. A shape in which not all sides and angles are equal.

legend. An explanation of figures used in a chart.

length. The measure from end to end.

linear units. A unit used to measure length.

measures of central tendency. Mean is commonly known as the average; median is the middle value; and mode is the number repeated most often.

metric system. International System of Units (French: Système international d'unités, SI) based on powers of ten.

mixed number. A number formed by an integer and a fraction.

multiples of a number. A number multiplied by various integers.

multiplication. Addition of a number to itself a specified number of times.

non-negative. Greater than or equal to zero (positive or zero).

numerator. The top number of a fraction.

operation. A mathematical action.

order of operations. The sequence of operations that must be followed to simplify an expression.

ordering numbers. Putting numbers in order of lowest to highest.

outlier. A data point that is distinctly separate from other data; an unexpected value.

percent decrease. The negative difference between two numbers, divided by the first number, multiplied by 100.

percent increase. The positive difference between two numbers, divided by the first number, multiplied by 100.

percent. Parts per hundred.

perimeter. The distance around a two-dimensional shape.

place value. Numerical value defined by position.

point on a graph. The location of a value expressed as (x, y).

proportion. An equality of two ratios.

range. The difference between the highest and lowest values in a set.

rate of change. A rate that describes how one quantity changes in relation to another.

rate. A ratio that compares quantities of two unit of measure.

ratio. A comparison of the sizes of two numbers.

rational number. A number that can be expressed as a fraction.

reciprocal. One divided by the original number, or, for a nonzero fraction a/b, the reciprocal is b/a.

repeat. Do again.

rounding. Simplifying a number by removing decimal places or changing those places to zero.

scale. Ratio of graphical representation to actual size.

shape. Symmetry, number of peaks, skewness, and uniformity of data distribution.

simplify. Reducing a fraction or an expression to a simpler form by actions such as cancellation of common factors and regrouping of terms with the same variable.

solution. The answer.

solve. Find the answer.

spread. The range of values in data distribution.

square units. The area of a square with sides that measure 1 unit.

subtend. Form an angle at a particular point on an arc.

subtraction. Removing one number from another; the inverse of addition.

sum. Total of two or more values.

surface area. The total area of a three-dimensional object's surface.

table. A set of data displayed in rows and columns.

terminate. To end.

unit conversion. Calculating equivalent values between systems of measurement.

unit rate. A rate which shows how many units of one quantity (in the numerator) correspond to one unit of the second quantity (in the denominator), such as miles/hour.

variable terms. Numeric values consisting of variables and coefficients or constants.

variable. A letter, often x, y, or z, that stands for an unspecified quantity.

whole number. The numbers used in counting and zero: 0, 1, 2, 3, 4, 5, 6, 7, ...

Practice Problem Answers

Chapter 20

1. Solutions worked out:

   - $3.25 \times 100\% = 325\%$
   - $0.215 \times 100\% = 21.5\%$
   - $62.9\% \div 100\% = 0.629$
   - $145\% \div 100\% = 1.45$
   - $0.265 = \dfrac{265}{1000}$, where 265 is the numerator and the last decimal place is the thousandths.
   - $1.39 = \dfrac{139}{100}$, where 139 is the numerator and the last decimal place is the hundredths.
   - $26 \div 10 = 2.6$.
   - $16 \div 25 = 0.64$.

2. Option D is correct. This is calculated by dividing 17 by 10 and multiplying by 100%.

3. Option A is correct. This is calculated by converting to a decimal (0.564) and then writing the 564 over the place value of the last digit in the decimal (1,000).

4. Option C is correct. This is calculated by dividing 3.75 by 100 and dropping the percent sign.

5. Option A is correct. This is calculated by dividing 16 by 50.

Chapter 21

1. Solutions worked out:

   - First, perform operations in parentheses: $12 - 9$
     Then multiply: 24
     Finally, add: 30
   - First, perform operations in parentheses: $9 \div 3$
     Then divide: 3
   - First multiply and divide from left to right.
     $28 + 8 \div 4 - 3 \times 6$
     $28 + 2 - 3 \times 6$
     $28 + 2 - 18$
     Then add and subtract from left to right:
     $30 - 18 = 12$
   - First simplify the numerator and denominator.
     Numerator: $50 - 14 = 36$
     Denominator: $6 + 12 = 18$
     Lastly, divide numerator by denominator:
     $36 \div 18 = 2$

2. Option C is correct. Multiply first: $3 + 12 - 4$. Then add: $15 - 4$. Then subtract: 11.

3. Option B is correct. Simplify both numerator and

denominator first: $\dfrac{25}{5} = 5$

4. Option A is correct.
   First complete the operation in parentheses: 24
   Then simplify the both the numerator and denominator: $15/3 = 5$
   Then add and subtract from left to right:
   $50 - 24 + 5 = 31$

5. Option B is correct. First complete the multiplication in the numerator: 6
   Then complete operations in the numerator:
   $18 - 6 = 12$
   Then simplify the fraction: $12/6 = 2$
   Then complete the addition: $17 + 2 = 19$

Chapter 22

1. If $8\dfrac{3}{4}$ is converted to a decimal, it becomes 8.75. Thus, the increasing order is -8, 8.43, $8\dfrac{3}{4}$.

2. Option B is correct. $9\dfrac{1}{6} = 9.17$ is larger than 9.14.

   - 9.14 is not larger than $9\dfrac{1}{6} = 9.17$.
   - 9.14 is not equal to $9\dfrac{1}{6} = 9.17$.
   - $9\dfrac{1}{6} = 9.17$ is not smaller than nor is it equal to 9.14.

3. Option D is correct. If $4\dfrac{1}{5}$ is written in decimal form, it equals 4.2. The decimals can be stacked to compare.

4. Option C is correct. The lowest common denominator for the fractions is 16.

   $\dfrac{1}{2} = \dfrac{8}{16}, \dfrac{3}{8} = \dfrac{6}{16}, \dfrac{3}{4} = \dfrac{12}{16}$. The ordered list is $\dfrac{3}{8}, \dfrac{1}{2}, \dfrac{11}{16}, \dfrac{3}{4}$.

5. Option A is correct. If $-1\dfrac{3}{5}$ is written as a decimal, it is -1.6. If $-1\dfrac{3}{4}$ is written as a decimal, it is -1.75. The decimals can be stacked to compare.

Chapter 23

1. Option A is correct. To isolate the variable on one side of the equation, you would add 17 to both sides of the equation.

2. Subtract 2x from both sides of the equation as shown.

$$2x - 2x - 6 = -4x - 2x$$

Next, divide by –6 on both sides of the equation as shown.

$$-6 = -6x$$

$$\frac{-6x}{-6} = \frac{-6}{-6}$$

$$1 = x$$

3. Divide both sides of the equation by 6 as shown.

$$6x = 19$$

$$\frac{6x}{6} = \frac{19}{6}$$

$$x = \frac{19}{6}$$

4. Multiply both sides of the equation by $\frac{5}{7}$ as shown.

$$\frac{7}{5}X = 35$$

$$\frac{5}{7}, \frac{7}{5}X = \frac{5}{7} \times \frac{35}{1}$$

$$x = 25$$

5. Option C is correct. Subtracting 3x from both sides gets the variables collected on the left side of the equation. This is an acceptable first step.

- Subtracting 9 from both sides still leaves constants on each side of the equation.
- Adding 12 to both sides of the equation still leaves constants on each side of the equation.
- Adding 5x to both sides of the equation still leaves variables on both sides of the equation.

Chapter 24

1. Step 1: Understand the problem.

How many pavers should Jayden buy?

The square pavers are 4 inches on each side. The garden is 8 feet long and 2 feet wide.

Step 2: Make a drawing of the garden. Recall that the opposite sides of a rectangle are equal.

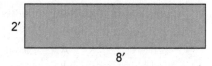

Because 1 foot equals 12 inches, it takes three 4-inch pavers to equal a length of 1 foot.

Add six pavers to both of the 2-foot sides in your drawing.

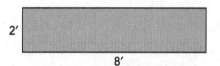

Next add 24 pavers to both of the 8-foot sides.

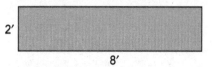

One extra paver is needed in each corner to surround completely the garden.

Step 3: Add up the pavers needed.

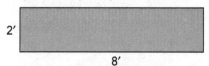

Length	Number of Pavers Needed
8 feet	24
2 feet	6
8 feet	24
2 feet	6
4 corners	4
TOTAL	64

Step 4: Visualize walking around the drawing, counting three pavers for each foot. Don't forget to step on each corner.

64 pavers is a reasonable solution.

2. Step 1: Understand the problem.

How many days will the bottle last?
The dosage is 2.5 mL twice a day. The bottle contains 200 cc.

Step 2: Because 1 cc is equivalent to 1 mL, the cat needs to take 5 cc per day (2.5 mL twice daily). Divide the bottle's volume by the dosage.

Step 3: Perform the division.
200 cc divided by 5 cc/day will equal the number of days.

Step 4: Evaluate for reasonableness.
40 days is a reasonable time period for a prescription. Each day requires 5 cc, and 200 is much more than 5, so you would expect an answer greater than 1. Two days requires 10 cc, 3 days 15 cc, and so on. So 40 days requires 200 cc of the vitamin overall.

- $\frac{200 \text{ cc}}{5 \text{ mL}/\text{day}} = 40 \text{days}$

3. Step 1: Understand the problem.
   Fluid intake: Monday: 1,800 mL, Tuesday: 2,350 mL
   Total fluid outtake: 1,775 mL

   Step 2: Add to determine total fluid intake.
   Total fluid intake = 1,800 + 2,350 = 4,150 mL

   Step 3: Determine net result by subtracting.
   Net result: Intake minus outtake
   = 4,150 mL − 1,775 mL = 2,375 mL

   Step 4: Check your answer for reasonableness.
   2,375 + 1,775 = 4,150, which was the total fluid intake, so the answer 2,375 mL is a reasonable solution.

4. Step 1: Understand the problem.

   1 batch of cookies requires $\frac{3}{4}$ cups of flour.

   Step 2. Use multiplication to determine the flour needed for $1\frac{1}{2}$ batches.

   Step 3: Multiply a fraction and a mixed number by renaming the mixed number as an improper fraction and then multiply the resulting numerators and denominators.

   $1\frac{1}{2} \times \frac{3}{4} = \frac{3}{2} \times \frac{3}{4} = \frac{9}{8} = 1\frac{1}{9}$ cups

   Step 4: Check for reasonableness.

   2 batches would require $\frac{3}{4}$ cups two times, or $1\frac{1}{2}$ cups. $1\frac{1}{2}$ cups is in the middle, which corresponds to $1\frac{1}{2}$ batches.

5. Step 1: Understand the problem.

   1,225 students take the bus. 1,955 students are enrolled in the school system.

   Step 2: Identify the part and whole.

   1,225 (part), 1,955 (whole)

   Step 3: Divide the part by the whole to determine the decimal equivalent. Then multiply the decimal by 100% to change to a percent.

   $\frac{1.225}{1.955} \approx 0.6266$; 0.6266 × 100% = 62.66%

   Step 4: Evaluate for reasonableness.
   Since 1,225 is a little more than half of 1,955, 62.66% is reasonable.

Chapter 25

1. Convert 4.5% to decimal form: 0.045. Multiply 0.045 × $55,000 = $2,475, which is your salary increase for next year.

2. Option A is correct. Convert 35% to a decimal (0.35), then multiply 0.35 × 900 = 315.

3. Option C is correct. Find 25% of $50 by multiplying 0.25 × $50 = $12.50. Subtract $50 − $12.50 = $37.50. Alternatively, you can subtract 100% − 25% to get 75%, rename 75% as 0.75, and then multiply 0.75 × $50 = $37.50.

4. Option D is correct. Find 6.5% of $550 by multiplying 0.065 × $550 = $35.75. Add $550 + $35.75 = $585.75. Alternatively, you can add 100% + 6.5% to get 106.5%, rename 106.5% as 1.065, and then multiply 1.065 × $550 = $585.75.

5. Option A is correct. Find 6% of $58,000 by multiplying 0.06 × $58,000 = $3,480.00. Add $3,480.00 and $900.00 to get $4,380.00.

Chapter 26

1. Option A is correct. Rounding each number to the nearest one is a good estimate.

2.

Number	Round to This Place	Your Answer	Number	Round to This Place	Your Answer
34.19	Tenths	34.2	$7\frac{4}{5}$	Ones	8
$\frac{6}{7}$	Ones	1	64.736	Tenths	64.7
7.219	Hundredths	7.22	547	Tens	550
933.74	Thousands	1,000	878	Hundreds	900
2.739	Hundredths	2.74	87.357	Hundredths	87.36
32.834	Tenths	32.8	32.95	Tenths	33.0
37.494	Tens	40	483.34	Hundreds	500
$\frac{23}{50}$	Ones	0			

- Rounding each number to different place values may introduce more error.
- You cannot ignore decimal place value and round to the first digit only.
- Rounding every number down to its smallest place value introduces more error than necessary.

3. Option B is correct. Meters and millimeters both measure length: however, since a meter is close to a yard, that unit would be too large to use. A paper clip is small, so millimeters is the best unit.

4. Option A is correct. A pet rabbit's weight may be measured in kilograms. Spilled water is a liquid and would be measured in liters or milliliters. A tablet of ibuprofen is very small and would be measured in milligrams. A piece of paper would likely be measured in length, such as centimeters.

MATHEMATICS

5. Option D is correct. In the numerator, round to the nearest hundred and nearest one, and then round to the nearest ten in the denominator. You will have a calculation you can do easily without a calculator.

Chapter 27

1. $$\frac{27 \text{ hours}}{3 \text{ weeks}} = \frac{x \text{ hours}}{7 \text{ weeks}}$$

   Multiplying both sides by 7 weeks yields

   $$\frac{27 \times 7}{3} = \frac{x \times 7}{7}$$

   Simplifying the left side leads to $x = 63$ hours

2. Option C is correct.

   $$\frac{2 \text{ sales}}{11 \text{ calls}} = \frac{x \text{ sales}}{55 \text{ calls}}$$

   Multiplying both sides by 55 calls will give

   $$\frac{2 \text{ sales} \times 55 \text{ calls}}{11 \text{ calls}} = x$$

   Simplifying the left side leads to $x = 10$ sales.

3. Option B is correct.

   $$\frac{4 \text{ defective}}{1000 \text{ TVs}} = \frac{x \text{ defective}}{95,000 \text{ TVs}}$$

   Multiply both sides by 95,000 TVs.

   $$\frac{4 \text{ defective} \times 95,000 \text{ TVs}}{1000 \text{ TVs}} = x$$

   Simplify the left side: $x = 380$ defective.

4. Option D is correct.

   $$\frac{1 \text{cm}}{75 \text{ miles}} = \frac{8.6 \text{ cm}}{x \text{ miles}}$$

   Multiply 75 by 8.6 cm to get $x = 645$ miles

5. Option C is correct. The remaining choices are in the form $y = mx + b$ where b is nonzero.

Chapter 28

1. $$\frac{\$900}{4 \text{ nights}} = \frac{\$223}{1 \text{ night}}$$ and $$\frac{\$1443}{7 \text{ nights}} = \frac{\$206.14}{1 \text{ night}}$$, so the 7-night deal is the better deal.

2. Option C is correct. The rate has been reduced correctly, and the denominator is one unit.
   - Option A: Nancy has written the reciprocal of the unit rate.
   - A unit rate should have 1 day in the denominator.
   - A rate must include units.

3. Option D is correct. The rate has been reduced correctly, and the denominator is one unit.
   - Option A is the reciprocal of the unit rate.
   - A unit rate should have 1 ounce in the denominator.
   - A rate must include units.

4. Option A is correct: The rate of change is
   $$\frac{\$1130 - \$360}{10 \text{ months}} = \frac{\$770}{7} = \frac{\$110}{\text{month}}$$

5. Option B is correct. The ratio has been reduced correctly.
   - Option A is the reduced ratio of black markers to total.
   - Option C is the ratio of red markers to black markers.
   - Option D is the ratio of red markers to black markers.

Chapter 29

1. The question asks how many weeks, so let w = number of weeks.

   The total number of cards over time would be $2w$. Seven cards to start with would be shown as $+ 9$. More than 35 cards would be shown as > 35. The inequality is $2w + 9 > 35$.

2. Option C is correct.
   - At least should be greater than or equal to ($\geq$).
   - The $15 is a one-time gift, not every week.
   - Option D gives Tom less than $255.

3. Option D is correct.
   - The taxi driver charges $2.00 before the taxi starts to move.
   - Option B ensures that the fare will be more than $25.
   - The $2.00 is only paid once, not every mile.

4. Option D is correct.
   - Grant has already driven 100 miles.
   - Option C ensures that Grant drives at most 350 miles.
   - At least means greater than or equal to.

5. Option B is correct.
   - 3 is not multiplied by 5 and 9 is not multiplied by 3.
   - Option C ensures that Grant drives at most 350 miles.
   - Greater than will not be equal to.
   - 9 is not multiplied by x.

Chapter 30

1. Option D is correct. The average rate of change on a graph is the same as the slope. Find the slope between year 4 ($800) and year 1 ($200).

   - The cost to maintain the car decreased between years 6 and 7. It is possible that a new car was purchased.
   - The graph shows the expense for each year individually. The total cost for the first 3 years is $800.
   - There are only 3 years between year 1 and year 4.

2. Option B is correct. The number of pounds of corn sold increased from day 1 to day 3.

   - The most zucchini was sold on Day 1.
   - The scale on the y-axis is 10 pounds and not 1 pound.
   - The most carrots were sold on day 1 and not day 3.

3. Dani's and Frank's tips:

Night	Dani's Tips	Frank's Tips
Monday	$15	$20
Tuesday	$20	$15
Wednesday	$30	$25
Thursday	$40	$35
Friday	$35	$50

   - On Friday night, Dani's tips decreased from $40 to $35.
   - On Friday night, Frank earned $15 more than Dani.
   - The average rate of change is
     $$\frac{\$50 - \$20}{4 \text{ nights}} = \frac{\$30}{4 \text{ nights}} = \$7.50 / \text{night.}$$

4. Option B is correct. The greatest increase in profits was $15,000 from 2016 to 2017.

   - There was a decrease in profits from 2015 to 2016.
   - Max earned $35,000, and not zero, in 2013.
   - There were three increases of $5000: from 2014 to 2015, from 2017 to 2018, and from 2018 to 2019.

5. Option C is correct. Most people chose rock as their favorite genre of music.

   - Country music was a favorite of 25% of people and not 25 people.
   - There was a difference of 5% of people and not 5 people for preference country music to pop music.
   - Neither rock nor country was chosen by 40% of people and not 40 people.

Chapter 31

1. Solutions:

   - Mean $\dfrac{0+1+2+2+3+5+6+7+8+16}{10} = \dfrac{50}{10} = 5$
   - Median $= \dfrac{3+5}{2} = \dfrac{8}{2} = 4$
   - Mode $= 2$

2. Option A is correct. When most of the data is in the center of a histogram, it is bell-shaped.

   - Bell-shaped is symmetric on both sides.
   - Normal is bell-shaped.

3. Option B is correct. As the value of x increases, the value of y increases.

4. Option B is correct. When a data set is skewed left, the data peaks closer to higher values.

5. Option B is correct. When one set of values increases and the other set of values decreases, there is a decreasing trend.

Chapter 32

1. Option A is correct. As the batting average goes up, the runs scored also goes up.

   - Variables represent quantities that are changing. They are not constant but instead representative of the time period from 2006 to 2012.
   - When graphing this, the batting average would come first and be the independent variable.
   - Because the values go in the same direction, they are directly related.

2. Option D is correct. For a direct relationship, as one variable increases so does the other. This would have a positive slope.

   - For any direct relationship, as one variable increases so does the other. This would have a positive slope.
   - The side of the square determines the area of the square, so it is the independent variable. When collecting data, it will not always be immediately known which variable is independent and which is dependent.
   - The relationship is not linear. Because the area is growing by multiplication, the graph would be curved.

MATHEMATICS

3. Options B and C are correct.
   - Option A: False. If there is no relationship between variables, there is no covariance. If sometimes one goes up while the other goes down and vice versa, there is no covariance.
   - Option B: True. The more you practice, the better you perform. This is a belief held by many musicians and music teachers.
   - Option C: True. This statement is usually heard in sports, exercise, and in medical or dental procedures.
   - Option D: False. The two variables are inversely (not directly) related. It is a good example of negative covariance. As your coughing increases, you will likely have difficulty running at a fast pace.

4. Option A is correct. The more snow on the ground, the less likely schools will be open.
   - Option B: False. This is a positive covariance because both quantities decrease. Option D is logically equivalent to this statement, too.
   - Option C: False. This is a positive covariance. The more likely school will be closed is logically equivalent to the less likely school will be open.
   - Option D: False. This is a positive covariance.

5. Options A, B, and D are all true. There is an inverse relationship, which suggests a negative covariance. This means that the rate of change between any two points is negative.
   - Option C: False. This is not a positive covariance.

Chapter 33

1. Find the areas of the rectangle and inner rectangle, and imagine "cutting out" the area of the inner rectangle. The area of the shaded region is the area left over after the subtraction. Therefore, $(12 \times 10) - (7 \times 2) = 120 - 14 = 106$ sq m.

2. Option D is correct. The missing horizontal segment is $34 - 20 - 7 = 7$ ft. The missing vertical segment is $20 - 8 = 12$ ft. The combined perimeter is $34 + 8 + 8 + 7 + 7 + 12 + 12 + 20 = 108$ ft.

3. Option B is correct. The height of the triangle is $12 - 8 = 4$ ft, and the base of the triangle is 24 ft. To find the area, add the area of the rectangle to the area of the triangle:
$$(24 \times 8) + \frac{1}{2}(24 \times 4) = 192 + \frac{1}{2}(96)$$
$$= 192 + 48 = 240 \text{ sq ft.}$$

4. Option C is correct. To find the area, add the area of the rectangle and the area of the semicircle.
$$(12 \times 8) + \frac{1}{2}(3.14 \times 6^2) = 96 + \frac{1}{2}(113.04) = 96 + 56.52$$
$$= 152.52 \text{ sq ft}$$

5. Option C is correct. To find the area, imagine the upper right corner is being cut off. Subtract that area from the total area.
$$(15 \times 10) - (6 \times 4) = 150 - 24 = 116 \text{ sq m.}$$

Chapter 34

1. Option D is correct. The answer would be rounded to 1 tsp in the kitchen.
   - The mL units do not factor out to leave tsp. This is not set up correctly.
   - Without units on the 5, it is hard to know if this is set up correctly.
   - This is the wrong conversion factor. Teaspoons are smaller than tablespoons.

2. Option C is correct: $\dfrac{€50}{1} \times \dfrac{\$1.20}{€1} = \$60.00$
   - Patricia did not use the unit conversion method.
   - $\dfrac{€50}{12} = €4.17$. There was no conversion.
   - To compare prices, they both must be in the same monetary unit.

3. Solution:

Original Unit	Equivalent Unit
750 mL	0.75 L
75 mL	75 cc
26.4 lb	12 kg
100°C	212°F
600 m	0.6 km
12.7 cm	5 in
40 mm	4 cm
720 g	0.72 kg

4. Option D is correct. $\dfrac{3 \text{ m}}{1} \times \dfrac{3.28 \text{ ft}}{1 \text{ m}} = 9.84$ ft.
   - The meters units do not factor out to leave feet. This is not set up correctly.
   - The conversion factor is incorrect; 1 m is not equal to 2.54 ft.
   - The conversion factor is incorrect; 1 ft is not equal to 2.54 m.

5. Option A is correct. $\dfrac{5 \text{ gal}}{1} \times \dfrac{3.8 \text{ L}}{1} = 19$ L;
   $19 \text{ L} + 35 \text{ L} = 54$ L.
   - You do not divide 35 L by 3.8.
   - Although 5 gal is equivalent to 19 L, you need to add 35 L to get the total.
   - You cannot add unlike units, such as gallons and liters. You need to first convert gallons to liters.

✅ Unit Quiz

1. Which of the following pairs is equivalent to 6.74%?

   A. $\dfrac{6.74}{100}$, 0.0674

   B. $\dfrac{674}{10}$, 6.74

   C. $\dfrac{6.74}{1000}$, 674

   D. $\dfrac{674}{1000}$, 67.4

2. Which of the following is the correct value of the given expression?

   $$\dfrac{22 + 14 + 7}{17 - 42 \times 3}$$

   A. $\dfrac{5.14}{-75}$

   B. $\dfrac{24}{109}$

   C. $\dfrac{24}{-109}$

   D. $\dfrac{5.14}{75}$

3. Which of the following choices arranges the numbers from least to greatest?

   $\dfrac{8}{11}$, 0.625, −1.33, $-1\dfrac{4}{5}$, $\dfrac{15}{13}$

   A. $\dfrac{15}{13}, \dfrac{8}{11}$, 0.625, −1.33, $-1\dfrac{4}{5}$

   B. 0.625, −1.33, $-1\dfrac{4}{5}, \dfrac{15}{13}, \dfrac{8}{11}$

   C. $-1\dfrac{4}{5}$, −1.33, 0.625, $\dfrac{8}{11}, \dfrac{15}{13}$

   D. −1.33, $-1\dfrac{4}{5}$, 0.625, $\dfrac{15}{13}, \dfrac{8}{11}$

4. Which of the following shows the correct steps to finding the solution for the given equation?

   $8x + 3x - 5 = 4x + 16$

   A. $8x - 3x = 11x$
   $11x - 5 = 4x + 16$
   $6x = 12x$
   $x = 2$

   B. $3x - 5 = 4x - 8x + 16$
   $-2x = -4x + 16$
   $-2x = 16x$
   $x = -8$

   C. $8x - 5 = 4x - 3x + 16$
   $-3x = x + 16$
   $2x = 16x$
   $x = 8$

   D. $8x + 3x = 11x$
   $11x - 5 = 4x + 16$
   $11x - 4x = 16 + 5$
   $7x = 21$
   $x = 3$

5. Jocelyn's doctor prescribed a medication for her; the dosing instructions were to take 37.5 mg daily for 45 days. The pharmacy only had the pills in a higher dosage. They needed to cut 15 pills to fill her prescription. Which of the following is the number of milligrams in 1 pill that the pharmacy had? How many parts were the pills cut into so that Jocelyn receives the correct daily dose of 37.5 mg?

   A. 112.5 mg, 3 parts
   B. 135 mg, 3 parts
   C. 112.5 mg, 2.5 parts
   D. 150 mg, 4 parts

6. Sharonda's company has announced that there will be performance bonuses given out this year. For employees who receive a high rating, their bonus ranges from 3% to 5% of their salary. Sharonda is excited because she earned a high rating, so she is eligible for a bonus. She is currently making a salary of $79,200.

   Which of the following is the range of possible bonuses Sharonda could receive?

   A. $2,400 to $4,000
   B. $2,376 to $3,960
   C. $2,187 to $3,645
   D. $2,250 to $3,750

The Percentage of High School Students Who:	2007 Total (%)	2009 Total (%)	2011 Total (%)	2013 Total (%)	2015 Total (%)	2017 Total
Watch streaming television	6.0	6.9	7.4	7.7	7.8	6.0
Use social media	45.5	56.0	66.9	67.1	77.6	6.7
Participate in sports	14.9	15.5	16.2	14.8	15.5	14.9
Play video games	20.0	19.9	20.1	19.6	19.2	19.0
Read comic books	7.5	7.4	7.5	7.3	7.5	7.4
Write poetry	13.4	12.6	11.7	10.3	9.6	8.0
Volunteer with an organization	11.3	10.8	10.7	10.4	10.6	6.9

7. Based on the data in the table, which of the following statements is correct?

   A. The percentage of high school students who play video games has increased consistently from 2009 to 2017.

   B. The percentage of high school students who read comic books has remained fairly consistent from 2007 to 2017.

   C. The percentage of high school students who use social media has decreased steadily from 2007 to 2017.

   D. The percentage of high school students who volunteer with an organization has declined more rapidly than those who write poetry.

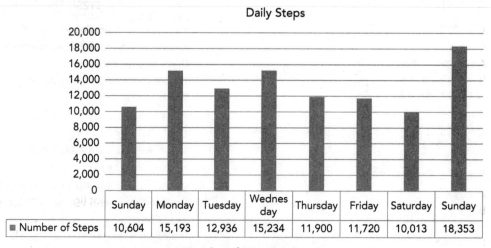

Daily Steps

	Sunday	Monday	Tuesday	Wednesday	Thursday	Friday	Saturday	Sunday
■ Number of Steps	10,604	15,193	12,936	15,234	11,900	11,720	10,013	18,353

■ Number of Steps ■ Column1

8. According to the graph, which of the following best represents the median of the data represented?

   A. 12,418
   B. 11,900
   C. 12,936
   D. 13,244

9. Which of the following examples would describe positive covariance?

   A. Because Samantha was able to streamline her morning routine, she was able to sleep longer.

   B. Juan tries to increase the number of miles he travels before refilling his gas tank. This helps to reduce his carbon footprint.

   C. Dimitri asked for more shifts at work because he is saving for a down payment on a new car. If he makes a higher down payment, he will have a lower monthly payment.

   D. Darnell owns an ice cream shop. He notices that as the temperature rises, he sells more ice cream.

10. You have been asked to order new carpet for the hallway and waiting room of your office. The hallway is 6 ft wide by 67 ft long. The waiting room is 20 ft wide and 35 ft long, with a semicircular area by the door measuring 10 ft in diameter.

    Which of the following is the amount of carpet that needs to be ordered? Round your answer up to the nearest foot.

    A. 1,102 ft²
    B. 1,181 ft²
    C. 1,140 ft²
    D. 1,142 ft²

11. Which of the follow expresses $\frac{5}{8}$ as a decimal and a percent?

    A. 0.0625 and 6.25%
    B. 1.6 and 160%
    C. 0.58 and 58%
    D. 0.625 and 62.5%

12. Solve the equation. Which of the following is correct?

    $9x + 4 = 3x - 8$

    A. $x = 2$
    B. $x = -2$
    C. $x = 1/2$
    D. $x = 1$

13. Max has five lawns to mow on Saturday. The first lawn is 20 ft by 30 ft. The second lawn is 200 ft by 45 ft. The third yard is 50 ft by 50 ft. The fourth yard is 90 ft by 60 ft. The fifth yard is 150 ft by 95 ft. He can mow 240 ft² every minute. Approximately how long will it take him to mow all five lawns?

    A. 2 hours and 12 minutes
    B. 2 hours and 20 minutes
    C. 1 hour and 9 minutes
    D. 6 hours and 58 minutes

14. A going-out-of-business sale has marked all items in the store at 55% off the listed price. You found a shirt for $17.50 and a pair of pants for $37. Which of the following is the reduced total you will pay?

    A. $34.15
    B. $44.87
    C. $24.52
    D. $54.50

15. The Junior Class is charge of planning the prom. They have been told that the budget comes from the number of tickets sold and ticket prices cannot exceed $45 per person. Knowing the current expenses are as follows:

Room rental	$3,967
DJ	$563
Decorations	$2,311
Security	$125/hr for 5 hours

    Which of the following is the best estimate of how many tickets will have to be sold before a profit is made?

    A. 150
    B. 125
    C. 100
    D. 175

16. The high school is adding 50 spaces to its parking lot. Knowing that a space is 8 ft by 12 ft, which of the following best estimates the area of the new parking lot (ignore driving lanes)?

    A. 4,800 ft²
    B. 5,000 ft²
    C. 2,000 ft²
    D. 7,500 ft²

17. You are having a dinner party for 22 guests. You have a recipe for Dijon Chicken that serves 6. The recipe instructions use ¾ of a tablespoon of brown sugar. Which of the following is the amount of brown sugar needed to make the recipe to serve 22 guests?

    A. 2 ½ tablespoons
    B. 3 tablespoons
    C. 2 ¾ tablespoons
    D. 1 ¾ tablespoons

18. The interest earned on $1,000 is $23. If the interest rate is the same, which of the following is the amount of interest earned on $750?

    A. $17.25
    B. $23
    C. $20.50
    D. $18

19. There are 3,400 students and 200 teachers in a high school. A new neighborhood is being built, and there is the expectation that an additional 250 students will be added to the school. How many new teachers will be needed to keep the ratio of students to teachers the same?

    A. 15
    B. 25
    C. 35
    D. 50

20. A student intern is helping the athletic director prepare water coolers for afternoon practices. Each cooler holds 5 gallons of water, which serves 40 athletes. There are 17 volleyball players, 25 soccer players, and 67 football players. Which of the following sets is the correct ratio of water for each team?

    A. $2\frac{1}{2}$ gallons, $3\frac{3}{4}$ gallons, $8\frac{2}{3}$ gallons
    B. 2 gallons, 3 gallons, 8 gallons
    C. $2\frac{1}{8}$ gallons, $3\frac{1}{8}$ gallons, $8\frac{3}{8}$ gallons
    D. 3 gallons, 5 gallons, 10 gallons

21. The Booster Club wants to earn at least $500 for the next year. They plan to hold a raffle with a item worth $100 as the winning prize. If each ticket (T) is $2, which of the following expressions shows how many ticket they need to sell?

    A. $2T ≤ $500
    B. $2T ≥ $500
    C. $2T < $600
    D. $2T ≥ $600

22. While on a Spring Break field trip in Italy, the class is trying to decide if the 1L cola on the fast-food menu priced at $1.99 is cheaper than the 16-oz cola on the fast-food menu priced at $0.99 back home. Which of the following describes how to solve this dilemma? (1 L ≈ 34 oz)

    A. Multiply 34 oz by 16 to find the number of 16-oz colas that are in a liter and then divide that number by $0.99.
    B. Divide 34 oz by 16 to find the number of 16-oz colas that are in a liter and then multiply that number by $0.99.
    C. Divide 34 oz by 16 to find the number of 16-oz colas that are in a liter and then multiply that number by $1.99.
    D. Multiply 34 oz by 16 to find the number of 16-oz colas that are in a liter and then divide that number by $1.99.

    $$7 \times 3 - 8 + 6 \div 2$$

23. Which of the following is the correct value if the given expression is simplified?

    A. 3.5
    B. 16
    C. 9.5
    D. 14

24. Simplify the given expression. Which of the following is the answer given as a fraction in the lowest terms?

    $$\frac{2}{3} \times \frac{5}{8} + \frac{17}{18}$$

    A. $\frac{180}{408}$
    B. $\frac{45}{102}$
    C. $\frac{15}{34}$
    D. $\frac{135}{136}$

25. Which of the following lists is in order from least to greatest?

$$\frac{5}{8}, \sqrt{9}, -\sqrt{4}, \frac{3}{5}$$

A. $-\sqrt{4}, \frac{3}{5}, \frac{5}{8}, \sqrt{9}$

B. $\frac{3}{5}, \frac{5}{8}, -\sqrt{4}, \sqrt{9}$

C. $-\sqrt{4}, \frac{5}{8}, \frac{3}{5}, \sqrt{9}$

D. $\sqrt{9}, -\sqrt{4}, \frac{3}{5}, \frac{5}{8}$

26. Solve the equation. Which of the following is correct?

$$\frac{x}{5} + 13 = 25$$

A. $x = 65$
B. $x = -8$
C. $x = 12$
D. $x = 60$

27. Samir is saving his allowance to buy a new laptop that costs $513.49. He has saved 1/3 of the money so far. Once he has saved 3/4 of the money, his grandfather will pay the rest. Which of the following is the amount of money Samir still needs to save to reach 3/4 of the cost of the laptop?

A. $128.37
B. $213.96
C. $385.12
D. $171.16

28. At a car wash, each minivan and SUV (x) washed earns a teen group $10 and each sedan (y) $5. Each minivan and SUV costs $3 in supplies and each sedan costs $2 in supplies. Which of the following expressions represents the amount of money the teen group will have earned at the end of the car wash?

A. $10x + 5x - 3y + 2y$
B. $10x + 3x + 5y + 2y$
C. $10x + 3x - 5y + 2y$
D. $10x - 3x + 5y - 2y$

29. Which of the following conclusions does the graph support?

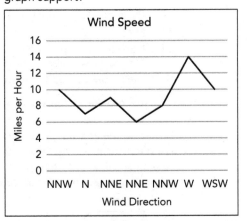

A. Winds from the NNE cause wind speeds to increase.
B. Wind speed is not impacted by wind direction.
C. The highest wind speed was recorded with winds from the W.
D. The lowest wind speeds were recorded with winds from the N.

30. Using the data represented, which of the following is the mean wind speed in miles per hour over the 7 days? (Round to the nearest tenth.)

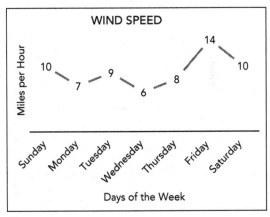

A. 9.1
B. 10.5
C. 10.7
D. 9.0

31. Which of the following shows a negative correlation?

    A. The more water I drink, the more energy I have.
    B. The more I sleep, the more I want to eat.
    C. The more I exercise, the more weight I lose.
    D. The longer I study, the more I remember.

32. You just brought home a new puppy and know that you will need to fence in your backyard. Which of the following is the perimeter if your yard has the following measurements? (Assume the angles that make the rectangle shape are right angles, and the triangle has 2 equal sides.)

    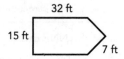

    A. 84.5 ft
    B. 108 ft
    C. 54 ft
    D. 93 ft

Ⓐ Unit Quiz Answers

1. Option A is correct because percent means parts per hundred. Therefore, 6.74% = 6.74/100 = 0.0674. Options B, C, and D are incorrect because 6.74% is not written as parts per 100.

2. Option C is correct because the order of operations was followed. The problem is solved by first dividing 14 by 7 to get an answer of 2. Then add the 2 to 22 for a total of 24 in the numerator. In the denominator, multiply 42×3 for an answer of 126. Then calculate $17 - 126$. This results in -109 in the denominator. The resulting fraction $\dfrac{24}{-109}$ is already lowest terms. Option A is incorrect because multiplication and division must come before addition and subtraction. Option B is incorrect because the order of operations was not performed correctly, and there is a computation error in the numerator. Option D is incorrect because the order of operations was not performed correctly, and there is a computation error in the numerator.

3. Option C is correct because they are ordered from least to greatest. This is easiest to see by converting all the numbers to decimals. The smallest number is $-1\dfrac{4}{5}$ because it is -1.8. Then $-1.33, 0.625, 0.727$ ($\dfrac{8}{11}$), and the largest is 1.154 ($\dfrac{15}{13}$). Option A is incorrect because the numbers are ordered from greatest to least. Option B is incorrect because a positive number is larger than a negative number. Option D is incorrect because -1.33 is greater than $-1\dfrac{4}{5}$ and $\dfrac{15}{13}$ is greater than $\dfrac{8}{11}$.

4. Option D is correct because the first step of combining $8x$ and $3x$ is correct. The second step uses inverse operations to get like terms on the same side of the equation. The third step correctly combines like terms on each side of the equation. The final step divides both sides by 7 to arrive at the correct answer of 3. Option A is incorrect because the second step does not combine like terms. Option B is incorrect because terms were not correctly combined in the first step; $3x$ and -5 are not like terms and cannot be combined. Option C is incorrect because terms were not correctly combined in the first step; $8x$ and -5 are not like terms and cannot be combined.

5. Option A is correct. The total number of milligrams that Jocelyn was prescribed was 37.5 mg per day $\times$ 45 days = 1,687.5 mg. The pharmacy needed 15 pills to fill her prescription, so the milligrams per pill can be calculated by the equation $15x = 1,687.5$ mg. Thus, $x = 112.5$ mg per pill. To figure out how to cut the pill, use the number of milligrams needed per day, which is 37.5 mg. Thus, the equation is $37.5x = 112.5$ mg, and $x = 3$. Each pill must be cut into 3 parts to give Jocelyn the proper daily dose of 37.5 mg.

6. Option B is correct. The range of her bonus will be between 3% and 5% of her salary of $79,200. So, the calculation of the range is 79,200 $\times$ 0.03 = 2,376 and 79,200 $\times$ 0.05 = 3,960. Option A is incorrect because the percentage of increase is calculated on an incorrectly rounded up salary of $80,000. Option D is incorrect because the percentage of increase is calculated on an incorrectly rounded down salary of $79,000 and not the actual salary. Option C is incorrect because a mathematical error is made.

7. Option B is correct because the data from 2007 to 2017 in the table showed little change (7.5, 7.4, 7.5, 7.3, 7.5). Option A is incorrect because the percentage of students playing video games has decreased overall. Option C is incorrect because the percentage of students using social media has increased steadily. Option D is incorrect because the decrease in writing poetry (5.4%) is greater than the decrease in volunteering (4.4%).

8. Option A is correct. First, the numbers must be ordered from least to greatest to find the median. Because there are two middle numbers (11,900 and 12, 936) they must be averaged: 11,900 + 12,936/2 = 12,418.

9. Option D is correct because as temperature increases, the ice cream sales increase. This is a positive covariance. Option A is incorrect because as Samantha decreased the time spent on her morning routine, her sleep time can increase, which is a negative covariance. Option B is incorrect because Juan is able to increase his miles and decrease his carbon footprint, which is a negative covariance. Option C is incorrect because as the down payment increases, his monthly payment decreases, which is a negative covariance.

10. Option D is correct. The area of the hallway (6 ft × 67 ft) is 402 ft². The area of the waiting room (20 ft × 35 ft) is 700 ft². The area of the semicircle is determined by using the formula for the area of a circle ($a = \pi r^2$) and then dividing that by 2 because a semicircle is half of a circle. The diameter of the area is 10 ft, so the radius is 5 ft. The equation is thus $\frac{\pi 5^2}{2}$ ft, which equals 39.35 ft². So, the total area of carpet needed is 402 ft² + 700 ft² + 39.25 ft² = 1,141.25 ft², which rounded up to the nearest square foot is 1,142 ft².

11. Option D is correct because 5 ÷ 8 = 0.625 and 0.625 × 100 = 62.5%. Option A is incorrect because it is the answer to 5 ÷ 80 and, therefore, that percentage. Option B is incorrect because it solved the equation 8 ÷ 5 and then gave that percentage. Option C did not convert the fraction to a decimal or a percentage, it just placed the numbers into the decimal and percentage format.

12. Option B is correct because like terms are first combined by subtracting 3x from both sides of the equation. Then 4 is subtracted from both sides of the equation. Finally, both sides are divided by 6. Option A is not correct because when subtracting 4 from both sides, there is a negative number on the right leading to negative number for x in the final division step. Option C is not correct because both sides are divided by 6 and not by 12. Option D is not correct because like terms must first be combined before solving the equation.

13. Option A is correct because the total area of all the lawns must be determined first and then divided by the area mowed in a minute:

$$\frac{(20 \text{ ft} \times 30 \text{ ft})^2 + (200 \text{ ft} \times 45 \text{ ft})^2 + (50 \text{ ft} \times 50 \text{ ft})^2}{240 \text{ ft}^2}$$

$$\frac{+ (90 \text{ ft} \times 60 \text{ ft})^2 + (150 \text{ ft} \times 95 \text{ ft})^2}{240 \text{ ft}^2} = x.$$

This number must then be converted to hours and minutes x = 2.20 converted is 2 hours and 12 minutes. Option B is not correct because 2.20 is incorrectly converted to hours and minutes. Option C is not correct because the perimeter, and not the area, is used. Option D is not correct because the total area was multiplied by 240 and then not divided by 60 minutes; its decimal form was used as hours and minutes.

14. Option C is correct because the new cost of the shirt is $7.87, and the pants are now $16.65. Added together $7.87 + $16.65 = $24.52. Option A is incorrect because you only took the 55% off of the pants and not the shirt. Option B is not correct because you only took the 55% off of the shirt and not the pants. Option D is not correct because you did not take off the 55% from the total price.

15. Option D is correct because all the expenses have to be rounded first, so room rental rounds to $4,000, DJ to $600, decorations to $2,000, and security would be $500 ($125 for 5 hours). That number, $7,100, is divided by $40 because the cost of tickets prices cannot be more than $45. Option A is incorrect because in the estimation, the exact amount of the ticket was used instead of rounding down. Option B is incorrect because the estimated numbers were all rounded down, security was only planned for 1 hour, and the exact ticket price was used. Option C is incorrect because the estimation does not use all the expenses.

16. Option B is correct because the area of 1 parking space is estimated to be 10 ft × 10 ft = 100 ft², for 50 spaces, that total is multiplied by 50: 100 ft² × 50 = 5,000 ft². Option A is incorrect because there was no estimation of the parking space. Option C is incorrect because it estimated perimeter instead of area. Option D is incorrect because it rounded 12 ft up to 15 ft instead of down to 10 ft.

17. Option C is correct because the proportion is ¾ tablespoons to 6 servings = x tablespoons to 22 servings or $\dfrac{\frac{3}{4} \text{ tablespoons}}{6 \text{ servings}} = \dfrac{x \text{ tablespoons}}{22 \text{ servings}}$.

    Simplifying the left side yields $\dfrac{\frac{3}{4} \times 22}{6} = x$, where $x = 2.75$ and then converted back to a fraction is 2 ¾. Option A is incorrect because in simplifying the proportion, both sides must by multiplied by 22 and then divided, and not multiplied, by 6. Option B is incorrect because the question asked for 22, and not 24, servings. Option D is incorrect because simplifying the proportion would be multiplying, and not dividing, both sides by 22.

18. Option A is correct because the interest rate stayed the same, so the proportion is set up as $\dfrac{23}{1000} = \dfrac{x}{750}$. Simplifying the left side yields $\dfrac{23 \times 750}{1000} = x$, where $x = \$17.25$. Option B is incorrect because even though the interest rate remained the same, the amount earned is not the same. Option C and D are incorrect because the proportion is set up incorrectly.

19. Option A is correct because the initial ratio is $\dfrac{200}{3400}$, which is simplified to $\dfrac{1}{17}$. The new ratio becomes $\dfrac{x}{3650}$. To keep the ratios the same, the equation is $\dfrac{1}{17} = \dfrac{x}{3650}$. Simplifying the left side yields $\dfrac{1 \times 3650}{17} = x$, where $x = 214.7$. However, because 0.7 or $\dfrac{7}{10}$ of a person is not feasible, the number needs to be rounded up. Hence, 15 additional teachers are needed to keep the ratio the same. Option B is not correct because the ratio would be $\dfrac{1}{16}$. Option C is not correct because the ratio would be $\dfrac{1}{15}$. Option D is not correct because the ratio would be $\dfrac{1}{14}$.

20. Option C is correct because the ratio is set up correctly by using the number of athletes per sport over the total number served by the 5 gallons, which is equal to the unknown needed gallons over the 5 gallons.

    For the volleyball team, where simplifying the left yields $\dfrac{17}{40} = \dfrac{x}{5}$, where $\dfrac{17 \times 5}{40} = x = 2.125$ or $2\frac{1}{8}$.

    For the soccer team $\dfrac{25}{40} = \dfrac{x}{5}$, where simplifying the left yields, where $\dfrac{25 \times 5}{40} = x = 3.125$ or $3\frac{1}{8}$.

    For the football team be $\dfrac{67}{40} = \dfrac{x}{5}$, where simplifying the left yields $\dfrac{67 \times 5}{40} = x$, where $x = 8.375$ or $8\frac{3}{8}$. Option A is incorrect because the ratios were not set up correctly or the calculations were not completed correctly. Option B is not correct because the problem did not ask for the answers to be rounded down. Option D is not correct because the problem did not ask for the answers to be rounded up.

21. Option D is correct because the income from the sales of the $2 tickets must equal or be greater than what the booster club wants to earn plus the amount of the winning prize. Option A is not correct because even though the amount of the tickets sales has to be great than or equal to the amount of the total sales, it does not include the cost of the winning prize. Option B is not correct because even though the amount of the tickets sales is more than or equal to the amount of the total sales, it does not include the cost of winning prize. Option C is not correct because the income from the sales of the $2 tickets is less than what the booster club wants to earn plus the cost of the winning prize.

MATHEMATICS

22. Option B is correct because determining how many 16-oz colas are in a 1-L cola must be done first, then that number is multiplied by $0.99, and finally compared to the price of the 1-L cola at $1.99 to see which is the better price. Option A is not correct because the number of colas at $0.99 should be multiplied, and not divided, by $0.99. Option C is not correct because the number of colas needs to be multiplied by the cost of the cola in ounces and not the cost of the cola in liters. Option D is not correct because the number of colas needs to be multiplied by the cost of the cola in ounces and not divided by the cost of the cola in liters.

23. Option B is correct because following the order of operations, the first step is to perform all multiplication and division, completing the operations as they occur from left to right. In this equation, $7 \times 3 = 21$, and $6 \div 2 = 3$. So the equation now reads $21 - 8 + 3$. The next step is to perform all addition and subtraction, completing the operations as they occur from left to right, which yields 16. Options A, C, and D are not correct because the order of operations was not properly followed.

24. Option C is correct because the fractions inside the parentheses must first be multiplied, which is $\frac{10}{24}$ and can be reduced to $\frac{5}{12}$. The next step is to divide by $\frac{17}{18}$, which means using the reciprocal and multiplying: $\frac{5}{12} \div \frac{17}{18} = \frac{5}{12} \times \frac{18}{17} = \frac{5}{2} \times \frac{3}{17} = \frac{15}{34}$. Options A and B are not correct because they are not simplified. Option D is not correct because cross multiplication was incorrectly used in the first step.

25. Option A is correct because they are ordered from least to greatest. This is easiest to see by converting all the numbers to decimals: $-\sqrt{4} = -2$, $\frac{3}{5} = 0.6$, $\frac{5}{8} = 0.625$, $\sqrt{9} = 3$. Option B is not correct because -2 is smaller than 0.6 and 0.625. Option C is not correct because 0.625 is greater than 0.6. Option D is not correct because $\sqrt{9} = 3$ and not -3.

26. Option D is correct because 13 is first subtracted from both sides of the equation, $\frac{x}{5} + 13 - 13 = 25 - 13$ and both sides are then multiplied by 5, $\frac{x}{5} \times 5 = 12 \times 5$, $x = 60$. Option A is not correct because although 13×5 was multiplied, the subtraction was not done. Option B is not correct because both sides were divided by 5 and then 13 was subtracted. Option C is not correct because the equation was not multiplied by 5 on both sides.

27. Option B is correct because 3/4 of the total amount, which is $385.12, and 1/3 of the total amount, which is $171.16, both need to be determined. Subtracting the two numbers is the total amount, $213.96, that Samir still needs to save. Option A is incorrect because that is how much his grandfather will pay toward the cost of the laptop. Option C is incorrect because that is how much Samir will have saved when he has 3/4 of the money and not how much he still has left to save. Option D is not correct because that is how much Samir has saved already and not how much he still has to save.

28. Option D is correct because this models $10 per minivan and SUV washed (x), subtracting $3 for the supplies and adding $5 for each sedan washed (y), subtracting $2 for the supplies. Option A is not correct because the problem gave the symbol of (x) for minivans and SUVs washed and (y) for sedans washed and not (x) for all cars washed and (y) for all supplies. Option B is not correct because all numbers are added, and there are no costs subtracted. Option C is not correct because the cost for supplies are added to money earned for the car wash, and then the amount of money earned from the two styles of car washed is subtracted.

29. Option C is correct because according to the line graph, the highest recorded wind speed occurred when the winds were from the W. Option A is incorrect because winds from the NNE caused wind speeds to both increase and decrease. Option B is incorrect because the line is not straight, so wind speed must be impacted by wind direction. Option D is incorrect because, according to the graph, the lowest wind speeds were recorded with winds from the NNE and not the N.

30. Option A is correct because it adds all the values together, which totals 64, and then divides it by the number of days, which is 7, to find the mean of 9.1. Option B is incorrect because it used the total value of 74 instead of 64. Option C is incorrect because the total value is only divided by 6, and not 7, days instead. Option D is incorrect because 9.0 is the median and not the mean.

31. Option C is correct because as one variable (exercise) increases, the other variable (weight) decreases. Options A and D are incorrect because they are positive correlations because as one variable increases, the other variable increases, too. Option B is incorrect because it is a positive correlation, even though eating more may seem to be a negative.

32. Option D is correct because all the sides are added together to determine the perimeter: 15 + 32 + 32 + 7 + 7 = 93. Option A is incorrect because the area of the triangle was calculated and added to the perimeter of the rectangle. Option B is incorrect because the base of the triangle was added into the perimeter. Option C is not correct because all the sides were not added together.

Science

The following 22 chapters cover the tasks from the ATI TEAS test plan for the Science unit. These are focused on assessment of knowledge and understanding of scientific information and concepts and are organized into three sections:

- Human anatomy and physiology
- Life and physical sciences
- Scientific reasoning

Each chapter in this unit introduces knowledge, skills, and abilities relevant to the Science task and provides an overview of some essential topics, along with specific examples to highlight important concepts. Practice questions at the end of each chapter will allow you to test your knowledge of select concepts. In addition, there are key terms included at the end of each section and a practice Science quiz at the end of the unit. This unit quiz includes the same number of questions as the Science unit on the ATI TEAS and matches the test plan task allocations (shown below). The quiz will give you a good idea of the number and types of sources you will encounter and the questions that will accompany those sources. Keep in mind that these chapters are a great starting point and guide to your studies, but they are not an exhaustive review of all concepts that might be tested in the Science unit of the ATI TEAS. You should use other sources (textbooks, online resources, etc.) for additional study and practice in areas that you haven't mastered.

Items in the human anatomy and physiology section area relate to describing the anatomy and physiology of a human and specifically the respiratory, cardiovascular, gastrointestinal, neuromuscular, reproductive, integumentary, endocrine, genitourinary, immune, and skeletal systems. Life and physical sciences has items related to describing the basic macromolecule and biological system, as well as comparing and contrasting chromosomes, genes, and DNA. Additionally, items cover Mendel's laws of heredity, basic atomic structure, properties of substances, and chemical reactions. Students are also asked to respond to items comparing and contrasting changes in states of matter. The scientific reasoning section is comprised of items related to identifying basic scientific measurements using laboratory tools; explaining relationships among events, objects, and processes; and analyzing the design of a scientific investigation, as well as using logic and evidence to critique a scientific explanation.

There are 47 scored Science items on the TEAS. These are divided as shown below. In addition, there will be six unscored pretest items that can be in any of these categories.

Section	Number of scored items on the ATI TEAS
Human anatomy and physiology	32
Life and physical sciences	8
Scientific reasoning	7

CHAPTER

35

Describe the general anatomy and physiology of a human

 This objective includes, but is not limited to, the following examples of knowledge, skills, and abilities.

- Identify basic cell parts.
- Describe the functions of the cell parts (e.g., obtaining and using energy, cell reproduction, cell productivity, cell growth, and metabolism).
- Know anatomical positions.
- Know anatomical planes.
- Identify anatomical direction.

This TEAS task requires an understanding of the general anatomy and physiology of the human body. You will need a general knowledge of cell parts and their functions and how cells form structures. You will also be required to locate body structures using anatomical positions, planes, and direction. There are many resources available on this subject, including print textbooks, online content and quizzes, and free online textbooks. These are excellent for both learning the concepts and committing them to memory. First, it is important to understand the hierarchy of structures and functions within the human body.

Biological Hierarchy

Biological hierarchy is a way to organize structures in living things from smallest to largest, as shown in the following diagram.

SCIENCE

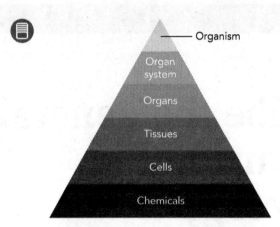

Chemicals build cells, which are the first structural organizational level. Key macromolecules important to living things include carbohydrates, proteins, lipids, and nucleic acids. The cell is the fundamental unit of life because all life functions can take place there. More than 200 different types of cells enable the human body to carry out life processes. The four basic types of cells are epithelial, connective, nervous, and muscular. Cells with the same function are collected into larger groups called "tissues," such as connective tissue. Tissues of different types can then form organs, which carry out a single task. For example, lungs are an organ whose task is to deliver oxygen to the bloodstream.

Organs work together in an organ system that performs coordinated, large-scale functions. In the nervous system, the nerves and brain work together to collect and process information. The nervous system then works with other systems in the body. For example, the nervous system sends signals to the musculoskeletal system to coordinate movement. Together, organ systems allow an organism to function. Chapters 36 to 46 explore the anatomy and physiology of the organ systems of the human body.

Cell Structure and Function

The cell is the building block of all living organisms. The basic parts of a cell are the nucleus, plasma membrane, and cytoplasm. Structures called "organelles" are found in a cell's cytoplasm. The following diagram shows the key organelles found in most cells.

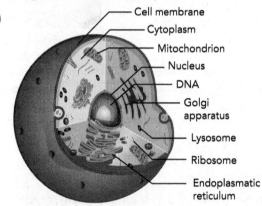

Each type of organelle performs a specific function. For example, the mitochondria is the site of energy production. The number and type of organelles vary depending on the cell type, although certain organelles are found in all cell types. Skeletal muscle cells contain high numbers of mitochondria because of the energy needed for movement. Organelles coordinate with other organelles to perform a cell's basic functions, such as energy processing, waste excretion, or protein synthesis. For example, several organelles such as ribosomes, the endoplasmic reticulum, and the Golgi apparatus work together to build proteins. The following chart lists the functions of key organelles in the cell.

Organelle	Function	Image
Cell Wall	Provides structural support and protection for the cell.	
Chloroplasts	Uses photosynthesis to produce ATP and other sugars.	
Cytoskeleton	Aids in the transferring of materials and movements of whole cells.	
Golgi Apparatus	Processes proteins.	
Lysosomes	Aids in digestion and recycling of old cell materials.	
Mitochondria	Manufactures ATP.	
Nucleus	Holds all genetic information such as DNA, and conducts the building of ribosomes	
Plasma Membrane	Maintains cell's environment through the process of selective permeability.	
Ribosome	Synthesizes proteins in the cell.	
Rough Endoplasmic Reticulum	Synthesizes and processes proteins in the cell.	
Smooth Endoplasmic Reticulum	Synthesizes and processes lipids in the cell.	
Vacuoles	Serves as storage for a variety of elements, such as water, toxins, and carbohydrates.	

SCIENCE

Anatomical Terminology

For the TEAS assessment, you will also need to describe the position and location of features in the human body. You will need to use standard anatomical terminology, as shown in the following diagram.

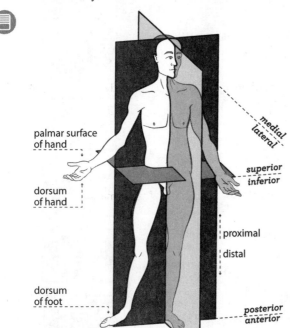

Anatomical Position

First, anatomical position describes the stance of an individual, and it gives a consistent frame of reference for the use of terminology. In anatomical position, the human body is erect and facing forward; arms are at the sides with palms forward. Feet are parallel, and arms and legs are slightly held away from the torso.

Anatomical Planes

Anatomical planes divide the body into two: Coronal or frontal plane is a front and back division, and transverse or cross-sectional plane is a top and bottom division. Sagittal or median indicates a left and right division. These planes also apply to organs, which can also be divided along planes.

Anatomical Direction

Anatomical direction identifies the location of structures in relation to other structures. Commonly used terms include superior and inferior, anterior and posterior, and lateral and medial. Sometimes two directional terms can be combined, such as posteroinferior. The terms "distal" and "proximal" are used to indicate which structure is closer (proximal) to the structure or farther away (distal). For example, the fingers are distal to the wrist because the wrist is closer to the main body. Lateral and medial are used to determine which structure is closer to the medial line, which divides a body into right and left sides. The rib cage is lateral to the sternum (breastbone), whereas the sternum is medial to the ribcage. Anatomical direction also includes "right" and "left." These terms reference the body's left and right rather the viewer's position.

CHAPTER 35 PRACTICE PROBLEMS

1. Which of the following describes the function of the ribosome?

   a. Protein synthesis
   b. Energy production
   c. Cell movement
   d. Storage of molecules

2. Because muscle cells require large amounts of energy to function correctly, which organelles would be prevalent in those types of cells?

   a. Ribosomes
   b. Mitochondria
   c. Cytoskeleton
   d. Cell membrane

3. Which of the following organelles is responsible for storing genetic information?

   a. Nucleus
   b. Ribosomes
   c. Cell membrane
   d. Lysosomes

4. In the human body, which of the following organs is in a superior position to the lungs?

   a. Stomach
   b. Brain
   c. Spleen
   d. Heart

5. In two to three sentences, describe the part of the arm that is most distal to the shoulder of the human body.

SCIENCE

Notes:

CHAPTER

36

Describe the anatomy and physiology of the respiratory system

 This objective includes, but is not limited to, the following examples of knowledge, skills, and abilities.

- Identify specific parts of the respiratory system from a list.
- Demonstrate knowledge of the function of the respiratory system.
- Demonstrate knowledge of the relationship between the respiratory and the circulatory systems.

The respiratory system's main function is to perform the critical tasks involved in transporting oxygen from the atmosphere into the body's cells and removing carbon dioxide from the body's cells. The respiratory system is specifically structured to maximize surface area for the exchange of oxygen and carbon dioxide. In fact, the surface area of the alveoli in a human lung is equivalent to half the size of basketball court! For the TEAS exam, you'll need to know the various parts of the respiratory system and how they contribute to the function of the respiratory system. You'll also want to be familiar with common respiratory problems and how they affect the system's function. Finally, the respiratory system works interdependently with the circulatory system, so you'll need to understand how these systems interact.

Structure of the Respiratory System

The respiratory system mediates the uptake of oxygen needed for metabolism and the release of carbon dioxide, which is a waste product of the human body, back into the atmosphere. The process of bringing oxygen into the lungs is known as ventilation or breathing. Several structures shown in the following diagram cooperate to form the respiratory system. Air enters through nasal openings, move into the nasal cavity, and travels past the pharynx (throat) and into the trachea, which is a large tube reinforced by cartilage rings that keep it from collapsing. Air continues to the first division of the trachea: the right and left bronchus. The air in the right bronchus continues to the right lung; the air directed to the left bronchus continues to the left lung. The right and left bronchi subdivide into smaller and smaller tubes called "bronchioles." Bronchioles terminate in alveoli, which are thin-walled structures that look like clusters of grapes. Alveoli are the sites of gas exchange. Alveoli are bathed in a layer of aqueous surfactant, a substance that serves as the medium for gas exchange and keeps the lung from collapsing on itself by maintaining surface tension.

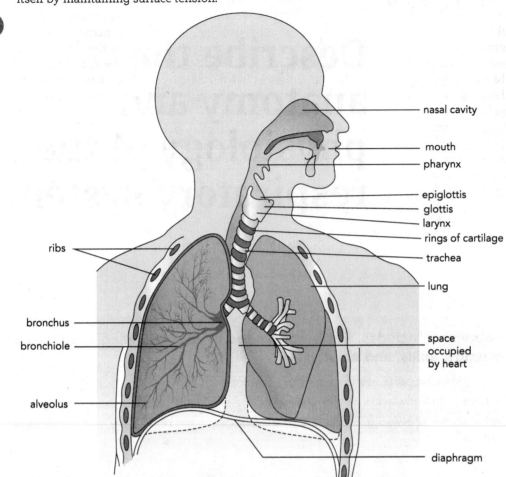

Interaction of the Circulatory and Respiratory Systems

The heart is located in the chest, marginally on the left side. This allows the right lung more space, and as a result, it is a little larger than the left lung. The right lung has three lobes: the superior, middle, and inferior. The left lung has two lobes: the superior and inferior lobes. Each lobe is divided into bronchopulmonary segments. Each segment receives air from its own bronchus and receives blood from its own artery.

Each lobe is contained within a tough, protective double membrane called the "pleura" and is surrounded by pleural fluid. The lungs are located in the thoracic cavity. Although the heart is not a part of the respiratory system, it has an important role when it comes to transporting oxygen and carbon dioxide throughout the body. The heart's pulmonary system sends blood low in oxygen and high in carbon dioxide to the lungs where oxygen is picked up and carbon dioxide is dropped off. This happens where capillaries of the circulatory system interact with alveoli of the lungs. This oxygenated blood is then returned to the heart where the systemic circulation sends it to all parts of the body. As oxygen is consumed by the cells, the blood becomes deoxygenated and is returned to the heart.

Function of the Respiratory System

The following diagram shows gas exchange in the lungs. Gas exchange in the lungs occurs by diffusion, which is a passive transport mechanism. The rate of diffusion is directly proportional to the surface area involved and the concentration gradient and is inversely proportional to the distance between the two solutions. For example, the rate of diffusion increases if the distance between the blood cells and the alveoli is decreased. During diffusion, oxygen in the lungs moves into the blood, and carbon dioxide in the blood moves into the lungs. The lungs then exhale the carbon dioxide back to the atmosphere. When the heart's pulmonary vessels enter the lungs, the blood has a low concentration of oxygen, whereas the recently inhaled air in the alveoli has a high concentration of oxygen in comparison to the capillaries. Molecules move from regions of high concentration to regions of low concentration. The thin alveolar epithelium allows the diffusion. Concentration of carbon dioxide is reversed in their location compared to oxygen levels. Capillaries contain a high level of carbon dioxide. Alveoli contain a low concentration; therefore, carbon dioxide diffuses into the alveoli. Exhalation releases the carbon dioxide. Inhalation brings in oxygen.

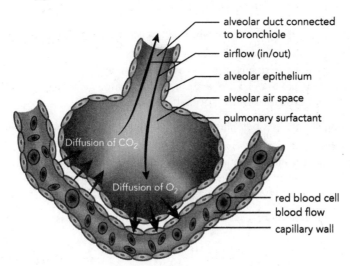

alveolar duct connected to bronchiole

airflow (in/out)

alveolar epithelium

alveolar air space

pulmonary surfactant

Diffusion of CO_2

Diffusion of O_2

red blood cell
blood flow
capillary wall

Ventilation occurs as a combination of muscle action and negative pressure. The diaphragm and the intercostal muscles of the ribs contract simultaneously to increase the volume of the lungs. This decreases the pressure in the lungs and draws in air. Subsequently, the diaphragm and the intercostal muscles relax, causing a reduction in lung volume and causing air to be pushed out. Periodic inspiration (inhalation of air) and expiration (expulsion of air) from lungs clear out air rich in carbon dioxide and replaces it with air rich in oxygen. The amount of air breathed in and out of the lungs is called the "tidal volume." A small amount of air rich in carbon dioxide, called the "residual capacity," remains trapped in alveoli after expiration and mixes with the air rich in oxygen brought in through inspiration. The breathing control centers of the brain's medulla oblongata control respiration through monitoring carbon dioxide levels and blood pH. If blood pH starts to decrease, then respiration rates will increase to balance carbon dioxide and oxygen levels.

Factors Affecting the Respiratory System

Many environmental conditions, genetic factors, and pathogens affect lung function. For example, asthma is a condition in which the airways of respiratory system narrow. This results from the swelling of the airways or from mucus buildup. Asthma can make it difficult to inhale and exhale normal amounts of air. This can lead to shortness of breath, difficulty breathing, and wheezing. Be aware of the effect of environmental pollutants such as chemicals, pollen, and smoke, which can impede lung function by damaging cilia or causing emphysema, allergies, and inflammation. Genetic conditions such as

SCIENCE

lung surfactant insufficiency, asthma, and cystic fibrosis can seriously impede lung action. There are also several pathogens that affect lung function and cause diseases such as influenza, tuberculosis, and pneumonia. For example, influenza is an infection caused by a virus that affects many parts of the respiratory system, including the nasal cavity, trachea, bronchi, and lungs. The virus uses cells in the respiratory system to make new viruses. The body's immune system attacks these cells infected by the virus, causing some of the symptoms, including mucus, pain, and coughing.

CHAPTER 36 PRACTICE PROBLEMS

1. Which of the following structures changes the volume of the lungs?

   A. Alveoli
   B. Heart
   C. Trachea
   D. Diaphragm

2. Which of the following statements best explains how the structure of alveoli relates to its function?

   A. Alveoli are large to maximize gas exchange.
   B. The walls the alveoli are thin to increase the rate of diffusion.
   C. The walls of the alveoli are thick to prevent pressure buildup.
   D. Alveoli are small to increase the transportation of cells.

3. Which of the following statements best describes the primary function of the respiratory system?

   A. It transports oxygen and carbon dioxide to cells all over the body.
   B. It involves the inhalation and exhalation of gases into the environment.
   C. It exchanges gases between the blood and the air in an environment.
   D. It maintains proper blood level pH.

4. Which of the following conditions causes a narrowing of airways in the respiratory system?

   A. Influenza
   B. Bronchitis
   C. Asthma
   D. Pneumonia

5. In two to three sentences, describe what will occur in the blood if the tidal volume in the lungs increases.

Notes:

Notes:

CHAPTER

37

Describe the anatomy and physiology of the cardiovascular system

 This objective includes, but is not limited to, the following examples of knowledge, skills, and abilities.

- Identify specific parts of the cardiovascular system.
- Demonstrate knowledge of the function of the cardiovascular system.
- Trace the blood flow through the cardiovascular system.

The cardiovascular, or circulatory, system is responsible for the movement of blood and lymph around the body. This system allows for nutrient distribution, waste removal, communication, and protection. To be successful at this task, it is important to know not only the structure of these two systems but also the functional components of each.

Parts of the Circulatory System

The circulatory system includes the closed system of blood pumped around the body by the heart through a network of arteries, veins, and capillaries, as well as the open lymphatic system, which comprises lymph that bathes the interstitial spaces between cells and is circulated through lymph vessels.

The heart is made up of muscle tissue and is split into four chambers. The upper chambers are called "atria" and the lower chambers are called "ventricles." The atria and ventricles are attached to veins and arteries that are connected to different parts of the body. One-way valves control the flow of blood into and out of the chambers of the heart. The diagram below shows key parts of the heart.

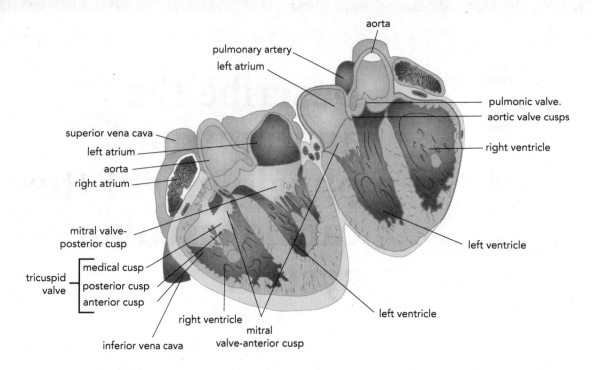

Functions of the Circulatory System

The cardiovascular system performs the vital functions of transporting nutrients, wastes, chemical messengers, and immune molecules. There are two well-integrated circulatory systems. The closed circulatory system is a double-loop system consisting of thick-walled arteries that transport blood away from the heart, thinner-walled veins that transport blood to the heart, and capillaries made of a single layer of endothelium that form a network that connect arteries to veins in tissues. The open lymphatic system circulates and filters interstitial fluid between cells and eventually drains into the circulatory system.

The closed, double-loop system transports blood. There are two parts of this loop: the pulmonary and the systole. The pulmonary loop carries deoxygenated blood from the right ventricle of the heart to the lungs where it is oxygenated and returns oxygenated blood to the left atrium. The systemic loop carries oxygenated blood from the left ventricle to the body, returning deoxygenated blood to the right atrium. The heart undergoes two cycles of contractions: systole and diastole. Systole indicates contraction of heart muscles, and diastole is relaxation of heart muscle. In a simplified overview of the heart cycle, the ventricles contract (i.e., ventricular systole), causing the atrioventricular valves (including the mitral and tricuspid valves) to close, making a "lub" sound. Subsequently, the empty ventricles are filled by blood pushed out during atrial systole. At the same time, the semilunar valves in the aorta and pulmonary arteries close, preventing blood from falling back into the ventricles, making a "dub" sound, and completing the "lub-dub" sound of the heart. These contractions are controlled by a "pacemaker" called the "sinoatrial node," which sends out electrical signals. Arteries have thick walls to withstand the pressure of blood pumped by the heart, whereas veins have walls with a thinner muscle layer and larger lumen.

Blood plasma contains nutrients, hormones, antibodies, and other immune proteins. Red blood cells contain hemoglobin and transport oxygen from the lungs to the rest of the body. Carbon dioxide dissolves in plasma and is removed by the lungs. White blood cells are divided into two main lineages: leukocytes and lymphocytes. White blood cells defend against pathogens.

The open circulatory system's capillaries drain interstitial fluid that fills the spaces between the cells and filter it through a system of lymph nodes that are enriched in lymphocytes and provide surveillance by the immune system. Lymph (essentially plasma with the red blood cells removed) eventually drains into the large veins leading back to the heart. Large numbers of leukocytes and lymphocytes are enriched in lymph nodes, where they monitor and respond to foreign molecules washed into the system. Typically, lymph nodes are enriched in oral, nasal, and genital regions where foreign entities enter the body.

You should have a general understanding of pathologies of the circulatory system, such as heart attacks, stroke, aneurysms, atherosclerosis, arrhythmias, and hypertension.

Blood Flow Through the Cardiovascular System

Blood flows throughout the cardiovascular system in a cyclic pattern as shown in the following diagram. Starting in the left ventricle, oxygenated blood is pumped to the body. As it flows through arteries to capillaries, it transports oxygen to tissues and picks up carbon dioxide. Then, the oxygenated blood returns to the heart through veins. This blood is now deoxygenated and concentrated with carbon dioxide. It enters the heart through the right atrium and then flows into the right ventricle. The right ventricle pumps the blood toward the lungs, where it picks up oxygen and loses carbon dioxide. Then, it returns to the heart through the left atrium and starts the cycle again.

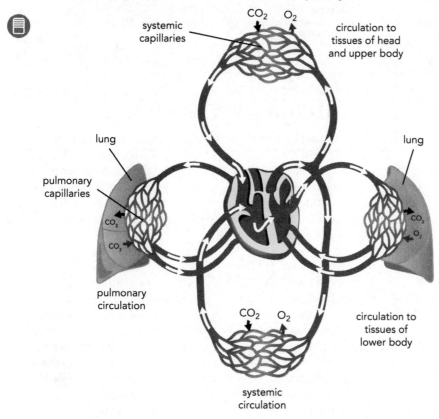

CHAPTER 37 PRACTICE PROBLEMS

1. Which of the following lists the primary parts of the heart?

   A. Blood cells
   B. Muscle tissue split into two chambers
   C. Muscle tissue split into four chambers
   D. Four ventricles

2. Which of the following blood components is responsible for transporting oxygen?

   A. Red blood cells
   B. Plasma
   C. Dissolved gases
   D. Leukocytes

3. Which of the following chambers pumps blood toward the lungs?

   A. Left atrium
   B. Right atrium
   C. Left ventricle
   D. Right ventricle

4. Which of the following statements best describes the function of veins?

   A. Veins carry deoxygenated blood.
   B. Veins carry oxygenated blood.
   C. Veins carry blood back to the heart.
   D. Veins carry blood away from the heart.

5. In two to three sentences, describe two chambers of the heart that have thicker walls. Why would these chambers be thicker?

Notes:

_____

_____

_____

_____

_____

_____

_____

_____

_____

_____

_____

_____

_____

_____

_____

_____

_____

_____

_____

_____

_____

_____

Notes:

CHAPTER

38

Describe the anatomy and physiology of the gastrointestinal system

 This objective includes, but is not limited to, the following examples of knowledge, skills, and abilities.

- Identify specific parts of the gastrointestinal system.
- Demonstrate knowledge of the function of the gastrointestinal system.
- Describe the role of enzymes in the gastrointestinal system.

The gastrointestinal system is also referred to as the digestive system. It begins with the mouth and then proceeds throughout the abdominal cavity to the anus. Its function is to break down food for absorption and distribution of nutrients to the rest of the body. Specialized regions and glands perform both mechanical and chemical (enzymatic) digestion. The smooth muscle involved in mechanical digestion and movement of food through the gastrointestinal system is controlled by the parasympathetic nervous system. Blood vessels located along the stomach and small and large intestines absorb digested nutrients. Undigested food is stored in the rectum for elimination. For this task, you need to be able to describe the structure and function of the digestive system organs, as well as the enzymes and hormones that control digestion.

Structure and Function of the Gastrointestinal System

The gastrointestinal system starts at the mouth and ends at the anus. Understanding the structure and function of the gastrointestinal system requires looking at specialized organs shown in the following diagram.

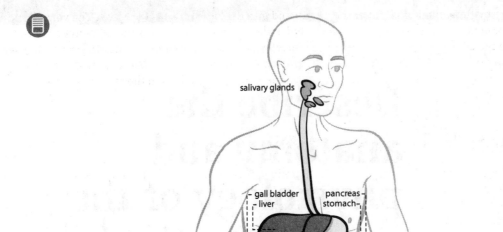

salivary glands

gall bladder
liver

pancreas
stomach

small intestine   rectum
large intestine   anus

First, food is ingested through the mouth where mechanical digestion begins. By chewing and grinding food in the mouth, food is broken down into smaller pieces, which increases the surface area. Mucus in saliva lubricates the food. Saliva also provides amylase and lipase to initiate chemical digestion of starch and lipids. Then, food then is packaged into small parcels called a "bolus" and swallowed (deglutition). As the bolus passes through the pharynx, the epiglottis closes the tracheal opening so that food does not enter the respiratory system, and the food passes into the esophagus. Peristalsis, which is the contractions of muscle in the esophagus, moves the bolus through the gastric sphincter to the stomach. The gastric sphincter prevents reflux of food back into the esophagus.

Once in the stomach, digestion continues. The stomach is a sac made up of smooth muscles. Stomach muscle contractions breaks down food even further into a substance called "chyme." There are three main secretions of the stomach: pepsinogen, mucus, and hydrochloric acid. Mucus lines the stomach, hydrochloric acid creates an acidic environment, and pepsin helps digest proteins in this acidic environment. Next, the chyme is pushed into the small intestine.

The first part of the small intestine is the duodenum. In the duodenum, chyme is neutralized by bicarbonate in pancreatic secretions. The duodenum receives alkaline bile juices from the gallbladder, which helps neutralize acidic chyme. In addition, the duodenum produces a large number "brush border" enzymes, including proteases, lactase and other disaccharidases, and bicarbonate. Villi and microvilli in the small intestine (largely the ileum) absorb polar-digested nutrients into blood, lipids into lacteals as chylomicrons, and vitamin B_{12}. From the small intestine, blood-carrying nutrients passes to the liver through the hepatic portal duct, allowing liver enzymes to deaminate amino acids, convert ammonia to urea, metabolize consumed toxins, and store glucose as glycogen.

The digested material then passes into the cecum and into the large intestine or colon. The vermiform appendix projects from the cecum, which is located at the junction of the small and large intestines. A lot of water and nutrients are absorbed in the small intestine, and the large intestine absorbs remaining water and salt from digested food. The waste from the small intestine is exposed to bacterial fermentation in the colon. Vitamin K is absorbed in the large intestine. The waste accumulates in the rectum and is ejected through the anus.

Hormones Involved in Digestion

Hormones regulate many aspects of nutrition. Ghrelin induces hunger, and leptin causes the sensation of satiety. Hormones induce secretions and speed up the movement of food through the small intestine. Insulin induces cellular uptake of glucose, and glucagon stimulates the breakdown of stored glycogen. Other hormones and nerve function modulate digestive action.

Enzymes Involved in Digestion

Many enzymes play a role in digestion. Enzymes are proteins produced by the body that catalyze and speed up the breakdown of food so that nutrients are available for the body. Enzymes are involved in chemical digestion of foods in the five organs listed in the following table. For example, digestion of proteins is initiated in the stomach by the action of the enzyme pepsin, which is activated by acid. Bile is a chemical that aids in digestion but is not an enzyme. The liver makes and releases bile into the small intestine, and bile is involved in the breakdown of lipids or fats.

Organ	Enzymes	Function
Mouth	Salivary amylase	Amylase breaks down starches
Stomach	Pepsin	Breaks down proteins
Pancreas	Pancreatic Amylase Trypsin Lipase (Pancreas makes and releases these enzymes into small intestine)	Amylase breaks down starch Trypsin breaks down protein Lipase breaks down fat
Small Intestine	Brush border enzymes (proteases, lactase)	Continue to break down molecules Carbohydrates break down into monosaccharides (simple sugars)
Large Intestine	None	None

CHAPTER 38 PRACTICE PROBLEMS

1. In which of the following organs does digestion begin?

   A. Mouth
   B. Stomach
   C. Small intestine
   D. Pancreas

2. In which of the following organs does the breakdown of proteins begin?

   A. Mouth
   B. Stomach
   C. Small intestine
   D. Pancreas

3. Which of the following structures absorbs nutrients in the small intestine?

   A. Mucus
   B. Microvilli
   C. Enzymes
   D. Hormones

4. Which of the following statements best describes peristalsis?

   A. The partly digested food moving from the stomach to the small intestine.
   B. The mechanical breakdown of food entering the stomach.
   C. Muscle contractions that move food through the digestive tract.
   D. Chemical digestion of food with the help of enzymes.

5. In a well-structured paragraph, describe the mechanical and chemical digestion of a starch or carbohydrate.

Notes:

Notes:

CHAPTER

Describe the anatomy and physiology of the neuromuscular system

 This objective includes, but is not limited to, the following examples of knowledge, skills, and abilities.

- Identify specific parts of the neuromuscular system.
- Demonstrate knowledge of the function of the neuromuscular system.
- Describe how the nervous system controls the muscles.

The neuromuscular system is a complex system that integrates muscles and nerves. This system affects every part of the body and is vital in controlling involuntary and voluntary movement. This TEAS task will ask questions about the specific parts of the neuromuscular system and how those parts contribute to the function of the system. You will also be required to know the structure and functions of muscles and nerves.

Structure and Function of the Nerves

Nerves and muscles comprise the neuromuscular system. Nerves are long bundles of axons that transmit signals from the central nervous system. These signals start as electrical impulses generated at the end of nerve cells. The impulse travels along the axon and then is transmitted to the next cell using chemical neurotransmitters secreted into the synapse from the axon terminals.

SCIENCE

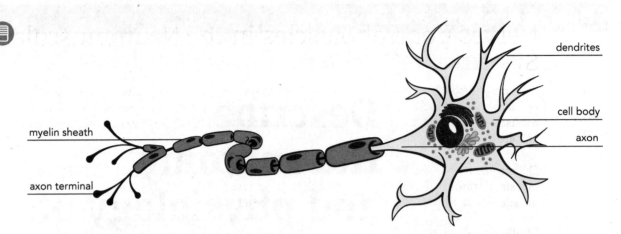

Nerves send and receive signals in the neuromuscular system. Sensory (afferent) nerves send messages to the central nervous system, and motor (efferent) nerves send messages out to the muscles. The autonomic (involuntary) nervous system controls involuntary actions involving cardiac and smooth muscle, such as heart rhythm, digestion, and breathing. Voluntary nerve signals make skeletal muscles do a deliberate action such as walking, throwing, or typing.

Structure and Function of Muscles

There are three types of muscles: skeletal, smooth, and cardiac. Skeletal muscles often attach to bone and are involved in the movement of bones. Smooth muscles can be found in the stomach, blood vessels, and intestines. Cardiac muscles can be found in the heart. Muscles contain long myofibrils made of sarcomere units, each consisting of long strands of proteins called "actin" (thin filaments) and "myosin" (thick filaments).

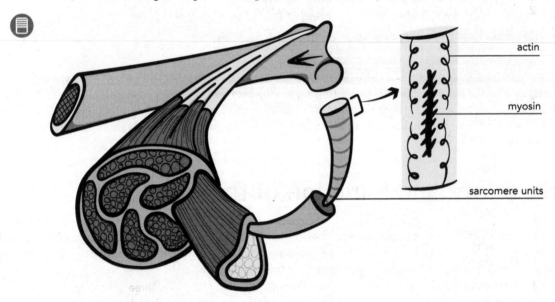

Nerves Control Muscles in the Neuromuscular System

Each muscle fiber is connected to a nerve fiber. For the entire muscle to move, it takes a concerted effort by many nerves and fibers and the use of adenosine triphosphate (ATP) to power the contraction. When a muscle is relaxed, myosin and actin filaments are not attached. When they contract, the filaments bind and are pulled together.

Skeletal muscles work by contracting. First, the nervous system sends a signal to a muscle. Actin and myosin proteins in the muscle slide past each other, creating either a contraction or a relaxation of the muscle. These two basic motions are responsible for all muscle movement.

Ideally, muscles respond to nerve impulses in specific ways. Receptors in muscles allow them to receive a signal and respond with the appropriate magnitude and movement. This signal and response can be disrupted by disorders ranging from muscle strain and sprain to muscular dystrophy.

CHAPTER 39 PRACTICE PROBLEMS

1. Which of the following actions is controlled by voluntary nerve signals?

   A. Walking
   B. Digestion
   C. Heart beating
   D. Breathing

2. Which of the following best describes the function of a nerve synapse?

   A. It carries a nerve impulse away from the nerve body.
   B. It is responsible for involuntary muscle movements.
   C. It allows for the passing of signals between neurons and muscles.
   D. It contains a bundle of fibers that transmit electrical impulses.

3. Which of the following types of muscle cell are often voluntary?

   A. Skeletal
   B. Smooth
   C. Cardiac
   D. Nervous

4. Which of the following types of nerves sends messages to the brain?

   A. Skeletal
   B. Smooth
   C. Sensory
   D. Motor

5. A person puts their hand on something hot but quickly removes it. In three to five sentences, describe the pathway of the signal and response through the neuromuscular system.

Notes:

_____

_____

_____

_____

_____

_____

_____

_____

_____

_____

_____

_____

_____

_____

_____

_____

_____

_____

_____

_____

_____

_____

_____

CHAPTER

40

Describe the anatomy and physiology of the reproductive system

 This objective includes, but is not limited to, the following examples of knowledge, skills, and abilities.

- Identify specific parts of the male and female reproductive systems.
- Demonstrate knowledge of the function of the reproductive system.
- Demonstrate knowledge of the relationship between the reproductive system and the endocrine system.

The male and female reproductive systems are complex and involve physical structures, hormones, and secretions. The reproductive system works in tandem with the endocrine system to influence many other parts of the body. This TEAS task will ask questions about the male and female systems that require knowledge of the various organs in the system and how they contribute to reproductive functions.

Male Reproductive System

The purpose of the male reproductive system is to generate male gametes (sperm) and deliver them to the female reproductive system. Major components of the male system include the penis, vas deferens, urethra, prostate, seminal vesicles, testis (plural: testes), and scrotum. The testes are the primary reproductive organ. Within the testes, there are lots of seminiferous tubules in which sperm are produced. The scrotum is a sac that houses the testes away from the body to lower their temperature during sperm production. This temperature helps sperm develop. The prostate and seminal vesicles produce the fluids necessary for lubricating and nourishing the sperm. The vas deferens, urethra, and penis form the conduit through which sperm is ejected. The vas deferens leads to the urethra, which leads sperm outside the body through the penis.

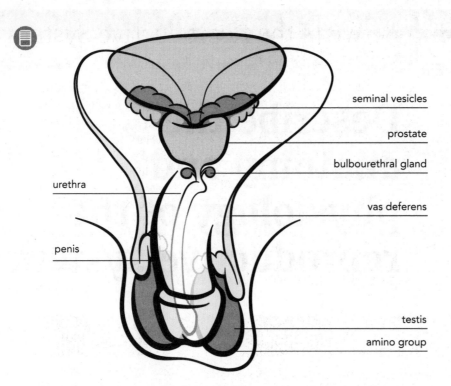

seminal vesicles

prostate

bulbourethral gland

urethra

vas deferens

penis

testis

amino group

Female Reproductive System

The female reproductive system's primary roles include generating female gametes (eggs) and incubating the fetus during pregnancy. The majority of the female reproductive system is internal: ovaries, Fallopian tubes, uterus, cervix, and vagina. The vagina leads from the external genitals to the cervix, which is the opening to the uterus. The Fallopian tubes connect the ovaries to the uterus. In response to changing hormone levels, the Graafian follicle in the ovary matures and releases an egg that then travels down the Fallopian tubes to the uterus. Fertilization normally occurs in the Fallopian tubes. If a released egg is fertilized by a sperm, the egg may embed itself in the uterine wall (endometrium). Here, the fertilized egg develops into a fetus and produces placenta that allows the fetus and parent blood supplies to network. The placenta nourishes the fetus and removes wastes. Once the fetus is ready for birth, the uterus contracts and the fetus is pushed out through the vagina.

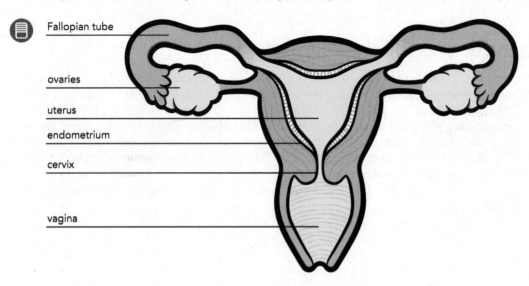

Fallopian tube

ovaries

uterus

endometrium

cervix

vagina

Relationship Between the Reproductive System and the Endocrine System

Hormones are part of the endocrine system and allow for cell-to-cell communication. This communication controls many processes in the reproductive system. Puberty is initiated by the production of two hormones: follicle-stimulating hormone (FSH) and luteinizing hormone (LH). In males, LH is released and signals the testes to produce more testosterone. Testosterone and FSH stimulate the production of sperm cells. In females, FSH signals the ovaries to produce more estrogen. Release of estrogen causes the egg to mature in the ovary's Graafian follicle and the uterine endometrium to thicken. A surge of LH from the pituitary causes the developing egg to be released. The empty Graafian follicle is now called the "corpus luteum" and produces large amounts of progesterone to prepare the endometrium for implantation of the fertilized egg. If implantation does not occur, the uterine lining sheds. This cycle of maturation and shedding of endometrium is called the "menstrual cycle." In males, testosterone production is not cyclical, so sperm, unlike eggs, are constantly produced and mature. Both male and female hormones help control secondary sexual characteristics, such as production of mammary glands, axial and facial hair, fat deposition patterns, and muscle growth.

CHAPTER 40 PRACTICE PROBLEMS

1. Which of the following organs produce female gametes?

   A. Ovary
   B. Testes
   C. Prostate
   D. Uterus

2. Which is the location where fertilization typically takes place?

   A. Vagina
   B. Penis
   C. Vas deferens
   D. Fallopian tubes

3. Which of the following best describes one function of estrogen?

   A. Production of sperm cells
   B. Maturation of eggs
   C. Release of egg
   D. Fertilization

4. Which of the following results from the production of luteinizing hormone (LH) in males?

   A. Bone growth
   B. Facial hair growth
   C. Testosterone production
   D. Sperm production

5. In three to five sentences, describe how the production of male and female gametes differs.

SCIENCE

Notes:

CHAPTER

41 Describe the anatomy and physiology of the integumentary system

 This objective includes, but is not limited to, the following examples of knowledge, skills, and abilities.

- Identify specific parts of the integumentary system.
- Demonstrate knowledge of the function of the integumentary system.
- Describe the role of the integumentary system in thermoregulation.

The integumentary system refers to the body's largest organ: the skin. The integumentary system contains organs and glands that are vital to protecting the body and regulating temperature. This TEAS task requires knowledge of the parts of the integumentary system and its function in both excretion and thermoregulation.

Structure of the Integumentary System

The integumentary system consists of skin, hair, and nails, as well as the sebaceous, sudoriferous, and ceruminous glands. Within the skin, there are hair follicles, sweat glands, and blood vessels.

The skin can be divided into the epidermis (outer layer), dermis (middle layer), and subcutaneous or hypodermis (inner layer) as shown in the following diagram. The epidermis is made up of dead cells on the outside, and it has an inner layer of living cells. The epidermis also includes cells known as "melanocytes." Melanocytes produce and distribute melanin, which has many functions such as skin pigmentation and sleep regulation. Beneath the epidermis is the dermis. The dermis contains collagen, blood vessels, glands, hair follicles, and nerve endings. The innermost layer is the hypodermis.

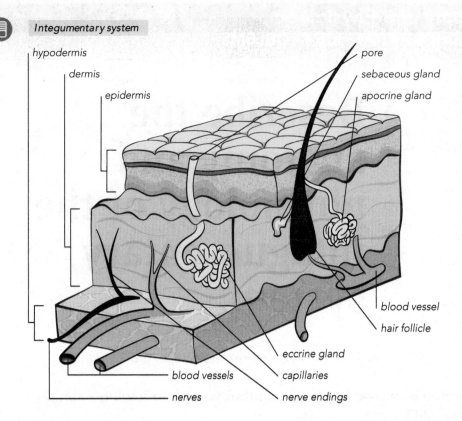

Integumentary system

hypodermis

dermis

epidermis

pore

sebaceous gland

apocrine gland

blood vessel

hair follicle

eccrine gland

blood vessels

capillaries

nerves

nerve endings

Functions of the Integumentary System

There are many functions of the integumentary system. The first is protection. The epidermis provides a barrier between the body and outside pathogens such as bacteria. It also prevents the body from drying out. The inner cells of the epidermis divide quickly, pushing older cells toward the surface. These old cells die and create a tough, waterproof outer surface. Melanocytes in the epidermis produce melanin, which helps to protect the body from ultraviolet radiation from the Sun. Skin cells also produce nails that protect the tips of fingers and toes.

Another function of the integumentary system is excretion. Along with water, minerals, including sodium, chloride, and magnesium, are excreted by glands. When these minerals build up in the body, they are excreted in higher amounts. Sweat can also contain trace amounts of urea, lactic acid, and alcohol.

The skin allows for the interaction between the body and the environment. The skin contains sensory nerve endings that allow the body to detect touch, change in temperature, and pain. Skin also produces vitamin D when ultraviolet light hits the skin. These nerve endings are found in the skin's dermis layer.

Thermoregulation and the Integumentary System

The integumentary system plays a vital role in thermoregulation. When the body becomes too warm, sebaceous glands produce sweat. The evaporation of the water on the skin creates a cooling effect. Blood vessels in the skin can also dilate when the body is warm. The dilated blood vessels carry more blood closer to the skin surface, and this can appear as flushed cheeks. The blood is then cooled and returned to deeper tissue at a cooler temperature. If the body is too cold, blood vessels constrict so that less blood is carried to the skin surface.

CHAPTER 41 PRACTICE PROBLEMS

1. Which of the following is the layer of skin that forms a protective, waterproof barrier?

   A. Dermis
   B. Sudoriferous
   C. Sebaceous
   D. Epidermis

2. Which of the following best describes the function of melanocytes?

   A. Secretion of substances like minerals and alcohol
   B. Production of melanin
   C. Absorption of vitamin D
   D. Sensing the environment

3. Which of the following layers of the skin contains hair follicles?

   A. Dermis
   B. Sudoriferous
   C. Sebaceous
   D. Epidermis

4. Which of the following layers of the skin contains a layer of dead cells?

   A. Dermis
   B. Hypodermis
   C. Sudoriferous
   D. Epidermis

5. In two to three sentences, describe how the integumentary system reacts to a rise in body temperature.

Notes:

CHAPTER

42

Describe the anatomy and physiology of the endocrine system

 This objective includes, but is not limited to, the following examples of knowledge, skills, and abilities.

- Identify specific parts of the endocrine system.
- Demonstrate knowledge of the function of the endocrine system.
- Demonstrate knowledge of the relationship between the central nervous system and the endocrine system.

The endocrine system is a set of organs that secrete hormones directly into the circulatory system. Hormones are various chemicals formed and then released by the body into the blood and act as signals to organs to perform various functions. Hormones are involved in regulating many of the functions in the human body, so understanding the endocrine system helps in understanding how the human body works. The TEAS task will require you to know about the parts of the endocrine system, hormones, and the regulatory functions provided by the endocrine system. In particular, you'll need to be familiar with the relationship between the endocrine system and the central nervous system.

Glands of the Endocrine System

The endocrine system is a complex network of glands and organs. A gland is a specific type of organ that secretes hormones into the blood to target and affect other organs. The following diagram shows the major glands in the endocrine system: pineal, pituitary, thyroid and parathyroid, thymus, and adrenal. Organs that contain endocrine tissue and produce hormones are the pancreas and the ovaries or testes. The hypothalamus is a part of the brain involved in the endocrine system, and it controls the pituitary gland that sits just below it. The pineal gland is located in the middle of the brain. The thyroid and parathyroid glands are found in the neck, and the two adrenal glands are located on the top of each kidney.

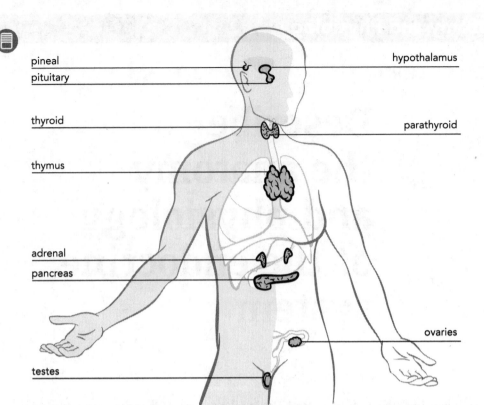

pineal

pituitary

thyroid

thymus

adrenal

pancreas

testes

hypothalamus

parathyroid

ovaries

Functions of the Endocrine System

The endocrine system regulates many body functions by controlling the timing and number of hormones released. All body systems are regulated by the endocrine system in some way. Examples include the regulation of blood production, appetite, reproduction, brain function, sleep cycle, electrolyte balance, growth, sexual development, and response to stress and injury. Glands and organs secrete hormones into the blood to be transported to target organs and tissues to control their function. For example, the pancreas releases the hormone insulin, which signals cells to uptake sugar. Without insulin's actions, sugar will not enter cells, resulting in high blood sugar levels. High blood sugar levels can result in insulin resistance and type II diabetes. When the pancreas cannot produce enough insulin, diabetes I results. The body's own immune cells mistakenly destroy insulin-producing cells in the pancreas. Another hormone, glucagon, is released from the pancreas when blood sugar levels drop. This hormone promotes the breakdown of glycogen, which is stored in the liver and in muscle cells. Glycogen is broken down into glucose, which raises blood sugar levels. Glucose can then be used by cells for energy. The pineal gland releases the hormone melatonin, which is involved in regulating sleep cycles.

Endocrine glands produce hormones that have different chemical structures, which are dependent on their function. Lipid-based hormones can enter a cell and regulate DNA. Some nonpolar, fat-soluble hormones, such as estrogen and progestogen, are released in a pattern set by age and development, and their effects are long lasting. Reproductive hormones are responsible for gamete production. For example, estrogen production increases at puberty and leads to the development of secondary sex characteristics.

Other polar, water-soluble hormones, such as epinephrine, are released in response to stress, and their actions are short lived. Hormone receptors on the cell membrane cause cellular changes to regulate and control body functions. When the adrenal glands secrete epinephrine into the bloodstream, heart rate, blood pressure, muscle strength, and metabolism increase. This response is called "the fight-or-flight" response. Hormone imbalance can cause metabolic diseases such as diabetes, hyperthyroidism, and gigantism. For example, in people with hyperthyroidism, the thyroid gland releases too much thyroxine. This can lead to an increase in both weight loss and heartbeat. To diagnose hyperthyroidism, doctors look for elevated levels of thyroxine in the blood. Gigantism occurs when the pituitary gland makes too much growth hormone, causing excessive growth. Hormone levels are often measured to determine if an endocrine-related disease is present.

The Central Nervous System and the Endocrine System

The nervous system is involved in rapid communication within the body as it detects stimuli and coordinates responses quickly. The endocrine system is generally involved with slower and more long-lasting responses to stimuli than the nervous system. The integration of these two systems is called the "activation of the neuroendocrine system." For example, the hypothalamus of the brain directs the activities of the pituitary gland. Certain biochemical levels send messages to the hypothalamus, which either stimulates or turns off messages to the pituitary gland, which sits just below the brain. Specialized cells in the hypothalamus secrete hormones called "releasing hormones" or "inhibiting hormones" to the pituitary. The pituitary gland then makes and sends specific hormones to target organs. For example, the pituitary gland secretes follicle-stimulating hormone (FSH), which functions in egg development in the ovaries.

Another example of the activation of the neuroendocrine system occurs in childbirth. During labor, the pressure of the fetus on the cervix sends signals through the nervous system to the hypothalamus, which results in oxytocin being secreted by the posterior pituitary gland. The hormone oxytocin stimulates contractions of the uterus that lead to childbirth.

CHAPTER 42 PRACTICE PROBLEMS

1. Which of the following best describes the kind of message sent in the endocrine system?
   A. Electrical signals between axons
   B. Chemical signals that travel through the bloodstream
   C. Physical sensory signals received through the integumentary system
   D. Audiovisual signals processed through the brain

2. Which of the following structures secretes releasing hormones?
   A. Hypothalamus
   B. Pituitary
   C. Pancreas
   D. Liver

3. Which of the following is a function of the pineal gland?
   A. Releasing growth hormone
   B. Releasing melatonin
   C. Releasing insulin and glucagon
   D. Releasing luteinizing hormone

4. Which of the following glands releases epinephrine during stress?
   A. Hypothalamus
   B. Adrenal glands
   C. Pancreas
   D. Pituitary gland

5. In three to five sentences, explain what happens to the levels of blood glucose and hormones after eating.

SCIENCE

Notes:

_____

_____

_____

_____

_____

_____

_____

_____

_____

_____

_____

_____

_____

_____

_____

_____

_____

_____

_____

_____

CHAPTER

43

Describe the anatomy and physiology of the genitourinary system

 This objective includes, but is not limited to, the following examples of knowledge, skills, and abilities.

- Identify specific parts of the genitourinary system.
- Demonstrate knowledge of the function of the genitourinary system.
- Demonstrate knowledge of the relationship between the cardiovascular system and the genitourinary system.

The organs in the genitourinary, or urogenital, system function in the excretory process. Some structures, such as the urethra and penis in the male, are also used by the reproductive system. This section of the TEAS will focus on the excretion process and its associated structures. Excretion is a necessary function for salt and water homeostasis and getting rid of wastes. It is important to know how the structures function and their contributions to the process of excretion and reproduction.

Parts of the Genitourinary System

The genitourinary system is composed of the kidneys, ureters, urinary bladder, and urethra. The kidneys lie against the dorsal body wall above the waist, superior to the lumbar region. Kidneys have two main regions or layers: the renal cortex and the renal medulla. The cortex is the outer layer of the kidney where blood vessels are located. The cortex also produces erythropoietin, a hormone that stimulates the production of new red blood cells. The renal medulla is the inner region of the kidney where the concentration of urine is regulated.

Kidneys have a renal artery, which allows oxygenated blood to enter the kidney, and renal veins, which allow filtered, deoxygenated blood to leave the kidney. Kidneys manufacture urine, which travels through the ureters to the urinary bladder where it is stored until it is excreted through the urethra. The ureters, urinary bladder, and urethra are parts of the excretory system. The ureters (one for each kidney) are small tubes that carry urine from the kidney to the urinary bladder, which holds the urine until elimination. In males, the urethra passes through the penis and also carries sperm. Females have a much shorter urethra.

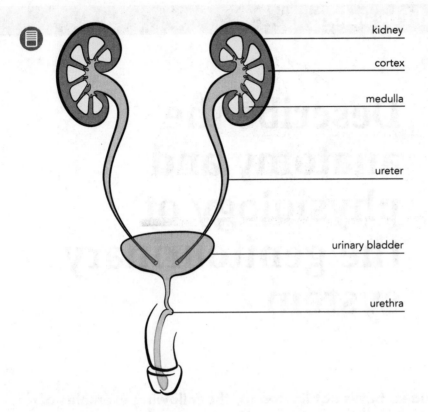

kidney

cortex

medulla

ureter

urinary bladder

urethra

Functions of the Genitourinary System

In the human body, it is important to maintain homeostasis. The genitourinary system is responsible in helping maintain this balance by getting rid of waste. Nitrogenous waste from protein digestion is toxic and must be removed because it will form ammonia. Kidneys, a major organ in this system, are primarily responsible for filtering blood, creating urine, stabilizing water balance, maintaining blood pressure, and producing the active form of vitamin D. The endocrine system also plays a vital role in several of these functions.

The functional unit of the kidney is the nephron. Nephrons are a system of microscopic tubes that use various pressure levels to remove wastes and reabsorb important molecules and water. Blood enters the kidney full of waste from metabolism, especially of protein metabolism. It enters a nephron capillary connected to the renal artery. It then flows to the glomerulus, a small, dense group of capillaries in the nephron. Here, material is filtered from the blood. This material is called "filtrate" and includes water, urea, glucose salts, and other small molecules. Then, the filtrate moves through the tubule. Water and other important substances to the body are reabsorbed through the capillaries back into the blood.

Finally, what remains in the tubule, urine, is emptied into a cavity in the kidney and drains from there to the ureter and then is stored in the urinary bladder. The urinary bladder is a hollow, muscular organ that holds 400 to 800 mL of liquid and has sensors that communicate with the central nervous system. For excretion to occur, both the internal and external sphincters of the bladder must relax. From the bladder, the urine is released through the urethra. Released urine is a waste product composed of 95% water, with urea, salts, and excess organic molecules.

Nephron

collecting duct

glomerulus

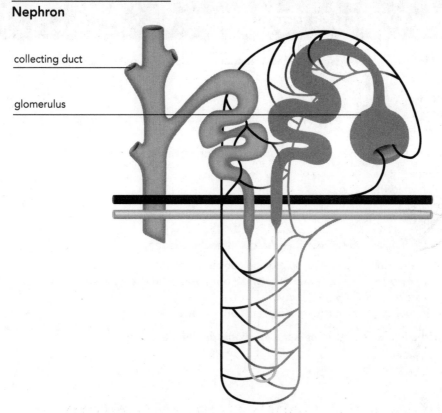

Relationship Between the Genitourinary System and Other Systems

Kidneys play a vital role in maintaining blood pressure by controlling the volume of the blood. Secreted hormones of the kidneys constrict or dilate blood vessels, causing the needed increase or decrease in blood pressure. Kidneys also help to control the production of red blood cells. The cardiovascular system pumps blood into the kidneys through the renal artery. The pressure of the blood helps the glomerulus filter out wastes and return vital nutrients through the renal vein to the blood. The kidneys also produce renin, a hormone that regulates blood pressure by retaining or removing water and salt.

SCIENCE

CHAPTER 43 PRACTICE PROBLEMS

1. Which of the following parts of the male genitourinary system also transports sperm?

   A. Ureter
   B. Urethra
   C. Uterus
   D. Urinary bladder

2. Which of the following waste products from digestion does the kidney remove?

   A. Nitrogen
   B. Sodium chloride
   C. Protein
   D. Carbon

3. Which of the following best describes the outcome if the kidneys stopped functioning?

   A. Blood would increase its carbon dioxide concentration.
   B. Blood would fill with waste and the human body would not be able to maintain homeostasis.
   C. The kidneys would fill with urine.
   D. The frequency in which a human excretes urine would increase.

4. Which of the following structures is the functional unit of the kidney?

   A. Renal capillaries
   B. Glomerulus
   C. Nephron
   D. Cortex

5. In two to three sentences, explain the purpose of blood pressure in the kidney.

Notes:

Notes:

CHAPTER

44

Describe the anatomy and physiology of the immune system

 This objective includes, but is not limited to, the following examples of knowledge, skills, and abilities.

- Identify specific parts of the immune system.
- Demonstrate knowledge of the function of the immune system.
- Demonstrate knowledge of the relationship between the immune system and all other systems.

The immune system functions like soldiers and fortifications in a battle to protect the body. For this TEAS task, you'll need to be familiar with the various parts of the immune system and how they contribute to that protection scheme. In particular, you'll need to understand how the immune system relates to the other body systems.

Parts of the Immune System

The immune system protects the body from disease-causing agents known as pathogens. The immune system is composed of both innate defense and adaptive defense systems. Innate defense is considered nonspecific response to pathogens, and adaptive defense is considered specific to a given pathogen. The innate immune system has three lines of defense: The first (skin, mucus, secretions) keeps pathogens from entering the body, the second (phagocytes, specific proteins, inflammatory response) fights pathogens that have entered the body, and the third is the adaptive immune system. Lymphocytes such as B cells and various types of T cells not only fight the pathogen but also retain a memory of the specific pathogen.

Functions of the Immune System

The immune system prevents entry of pathogens through the presence of barriers (much like walls and moats) composed of the skin and secretions such as acid, enzymes, and salt. If the external barriers are breached, there are cells and chemicals that act as soldiers to attack the pathogens. If that barrier fails, then the adaptive immune system specifically identifies, targets, and remembers the pathogen. Visualize the immune system as layers of protection that include barriers to prevent entry, signaling, and targeting. The ultimate function is to protect the body from a pathogen attack while allowing harmless molecules to enter the body.

The immune system functions through interactions with several others through which pathogens can enter the body. Pathogens enter through body openings of the digestive, urinary, and reproductive systems; injuries can also create ways for pathogens to enter. The lymph system is critical to the functioning of the immune system because pathogens from the blood circulate through the lymph also. B cells and T cells reside in the lymph nodes and are activated when a pathogen is encountered.

The Innate Immune System

The innate immune system is a series of nonspecific barriers—physical, cellular, and soluble components—that impede pathogens from entering the body or from multiplying. External barriers include the physical barrier of the skin and mucus secretions; chemical barriers, such as low pH, salt, enzymes; and cellular barriers of commensal microorganisms. If the pathogen breaches the barriers and enters the blood or tissues, a second line of defense is activated. For example, when a pathogen makes it into your body through a cut in the skin, mechanisms will go into effect to prevent the pathogens from affecting your body. One of the first responses is called the "inflammatory response." In an inflammatory response, histamines are released that increasing not only blood flow to the area but also the number of white blood cells known as phagocytes to the area. These phagocytes destroy bacteria. Interferons, which are proteins that interfere with the production of new viruses, are released if a virus enters the body. Fevers are also sometimes used by the body to speed up the immune response. Other internal barriers include antimicrobial peptides and "natural killer" (NK) lymphocyte cells that attack host cells that harbor intracellular pathogens.

The Adaptive Immune System

The adaptive immune system has two general responses to specific pathogens: cellular or humoral. A cellular response destroys the infected cell, and the humoral response destroys pathogens found in body fluids using antibodies secreted by B cells.

The adaptive immune system responds by remembering signature molecules, called "antigens," from pathogens to which the body has previously been exposed. The adaptive immune system's functional cells are lymphocytes called "T cells" and "B cells." Antigen-presenting cells (APCs) such as macrophages digest pathogens and present the pathogen's antigen signature to "helper" T cells. Depending on the type of antigen presented to the helper T cell, either a B cell or a cytotoxic T cell is activated. Helper T cells produce cytokines to activate a cytotoxic T cell. The cytotoxic T cell then searches out and destroys any cell that contains the pathogen's antigen signature. The helper T cell can also activate B cells in response to a specific antigen. The helper T cell induces the B cell to multiply rapidly into secretory cells called "plasma cells." These plasma cells will then produce large amounts of an antibody that can bind the antigen. B cells also clone into memory cells at the same time. This allows the body to remember a specific antigen. When that antigen appears again in the body, this triggers the memory cells to form plasma cells, which quickly produces the specific antibody to the antigen.

Passive and Active Immunity

Passive and active immunity are the two ways to protect the body through either passive introduction of antibodies as a protective agent or its active production by the body. Both passive and active immunity can be induced artificially. Vaccinations introduce antigens, which are weakened or killed, to elicit an immune response. Passive immunity introduces antibodies from another source that can rapidly neutralize toxins. Rapid treatment for a snakebite is an example of passive immunity.

Many diseases are caused by a malfunction of the immune system. Underactivity of the immune system can cause components to be ineffective. Acquired immune deficiency syndrome (AIDS) is caused by the human immunodeficiency virus (HIV), which infects helper T cells and prevents them from activating cytotoxic T cells and B cells and prevents the adaptive immune system from operating. Conversely, overactive immune systems can target innocuous foreign particles like pollen, causing the body to overproduce huge amounts of antibodies that trigger a histamine release from mast cells, which results in allergy symptoms, such as sneezing and mucus secretion. Alternately, the immune system can mistakenly target a host molecule as a foreign antigen, leading to autoimmune disease, a condition in which the immune system mistakenly attacks the body. Examples include type I diabetes, rheumatoid arthritis, and multiple sclerosis.

The Immune System and Other Body Systems

The immune system works hand in hand with other body systems to transport immune cells, signaling molecules, and antibodies throughout the body. For example, the circulatory system transports white blood cells throughout the body. The lymphatic system produces white blood cells or lymphocytes. The vessels in the lymph system drain fluid from body tissues and deliver foreign material to the lymph nodes to be processed by lymphocytes. Red bone marrow, found in many bones of the skeletal system, also produce white blood cells. In addition, the integumentary system functions as the first line of defense for most of the body.

CHAPTER 44 PRACTICE PROBLEMS

1. Which of the following helps to prevent pathogens from invading the body?

   A. Histamines
   B. Mucus
   C. T cells
   D. Macrophages

2. A bacteria cell enters the body through a cut in the skin. Which of the following describes the immune response that would occur next?

   A. Cytotoxic T cells form.
   B. Histamines are released.
   C. Antigens are released.
   D. Helper T cells are activated.

3. Which of the following types of cells produce antibodies?

   A. T cells
   B. Plasma cells
   C. Memory cells
   D. Macrophages

4. Which of the following best describes the purpose of a vaccine?

   A. To produce extra inflammatory responses such as the release of histamines
   B. To practice passive immunity
   C. To produce antibodies in case of future infection
   D. To increase macrophage production

5. In three to five sentences, describe what occurs in the immune system when it encounters an allergen.

Notes:

CHAPTER

45

Describe the anatomy and physiology of the skeletal system

 This objective includes, but is not limited to, the following examples of knowledge, skills, and abilities.

- Identify specific parts of the skeletal system.
- Demonstrate knowledge of the function of the skeletal system.
- Demonstrate knowledge of the relationship between the skeletal system and the neuromuscular system.

The skeletal system has three main functions: movement, protection, and storage of minerals and fat. To be successful at this task, you should know the names of the major bones of the human body, particularly those that help with movement, protection, and synthesis of blood cells. Study the structure of bone, including cells involved in bone synthesis and breakdown. You will also want to be familiar with diseases of the skeletal system, such as osteoporosis and arthritis.

Structure and Function of the Skeletal System

The skeletal system is the scaffold against which muscles pull for movement, and it provides protection for delicate organs. For example, the brain is protected by the skull. Bones also provide support and shape to the human body. Bones have other functions that you may not think of right away. They synthesize blood and immune cells, as well as store calcium, phosphate, and lipids. Bone is a dynamic tissue that is made and broken down according to need. Bones come in four major types: long, short, flat, and irregular. Long bones have longer lengths than widths and make up most of the bones in the arms and legs. The femur, or upper leg bone is an example of a long bone. Other examples of long bones are humerus, ulna, radius, tibia, and fibula. The marrow in a long bone is called "yellow marrow" and stores lipids. Red bone marrow is found at the ends of long bones and is the site of blood cell production. The ends of long bones have growth plates, and this is where the bone lengthens if it is growing.

Short bones have the same length and width. Examples of short bones are the square bones of the wrist and ankle. Flat bones are thin and flat and are used to protect vital organs. For example, ribs are flat bone that protect the heart and lungs. Flat bones also contain red bone marrow and produce blood cells. Irregular bones, such as the hip bones and parts of the skull, have other shapes.

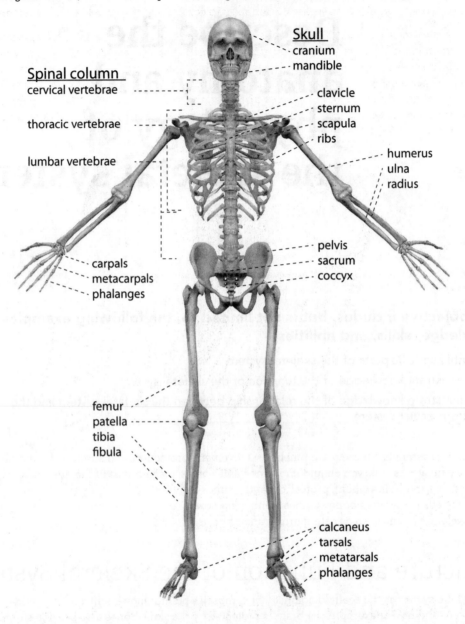

Joints are places where bones meet other bones. Some joints are movable, like the ball-and-socket joint of the hips and shoulders. There are other joints, such as those in the skull, that are immovable because the bones are fused together. Typically, bones are attached to other bones through ligaments. The hyoid bone, which supports the tongue, is the only bone in the body to not connected to other bones and is held in place only by muscle. The articulating surfaces of bones are covered in hyaline cartilage, which prevents them from grinding against each other. Synovial joints, such as the knees' hinges, also contain lubricating synovial fluid. Synovial joints, such as the pivot, ball-and-socket, and hinge, are usually capable of movement.

Bone is synthesized in tubular structures called "osteons," which is composed of calcium and phosphate-rich hydroxyapatite embedded in a collagen matrix and are the functional units of compact bone. Osteons are also called "Haversian systems." The osteon includes the matrix that forms in a concentric ring and the osteocytes that are in small cave-like spaces in the matrix, which are called "lacunae." The matrix forms around the central canal that contains blood vessels and nerves. Bone is covered by a fibrous sheath called the "periosteum," which contains nerves and blood vessels. Just like other cells of the body, bone cells need to be supplied with oxygen and nutrients and need to communicate with other body systems.

There are two main types of bone cells: multinucleate osteoclasts and mononucleate osteoblasts. Osteoblasts replace cartilage and secrete mineral deposits that form the matrix, the nonliving substance of the bone. Osteoblasts also develop into osteocytes, which strengthen bone tissue and carry out metabolic functions. Osteoclasts break down bone minerals of the matrix. This building up and breaking down of bone is important for strengthening bones. However, this can sometimes lead to problems. If osteoclasts break down bone faster than osteoblasts deposit minerals, the bones become weakened and brittle. This is what happens in osteoporosis.

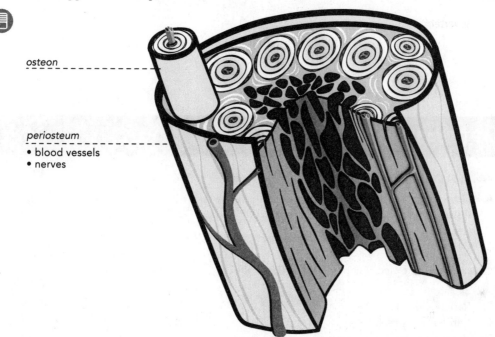

osteon

periosteum
• blood vessels
• nerves

There are several common diseases of bone. Excessive withdrawal of minerals from bone can cause the bone's rigidity to be lost and lead to osteoporosis. Arthritis damages the cartilage that articulates between joints. Brittle bone disease (osteogenesis imperfecta) results from a genetic defect in the collagen matrix. In osteogenesis imperfecta, the gene that codes for a necessary collagen needed to form the matrix of the bone is missing and causes bones to break easily.

The Skeletal System and Neuromuscular System

The skeletal muscles of the neuromuscular system and the bones involved in movement must work together in the body. Skeletal muscles attach to bones, and these muscles are connected to and communicate with the central nervous system. When the muscle receives a signal to contract from the central nervous system, the muscle contracts, moving a bone it is connected to. Muscles connect to bones with tendons, which is a connective tissue. For example, tricep and bicep muscles control the movement of the elbow. Biceps and triceps connect to the arm bones, and when contracted, they move the arm bones into different positions. Muscles work in tandem in pairs. As one of the pair relaxes, the other contracts for one type of movement as shown in the following diagram. The contracting muscle is called the "prime mover," and the relaxed muscle in the pair is called the "antagonist."

SCIENCE

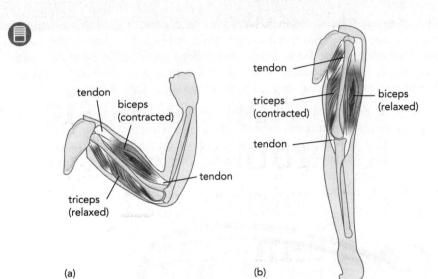

tendon

biceps
(contracted)

tendon

triceps
(relaxed)

tendon

(a)

tendon

triceps
(contracted)

tendon

biceps
(relaxed)

(b)

CHAPTER 45 PRACTICE PROBLEMS

1. Which of the following breaks down bone material?

    A. Osteoclasts
    B. Osteoblasts
    C. Canaliculi
    D. Osteocytes

2. Which of the following is considered a short bone?

    A. Skull bone
    B. Radius and ulna
    C. Carpals and tarsals
    D. Humerus and scapula

3. Which of the following best describes the purpose of hyaline cartilage in the skeletal system?

    A. It forms the matrix of a bone.
    B. It develops into osteocytes.
    C. It strengthens the entire skeletal system.
    D. It reduces friction at joints.

4. Which of the following best explains the cause of osteoporosis?

    A. Pathogens eat away at bone tissue.
    B. Ligaments degrade, causing joints to malfunction.
    C. Osteoclasts break down bone faster than osteoblasts deposit minerals.
    D. Osteoclasts break down bone slower than osteoblasts build them up.

5. In three to five sentences, describe how the skeletal and muscular system work together.

CHAPTER

46

Describe the basic macromolecules in a biological system

SCIENCE

 This objective includes, but is not limited to, the following examples of knowledge, skills, and abilities.

- Demonstrate knowledge of carbohydrates.
- Demonstrate knowledge of lipids.
- Demonstrate knowledge of proteins.
- Describe how basic macromolecules function in a biological system.

Living organisms are composed of chemical elements bonded together to form organic macromolecules. Monomers from food are used to build these macromolecules in biological systems. Monomers are also used to fuel production of energy in the form of adenosine triphosphate (ATP). In this TEAS task, you will identify the structure of each type of macromolecule and explain how the chemical structure of each macromolecule is related to its function. You will also recognize how reversible chemical reactions build macromolecules and break them down into their monomers. Finally, you should be able to recognize the macromolecule category of familiar food items.

Macromolecules

Macromolecules are large polymers. A "polymer" is a chemical compound formed when covalent bonds link monomers in long, repeating chains. Covalent bonds in macromolecules are formed by an endergonic removal of a water molecule. This chemical reaction is known as "dehydration" or "condensation synthesis." This reaction requires energy. Conversely, these bonds can be broken by an exergonic addition of water, which is known as "hydrolysis." Hydrolysis releases energy as bonds break between monomers.

The structures of macromolecules give them unique properties that allow them to perform different functions in biological systems. Macromolecules are classified into four groups: carbohydrates, lipids, proteins, and nucleic acids. The following chart shows the monomers that are joined by dehydration synthesis to form each type of macromolecule.

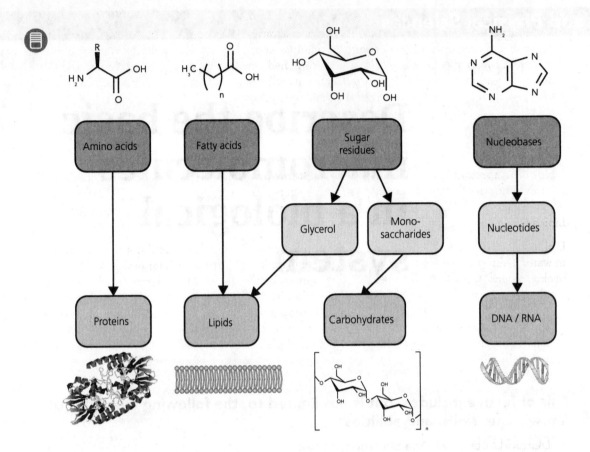

Carbohydrates

Carbohydrates, also known as "sugars" or "starch," are found in all living organisms. The monomers that join together to form carbohydrates have the general formula $C_nH_{2n}O_n$. Carbohydrate monomers are typically 3, 4, 5, or 6 carbons long. They are also known as "monosaccharides," or "simple sugars." For example, $C_6H_{12}O_6$ is a common monosaccharide known as "glucose." Two monosaccharides join by dehydration synthesis to form disaccharides. Sucrose is a common disaccharide shown in the following figure. Sucrose is made up of two monosaccharides joined together: one glucose monosaccharide and one fructose monosaccharide.

Polysaccharides are carbohydrate molecules formed by large numbers of linked monosaccharides. Animals store the monosaccharide glucose in the polysaccharide glycogen. Glycogen is formed by dehydration synthesis and is stored mainly in the liver and the muscles. When glucose is needed for energy production by a cell, glycogen is hydrolyzed into glucose. Plants store carbohydrates as the polysaccharide starch. Oligosaccharides contain a small number of monosaccharides. They are found on the surface of the cell membrane and function in cell recognition.

Carbohydrates can take many forms and perform a variety of functions. They can be linear, branched, or helix shaped. Linear carbohydrates such as cellulose and chitin often form structures. Cellulose is a major component in the rigid cell walls in plants. Branched carbohydrates such as glycogen and amylopectin function in energy storage. Glycoproteins and glycolipids are molecules that contain carbohydrates and other macromolecules, and they function in cell recognition.

Lipids

Lipids are important macromolecules but are not true polymers. They are not polymers because they are not formed from one type of repeated monomer. Instead, lipids are formed from a linear arrangement of carbon atoms and hydrogen atoms called "fatty-acid chains" that are attached to a glycerol molecule. Lipids tend to be hydrophobic and nonpolar.

Lipids are subdivided into four groups: fats and oils, waxes, phospholipids, and steroids, and all are insoluble in water. Each group of lipids has unique characteristics and functions. A fat molecule consists a glycerol backbone and three fatty acid chains. The human body uses fats for energy storage, cushioning, and insulation. Fats are a dietary component found in oils, butter, and meat. Waxes usually contain long fatty acid chains connected to alcohols. Waxes are hydrophobic and are used by living things to stay dry. Waxes cover the feathers of some birds and the leaves of many plants. Phospholipids are two fatty-acid chains attached to a phosphate molecule. One function of phospholipids is to form a semipermeable membrane around cells. Phospholipids help to separate aqueous compartments in living things. Steroids have a four-ring structure and include cholesterol, sex hormones, and hormones of the adrenal cortex. Steroids often function as chemical messengers.

Proteins

Proteins are polymers of long chains of amino acid monomers. Amino acids are composed of a central carbon, an amine group, a carboxylic acid, and a side group. The side group shown as the R side chain in the following diagram provides the variation that creates the 20 different types of amino acids. Each of amino acid has different properties because of its different side group. In proteins, the link between amino acids is a covalent bond called a "peptide bond."

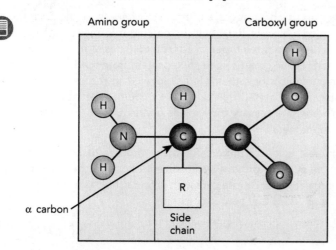

Proteins have a variety of shapes and functions. Fibrous, hydrophobic proteins like keratin and collagen have hydrophobic amino acids on their surface and are not soluble in water. They function as structural molecules in hair and nails. Globular proteins have hydrophilic surface amino acids and are soluble in water. They function as carrier molecules like hemoglobin, as antibodies, and as enzymes. Proteins associated with the cell membrane have a layer of hydrophobic amino acids sandwiched between layers of hydrophilic amino acids. Proteins are also imbedded in membranes where they function in transport or signal transfer. Proteins can be found in foods such as eggs, meat, and beans.

Enzymes are an important class of proteins that catalyze biochemical reactions without being consumed in the reaction. Enzymes speed up reactions by lowering the energy required by the system to initiate the reaction. Reactions can be exergonic (release energy) or endergonic (require energy). Energy in living organisms is typically supplied and released as ATP. Different cell types have a different enzymes present based on the metabolic function of the cell. Enzyme activity is affected by environmental conditions such as temperature and pH level. Enzymes typically have an active site into which the substrate or molecule being acted on fits. The active site is where catalysis occurs. One example of an enzyme is pepsin. Pepsin is produced and secreted by stomach cells and initiates protein digestion in the stomach.

Nucleic Acids

Nucleic acids are polymers made of linked nucleotides that contain hydrogen, carbon, oxygen, nitrogen, and phosphorus. Nucleotides have three components: a nitrogenous base, a sugar, and a phosphate group. The adenine nucleotide is shown in the following figure. The two nucleic acids in living systems are deoxyribonucleic acid (DNA) and ribonucleic acid (RNA).

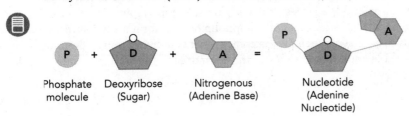

Phosphate molecule   Deoxyribose (Sugar)   Nitrogenous (Adenine Base)   Nucleotide (Adenine Nucleotide)

DNA is a double-stranded helix that stores genetic information. Genes are made up of DNA. Some genes provide the instructions to make molecules called "proteins." In humans, genes can contain a few hundred DNA bases to more than a million bases. Genes made of DNA are located on larger structures called "chromosomes." Chromosomes made of DNA and proteins are located in the nucleus of the cell. DNA contains nucleotides composed of a deoxyribose sugar, one of four nitrogenous bases (adenine, guanine, cytosine, or thymine), and a phosphate molecule.

RNA consists of ribonucleotides containing a ribose sugar, a nitrogenous base (adenine, guanine, cytosine, or uracil), and is typically a single-stranded molecule. RNA helps to convert information stored in the genes composed of DNA into the proteins. There are three types of RNA molecules. Messenger RNA (mRNA) located in the nucleus of the cell transcribes the genetic code for a protein from the DNA template. It then carries the genetic code out of the nucleus to ribosomes (rRNA) located in the cell's cytoplasm. There, transfer RNA (tRNA) brings the amino acid dictated by the mRNA's code to the ribosome (rRNA). The ribosome provides the catalytic environment necessary for peptide bonds to form. Ribosomes are the site of protein synthesis from amino acid monomers.

The sequence of nucleotides in a nucleic acid are important in the process of building proteins. The sequence of nucleotides determines the specific protein synthesized. Errors in the precise sequence of nucleotides are referred to as mutations that typically interfere with protein structure and function. Nucleic acids can be found in small amounts in all foods that contain proteins.

CHAPTER 46 PRACTICE PROBLEMS

1. Which of the following groups is synthesized from monosaccharides like glucose?

   A. Carbohydrates
   B. Lipids
   C. Protein
   D. Nucleic acid

2. Which of the following macromolecules stores genetic information?

   A. Carbohydrates
   B. Lipids
   C. Protein
   D. Nucleic acid

3. Which of the following monomers form enzymes?

   A. Glucose and fructose
   B. Amino acids
   C. Nucleotides
   D. Fatty acids

4. Which of the following foods contain mostly lipids?

   A. Potatoes
   B. Oil
   C. Chicken
   D. Lettuce

5. In 8 to10 sentences, explain why each type of macromolecule is important to the human body.

Notes:

CHAPTER

47 Compare and contrast chromosomes, genes, and DNA

 This objective includes, but is not limited to, the following examples of knowledge, skills, and abilities.

- Understand the function of chromosomes.
- Understand the function of genes.
- Understand the function of DNA.
- Explain the relationship between chromosomes and genes.
- Differentiate among the structures of chromosomes, genes, and DNA.

The hereditary material of most organisms is contained in DNA molecules. Genes are segments of DNA which can code for specific proteins. Genes are located on larger structures called chromosomes. Offspring inherit traits by inheriting their parents' DNA. In this TEAS task, you will explain the structure and function of DNA, genes, and chromosomes.

Chromosomes

Genetic information is contained in structures called "chromosomes." Chromosomes consist of DNA that winds around histone proteins as shown in the following figure. The winding process condenses the DNA and allows regulation of genes located on the particular chromosome. Each species of living things has a particular number of chromosomes. Organisms like bacteria have a single circular chromosome, whereas organisms that are eukaryotic (cells with nuclei) have many linear chromosomes. For example, humans have 46 chromosomes, and dogs have 78 chromosomes.

Genetic code in DNA and chromosomes within the nucleus

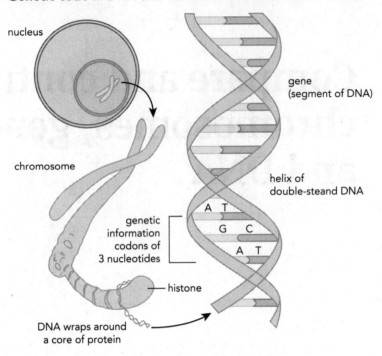

Genes

Genes are the primary unit of heredity. They are sequences of DNA located on chromosomes. Most genes contain the information needed to synthesize proteins. A few genes sequence code for other molecules that help the cell assemble proteins or regulate the making of proteins. Interestingly, genes tend to be clustered in areas in between regions of DNA with unknown function. Genes vary in size from a few hundred DNA bases to more than a million bases. Researchers estimate that humans have about 25,000 genes.

Genes can have structural or regulatory functions. Structural genes are converted into a short-lived RNA message (mRNA) that is decoded by the ribosome and assembled into proteins that build structures in living things. Regulatory genes control the expression of protein-coding genes by turning on or off activity, either directly or through a protein intermediate. In this way, regulatory genes control the expression of different subsets of structural genes in different cell types. Not all cells will express the same genes; therefore, they will make different proteins. For example, skin cells produce the protein keratin. Other cell types may not need keratin. Regulatory genes in these other cell types will "turn off" the genes that code for keratin. In this way, only the genes coding for needed proteins in a given cell are "turned on" or expressed.

DNA

Deoxyribonucleic acid (DNA) is a macromolecule that contains genes that are the coded instructions for a cell to produce proteins. The structure of DNA is a twisted ladder, or double helix. The sides of the ladder are made of phosphate and sugar molecules. The rungs of the ladder are composed of four nucleotide bases. The four nucleotide bases represented by letters: A (adenine), T (thymine), G (guanine), and C (cytosine). These bases are arranged in three-letter combinations. A "codon" is a sequence of three nucleotides that codes for a specific amino acid or stop signal during protein synthesis. A gene for a specific protein can be thousands of codons long. The gene will end with a "stop signal" codon. Ribosomes are the organelles that assemble proteins. They assemble proteins from amino acids in the order specified by the codons of the gene.

The DNA molecule is composed of two strands (or two sides of the ladder). The two strands of DNA are complimentary. This means that the nucleotide bases of the two strands are paired correctly and specifically. The base A (adenosine) always pairs with T (thymine) on the other strand, and G (guanine) always pairs with C (cytosine). Thus A-T and G-C are referred to as complementary base pairs. Complementary bases are linked by two hydrogen bonds between A and T and three hydrogen bonds between G and C Although an individual hydrogen bond is weak, these bonds are strong in DNA because they occur in large numbers and maintain DNA's integrity. However, these bonds are easier to break than covalent bonds. This allows the two strands to be separated for DNA replication and transcription. Before a cell replicates, chromosomes containing DNA must be copied to make two identical copies called "chromatids." Chromatids can then be separated, and the two new cells will have identical copies of DNA.

The two strands of DNA "run" in opposite directions as shown in the following figure. This makes the strands anti-parallel. Information is coded in DNA in the 5' to 3' direction, so this strand is called the "sense strand." The other strand going in the 3' to 5' direction is called the "anti-sense strand." The anti-sense strand is used in DNA replication and transcription.

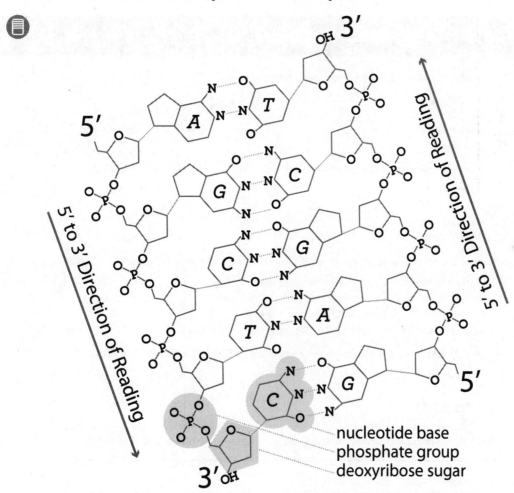

nucleotide base
phosphate group
deoxyribose sugar

DNA, Genes, and Chromosomes

Understanding the relationship among DNA, genes, and chromosomes can be confusing. Let's use the human genome as an example. Humans have 23 pairs of chromosomes, for a total of 46 chromosomes. Chromosomes are composed of DNA wrapped around a histone protein. Specific regions of the DNA molecule are called "genes." Genes contain the instructions for proteins or other regulatory molecules. Genes are made of codons that are three DNA nucleotide bases long. A gene can be thousands of codons long.

Human chromosomes vary in length, and each chromosome has a DNA molecule that has a specific number of genes. For example, the eighth human chromosome has DNA composed of billions of nucleotide bases. Certain regions of DNA on this chromosome make up genes. On the eighth chromosome, there are hundreds of genes. Some of the genes on this chromosome code for proteins important to brain development and function.

CHAPTER 47 PRACTICE PROBLEMS

1. Which of the following nucleotides pairs with adenine?

   A. Guanine
   B. Adenine
   C. Cytosine
   D. Thymine

2. Which of the following is the number of chromosomes found in a human cell?

   A. 1 circular chromosome
   B. 22 (11 pairs)
   C. 46 (23 pairs)
   D. 50 (25 pairs)

3. Which of the following statements about nucleotides and genes is correct?

   A. A gene contains thousands of chromosomes.
   B. A nucleotide contains many genes and chromosomes.
   C. Nucleotides form strings of DNA that make up genes.
   D. Nucleotides form strings of chromosomes that make up DNA.

4. Which of the following is the name for a segment of DNA that codes for a protein?

   A. Nucleotide
   B. Gene
   C. Chromosome
   D. DNA

5. In your own words, explain the relationship among chromosomes, DNA, and genes.

Notes:

Notes:

CHAPTER

48

Explain Mendel's laws of heredity

 This objective includes, but is not limited to, the following examples of knowledge, skills, and abilities.

- Describe the differences between a dominant and a recessive trait.
- Explain how gene pairs are inherited from parents.
- Describe the difference between inheritable and noninheritable traits.
- Use a Punnett square to predict traits of offspring.

Laws of heredity refer to principles regarding how traits are passed on to offspring. Mendel's three Laws of Heredity refer to Gregor Mendel's generalizations about how traits are inherited. Mendel was a 19th-century monk who grew and studied pea plants to determine how their characteristics were passed onto the next generation of plants. By crossing pea plants with different characteristics, Mendel was able to discern patterns in the inheritance of traits. In this TEAS task, you will need to explain Mendel's laws and describe differences in how traits are inherited. You will use a chart called a "Punnett Square" to make predictions about the likelihood of a trait being passed on to offspring.

Dominant and Recessive Traits

One of Mendel's observations was that there are differences in the prevalence of traits. This means that some traits are more likely to be passed on than others. He hypothesized that offspring inherit "factors" from their parents. Today we know that Mendel's factors are genes. Each gene for a trait comes in varieties called "alleles." For example, the gene for seed color in pea plants has an allele for green and another for yellow. Mendel found that for two alleles for a gene, the dominant trait is always expressed or shown by the organism if it is present, because it masks the recessive allele. The recessive allele is only expressed when both alleles are recessive. This is Mendel's third law, The Law of Dominance. For seed color, the green allele is dominant, and the yellow allele is recessive.

Inheritance of Gene Pairs

Most living things inherit one of each pair of chromosomes from each parent. For example, humans have 23 pairs of chromosomes for a total of 46 chromosomes. Each parent contributed 23 chromosomes. Therefore, offspring inherit two copies of each gene, one from each parent. They will have two alleles for each gene. This combination of two alleles is called a "genotype." If a chromosome contains two alleles that are the same, that genotype is called "homozygous." If the chromosome contains two different alleles, that genotype is called "heterozygous." The alleles that are present in an organism determine the phenotype of the organism; a "phenotype" is the expression of the genes for that trait. Phenotypes are visible traits such as seed color and unseen traits such as blood type.

Offspring express either a dominant or recessive phenotype based on the two alleles inherited for a trait. Only inherited traits are determined this way. Inherited traits are passed from parent to offspring through gametes (eggs or sperm). Each gamete carries 1 chromosome of the chromosome pair (and only one copy of each gene). For example, human gametes contain 23 chromosomes. When an egg and sperm fuse together (fertilization), a cell with two copies of each chromosome (and two copies of each gene) results. For humans, the zygote contains 46 chromosomes. Traits, such as culturally influenced behavior, are not inherited as part of the genome. These are nonheritable traits not coded for in genes. Mendel's Laws of Heredity focus on inherited traits.

Using Punnett Squares

One way to predict the likelihood of traits in offspring is to use a Punnett square. A Punnett square is a chart that can be used to determine the ratios of the genotypes of offspring from a reproductive cross. To use a Punnett square, you must know the genotypes of the parents. Genotypes are represented by two letters. Capital letters will represent dominant alleles, and small letters will represent recessive alleles. In pea plants purple (P) is the dominant flower color, and white (p) is recessive. The following graphic shows the genotypes of two parent pea plants. The first parent plant has a genotype of "PP," which means two dominant alleles. This plant would express the dominant trait or phenotype of purple flowers. This parent is homozygous dominant for this trait. The second individual has the genotype "pp." This second parent plant would express the recessive phenotype of white flowers because there is not dominant allele present. This parent is homozygous recessive for this trait. When these two parents (the P_1 generation) are crossed, each parent contributes one allele. The "PP" parent can only contribute a "P" or dominant allele. The "pp" parent can only contribute a "p" or recessive allele. All offspring of this cross (the F_1 generation)

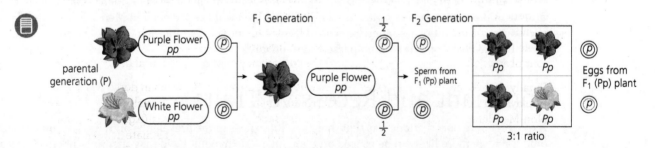

will have the heterozygous genotype "Pp." The will all have the phenotype of purple because they contain a dominant allele.

Now consider a cross between two heterozygous flowers (F_2 generation) using a Punnett square. The genotype of the sperm from one plant, "Pp," is placed at the top of the square. The genotype of an egg from another plant, "Pp," is placed at side. The F_2 genotypes can then be calculated. The Punnett square helps us to predict that 25% of offspring will be PP, 50% of offspring will be Pp, and 25% will be pp. This means that it is likely that 75% of the offspring will have purple flowers, and 25% will be homozygous recessive and have white flowers.

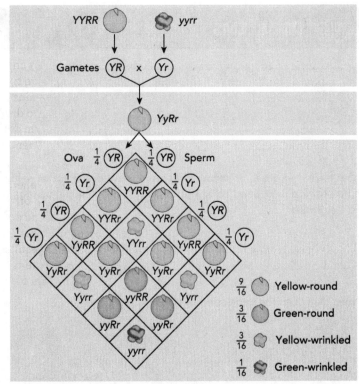

These results hold true only if parental genes for a trait must segregate or separate equally and randomly into haploid gametes (sperm or eggs). That way offspring have an equal chance of inheriting either allele. Offspring inherit one allele from each parent for a trait, and no allele is favored or has an advantage over the others. This is Mendel's Law of Segregation.

The inheritance of two traits can also be studied using a Punnett square. This is called a "dihybrid cross" as shown in the following image. A dihybrid cross illustrates Mendel's Law of Independent Assortment. A dihybrid cross tracks the inheritance of two different traits and starts with a parental cross of two true-breeding or homozygous organisms. One parent is homozygous dominant for both traits, and the other parent is homozygous recessive for both traits. The offspring (F_1 generation) are all heterozygous (YyRr) and show only two dominant traits—in this case round, yellow seeds. When an F_1 cross is performed, the F_2 generation shows both dominant and recessive traits. The result is a ratio of 9:3:3:1. This illustrates Mendel's Law of Independent Assortment because it shows that alleles are not inherited together. Each allele (Y, y, R, and r) are inherited separately, or independently assorted. This is supported by the fact that four phenotypes appear, rather than only the two phenotypes of the parental generation.

Finally, non-Mendelian inheritance occurs when there are factors other than dominant and recessive alleles in play. Mendelian ratios occur when simple dominance-recessive relationship exists between two alleles. Non-Mendelian inheritance results from factors such as multiple alleles (e.g., blood groups A, B, and O), incomplete dominance-recessive relationships that lead to an intermediate (e.g., red and white alleles making pink flowers), co-dominance (AB blood group express both A and B proteins), and interactions between genes called "epistasis." If the 3:1 or 9:3:3:1 relationship is not obtained when the F_2 phenotypes are analyzed, it is indicative of non-Mendelian inheritance.

CHAPTER 48 PRACTICE PROBLEMS

1. A pea plant has a dominant homozygous genotype. Which of the following letters best represent this genotype?

   A. WW
   B. Ww
   C. ww
   D. WX

2. Pea plants have seeds that are either green or yellow. Green seeds are dominant to yellow seeds. Two pea plants that are heterozygous for seed color are crossed. Predict the percentage of their offspring that will have green seeds.

   A. 0%
   B. 25%
   C. 50%
   D. 75%

3. Which of the following best describes the expression of alleles?

   A. Heritable trait
   B. Genotype
   C. Phenotype
   D. P generation

4. Which of the following best describes non-Mendelian inheritance patterns?

   A. Occurs when there are factors other than dominant and recessive traits
   B. Each trait has one dominant and one recessive allele
   C. Heterozygous monohybrid crosses result in a 1:1 ratio of dominant-to-recessive phenotypes
   D. Traits are only inherited on the somatic chromosomes

5. Use a Punnett square to show the likely phenotypes of crossing two heterozygous tall pea plants. The allele for tall plants is dominant.

Notes:

Notes:

CHAPTER

49

Recognize basic atomic structure

 This objective includes, but is not limited to, the following examples of knowledge, skills, and abilities.

- Label the parts of the atom.
- Know the basic structure of the atom.
- Describe an ion.
- Using a periodic table, identify the number of electrons and protons.

The atom is the fundamental constituent of matter that retains the properties of an element. As such, the atom is the smallest unit that has a unique identity. There are 118 elements arranged in the periodic table, starting with hydrogen, which has one proton, and increasing proton numbers for each element. Although atoms have distinct properties, all are composed of the same three subatomic particles: protons, neutrons, and electrons.

To be successful in this TEAS topic, it is important to understand the structure of an atom and the arrangement of electrons that determine an atom's chemical properties. Atoms undergo chemical reactions by gaining or losing electrons to achieve stability. An atom's properties can be inferred by its position on the periodic table, which relates to the number of valence electrons in its outermost shell. Atoms can lose, gain, or share electrons to make a variety of chemical bonds of varying strengths and properties. Familiarize yourself with the periodic table, get comfortable with identifying the valence of an atom based on its position, and infer the number and type of bonds that an atom would make.

Parts of an Atom

All atoms have a similar structure of a central nucleus containing positively charged **protons** and neutral **neutron. Surrounding the nucleus are** negatively charged **electrons. Electrons exist in an electron cloud surrounding** the nucleus. The negative electrons are held in orbit by their attraction to the positively charged protons in the nucleus and increase in energy with distance from the nucleus. Each type of atom will always have the same number of protons. Carbon, for example, has 6 protons. The numbers of neutrons in different atoms of the same element can vary, and these atoms are called "**isotopes**." The atomic mass of an atom is determined by the number of protons and neutrons found in the nucleus. Electrons are so small that their mass does not significantly add to the mass of the atom. For the carbon atom in the following figure, the atomic mass is determined by adding the protons and neutrons: 6 protons + 6 neutrons = 12 atomic mass units (or amu). Another isotope of carbon might have 7 neutrons. All carbon atoms have 6 protons. This isotope would have an atomic mass of 13 amu (6 protons + 7 neutrons).

 Carbon atom: 6 protons + 6 neutrons

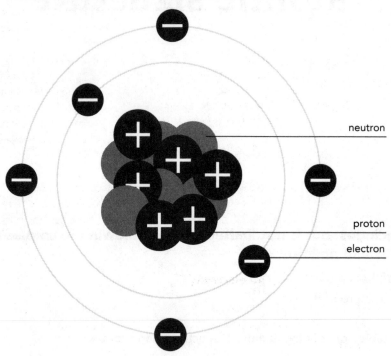

Subatomic particles have masses and charges related to their identity. The number of protons gives the atomic number of an atom. The number of protons plus neutrons equals the atomic mass of the atom. Neutral atoms have equal numbers of protons and electrons. The carbon atom illustrated previously would have a charge of 0 (neutral) because it has six positively charged protons and six negatively charged electrons. Neutrons do not change the charge because they are not charged particles.

SUBATOMIC PARTICLES	CHARGE	MASS (atomic mass units)
Proton	+1	1
Neutron	0	1
Electron	−1	0

Ions

Ions are atoms with a positive or a negative charge. A sodium (Na) atom is made up of 11 protons and 12 neutrons in its nucleus and 11 electrons in the cloud surrounding the nucleus. Because it has a single electron in its outer shell, sodium is likely to lose an electron. A sodium atom that has lost an electron becomes a charged sodium ion and is written Na^+. It has a positive charge because it now has more protons than electrons. A chlorine atom has 17 protons and either 18 or 20 neutrons in its nucleus, and

17 electrons in the cloud around its nucleus. Because a chlorine atom has a nearly full outer shell, it is likely to gain an electron. A chlorine atom that has gained an electron becomes a charged chlorine ion and is written Cl^-.

Using the Periodic Table

The periodic table arranges atoms by increasing **atomic number** (number of protons). Atoms are neutral, so the number of protons equals the number of orbiting electrons. The atomic number is shown as an integer in the periodic table. To identify the number of electrons and protons, look at the integer shown with the element. **Atomic masses** on the periodic table are shown in decimal form to account for the natural abundance of the element's various isotopes. The atomic mass shown on the periodic table is determined by the percentage of each isotope found in nature for that particular atom.

Because atomic properties are cyclic, the **periodic table** is arranged to highlight these shared properties, grouping similar atoms into vertical columns. Atoms with similar properties have the same number of **valence** (bonding) electrons. Depending on the number of the period, there are different numbers of orbitals that can accommodate different electron numbers. Note that an "s" orbital can accommodate a maximum of two electrons at a time. The s orbital is closest to the nucleus. Hydrogen and helium only have an s orbital that can hold a total of two electrons.

Periods represent large electron "highways" with multiple orbital "lanes." For example, the lower energy Period 1 has one "s" orbital with a maximum of two electrons allowed. Period 2 has two orbitals: "s" and "p." The "s" orbital can only accommodate two electrons, but "p" can accommodate six electrons. Therefore, Period 2 can contain a maximum of eight electrons. Study the following chart and periodic table to familiarize yourself with atomic mass, atomic number, orbitals, and periods.

Relationship among periods, orbitals, and electrons

PERIOD NUMBER	1	2	3	4
ORBITAL NAMES	s	s p	s p d	s p d f
MAXIMUM NUMBER OF ELECTRONS	s = 2	s = 2 p = 6	s = 2 p = 6 d = 10	s = 2 p = 6 d = 10 f = 14

Valence electrons are in the outermost shell of an atom and participate in chemical reactions (or bonding). Because atoms are most stable when they have a full valence shell, atoms are most likely to move toward stability. Noble gases, like helium and neon, have full valence shells and are quite stable. They do not react with other atoms because they are so stable. Because they are stable, they are also called "inert gases."

Periodic table of elements

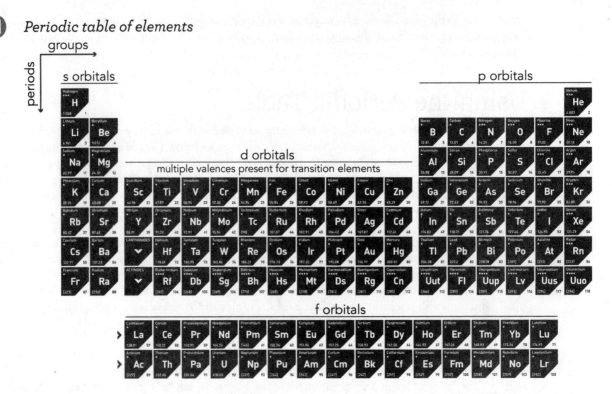

Image credit: Getty Images/iStockphoto

Other atoms gain or lose electrons to achieve full valence shells, forming charged atoms called **"ions."** Gaining electrons typically happens in atoms with valences greater than 4, and losing electrons typically happens in atoms with valence less than 4. Observe that all the elements in group 15 will gain 3 electrons and become **negatively charged ions (called "anions")**. For example, nitrogen, which has 7 protons and 7 electrons in a neutral atom, will gain 3 electrons to fill its valence shell. It will have a -3 charge (7 protons and 10 electrons). Electrons are donated by atoms that prefer to lose electrons, becoming **positively charged ions (called "cations")**. Bonds that are formed by transfer of electrons between atoms are called **"ionic bonds,"** and compounds with **ionic bonds** are soluble in water and conduct electricity. These compounds are called "ionic compounds." Let's look at an example. Sodium loses 1 electron to fill its outer shell, giving it a +1 charge. Chlorine gains an electron to fill its outer shell (taking 1 electron from sodium) giving it a –1 charge. The now positively charge sodium ion is attracted to the positively charged chloride ion.

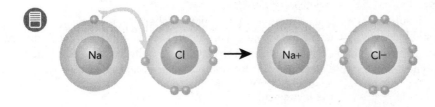

Atoms can also share electrons to achieve stability. For example, two oxygen (O) atoms have six valence electrons each. If they each shared two electrons, they would both resemble neon in their electron number. This is simpler to understand when visualized. It takes two electrons to make one bond, so there are two bonds between the O atoms in O_2. These shared bonds are known as "**covalent bonds.**" They are typically formed between two p-block elements. The following diagram shows four electrons creating two bonds between oxygen atoms.

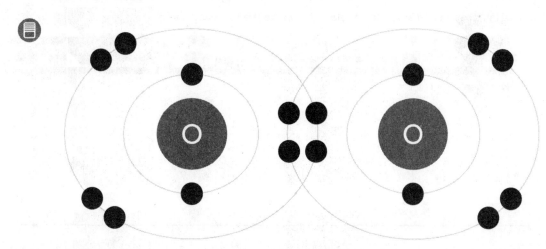

CHAPTER 49 PRACTICE PROBLEMS

1. Which of the following is neutral atom would have 10 protons, 11 neutrons, and 10 electrons?

   A. Neon
   B. Sodium
   C. Calcium
   D. Boron

2. Two isotopes of carbon are found, one with an atomic mass of 12 and the other 14. Which of the following best describes how these isotopes differ?

   A. The number of protons and electrons is different.
   B. Carbon 12 has fewer protons than carbon 14.
   C. Carbon 14 has more neutrons than carbon 12.
   D. Carbon 12 has two fewer electrons than carbon 14.

3. A neutral atom of calcium has two electrons in its outer shell. Which of the following will occur when calcium forms an ion?

   A. Calcium will lose two electrons to have a full valence shell.
   B. Calcium will gain two electrons to have a full valence shell.
   C. Calcium will add two protons to become neutral.
   D. Calcium will add six electrons to have a full valence shell.

4. Which of the following best describes an oxygen atom with 8 neutrons and 10 electrons?

   A. An anion with a −2 charge
   B. A cation with a 2 charge
   C. An anion with an atomic mass of 18
   D. A cation with a positive charge of +2

5. Use information in the periodic table to complete the following chart.

Element name	Element symbol	Proton number	Neutron number	Electron number	Atomic number	Atomic mass (amu)
Hydrogen						
	N	7				14
		78	117			
Chlorine						35
	K			19		39
	He				2	4

Notes:

Notes:

CHAPTER

50

Explain characteristic properties of substances

 This objective includes, but is not limited to, the following examples of knowledge, skills, and abilities.

- Demonstrate knowledge of density.
- Demonstrate knowledge of properties of water (e.g., solubility, cohesion, adhesion).
- Identify a substance using characteristics from a chart of given properties.
- Compare and contrast osmosis and diffusion.

Chemical substances have unique properties that allow them to be distinguished from other substances. To be successful in this TEAS task, recognizing physical characteristics such as density, melting point, boiling point, and polarity are necessary. This task requires a proficient understanding of the characteristics of common substances, particularly those of water. You will also use a chart of properties to identify different substances and compare the different ways that molecules move.

Chemical Properties

All substances have physical and chemical properties. Physical properties refer to observed properties of the substance and those that can change the state without changing the identity of the substance. An example is boiling liquid water. The steam (vapor) that is produced is a gaseous state of water with the same molecular formula as liquid water. The molecules in liquid water and vapor are both made up of two hydrogen atoms and one oxygen; its identity has not changed. The vapor can be condensed to form liquid water once again. Other physical properties include density, melting point, boiling point, malleability, specific heat capacity, and conductivity. Intensive physical properties (e.g., boiling point, melting point, luster) do not depend on the amount of the substance present. Extensive physical properties (e.g., mass and volume) can change depending on the amount of matter present.

Chemical properties depend on the chemical reactivity of the substance. When a substance chemically reacts with another substance, it results in formation of a new substance with a different composition and identity. A sugar cube can be cut in half, changing the volume of each half (an extensive physical property).

SCIENCE

But if the sugar cube is burned, the sugar combines with oxygen, converting sugar to the new substances carbon dioxide and water. How sugar reacts is considered a chemical property.

Atomic number	Symbol	Name	First ionization energy (kJ/mol)	Electro-negativity	Melting point (K)	Boiling point (K)	Density (g/cm³)	Atomic radius (pm)
1	H	hydrogen	1312	2.2	14	20	0.000082	32
2	He	helium	2372			4	0.000164	37
3	Li	lithium	520	1.0	454	1615	0.534	130
4	Be	beryllium	900	1.6	1560	2744	1.85	99
5	B	boron	801	2.0	2348	4273	2.34	84
6	C	carbon	1086	2.6				75
7	N	nitrogen	1402	3.0	63	77	0.001145	71
8	O	oxygen	1314	3.4	54	90	0.001308	64
9	F	fluorine	1681	4.0	53	85	0.001553	60
10	Ne	neon	2081		24	27	0.000825	62

Density

Physical properties can be used to identify substances. For example, density is the ratio of mass to volume. This ratio is not dependent on the size of the sample but rather the unique structure of the substance. This means that a sample of liquid water has a density of 1 gram per cubic centimeter (1 g/cm³) independent of the sample size. Denser substances will sink, whereas less dense substances will float. For example, solid water (ice) is less dense than liquid water. That is why ice floats in liquid water; think about icebergs and ice cubes. Density can be used to identify a substance. For example, let's say we have a 100-g sample of an unidentified metal. The sample takes up about 187 cm³. According to the preceding table, what element could it be? The density of this metal is 100 g/186 cm³ or about 0.534g/cm³ which happens to be the density of lithium. Other physical properties can be used to identify substances. For example, using the data table provided, it can be determined that an element with a melting point of 63 K and a boiling point of 77 K is nitrogen.

Properties of Water

Water has several unique properties. It is a polar molecule, which means it has negatively charged (oxygen end) and positively charged (hydrogen end) sides. The polarity of water allows it to form hydrogen bonds and demonstrate both cohesive and adhesive properties. Cohesion is a measure of how well similar molecules stick to each other or group together. Water molecules are cohesive because they are attracted to other water molecules. The cohesiveness of water allows it to travel through small capillaries without using energy. Cohesiveness also creates surface tension by creating a tight-knit layer of water molecules on the surface of any body of water. Breaking up the multitude of hydrogen bonds between water requires a lot of energy, so water is said to have high specific heat and high heat of vaporization. Water boils at 100°C (212°F). Ice floats on water because it has lower density than liquid water. Most substances have greater densities in solid form. Adhesiveness is a measure of how well dissimilar particles or surfaces cling to one another. The adhesiveness of water allows it to stick to other molecules because of water's polarity. Water is also considered the universal solvent, meaning many substances dissolve in water.

Osmosis and Diffusion

Diffusion and osmosis are key processes for the transport of molecules through substrates and across membranes. Diffusion is the movement of any substance from areas of high concentration to areas of low concentration. One example of this is when perfume is sprayed in a room. The molecules of perfume will at first be concentrated in the area where it was sprayed. However, over time, the molecules of perfume will spread out until the concentration of perfume molecules is the same in all areas of the room. Another example is the molecules in the capillaries of your lungs. The blood in the capillaries moving from the heart to the lungs has a high concentration of carbon dioxide. This carbon dioxide will move out of the capillaries and diffuses across a thin layer into the lungs. This decreases the carbon dioxide in the blood. The air in the lungs, which is rich in carbon dioxide, is then exhaled.

Osmosis is a specific type of diffusion referring to water moving from an area of high concentration to low concentration. Water moves passively across a membrane through pores made of aquaporin proteins. Remember that water is a solvent, meaning substances (solutes) dissolve in it. Water moves from regions where solvent concentration is high to areas where solvent concentration is low. One example of osmosis is how plants take in water through their roots. Root cells contain minerals, sugars, and salts dissolved in water. So, when water is available in soil, osmosis causes water to flow through the cell walls to the root interior where there is a lower concentration of water.

However, sometimes cells need substances to move from areas of low to high concentrations. To move from regions of low to high concentrations, energy must be used. Movement against the concentration gradient that requires energy is called "active transport." Diffusion and osmosis do not require energy, other than the kinetic energy of moving molecules.

SCIENCE

CHAPTER 50 PRACTICE PROBLEMS

1. Which of the following is the density of a substance that has a mass of 22.5 g and a volume of 5 cm³?

   A. 0.22 g/cm³
   B. 4.5 g/cm³
   C. 15 g/cm³
   D. 27.5g/cm³

2. Iron reacts with oxygen to form iron oxide, or rust. Which of the following describes the property of rust?

   A. A physical property
   B. A chemical property
   C. An ionic property
   D. Specific heat

3. Which of the following describes the process of diffusion?

   A. It is the movement of substances from a solid to liquid state.
   B. It is the movement of a substance from high concentration to low concentration.
   C. It requires a large amount of energy.
   D. It is specific to the movement of water only.

4. Concentrations of sodium dissolved in water are higher inside the cell than outside. Which of the following best predicts which way the water will flow?

   A. Water will remain in equal concentrations on both sides of the cell membrane.
   B. Water will move from its low concentration (outside the cell) to the higher concentration (inside the cell).
   C. Water will move from its high concentration (outside the cell) to the lower concentration (inside the cell).
   D. Water will increase in concentration inside and outside the cell.

5. In three to five sentences, explain why ice floats in liquid water. Use the concept of density in your answer.

Notes:

Notes:

CHAPTER

51

Compare and contrast changes in states of matter

 This objective includes, but is not limited to, the following examples of knowledge, skills, and abilities.

- Describe the states of matter.
- Demonstrate knowledge of the movement of molecules in the states of matter.
- Discriminate among the different phases of matter.
- Explain changes between states of matter (e.g., melting, freezing, evaporation, condensation).

Matter can exist in different states determined by environmental conditions. In this TEAS task, you will need to distinguish between states of matter. You will also need to be able to explain how the movement of the molecules is related to the state of matter and explain the transition between different phases of matter. The TEAS test uses examples of different substances changing between states of matter, so knowing how the processes work is important.

States of Matter

Molecules make up all matter. Matter exists in four phases: solid, liquid, gas, and plasma. Above absolute zero (0 K or –273°C), molecules are in constant motion. According to the Kinetic Molecular Theory, molecular motion changes as heat is added or removed. Heat overcomes the forces that hold matter together. As the temperature of a substance increases, the intermolecular forces that hold the molecules together are broken, causing the molecules to move away from each other. The amount of heat required for a phase change will not break the bonds within a molecule. In solids, the molecules are packed together in a tight, orderly pattern; there is vibrational motion but no translational motion experienced by the molecules. The molecules in liquids are less ordered and exhibit both translational and vibrational motion. Gas molecules are rapidly moving and spread far apart.

SCIENCE

The phase of a substance depends on two conditions: temperature and pressure. Increasing temperature has a tendency to move the particles of matter apart, and increasing pressure has a tendency to pack them closer together. In the phase diagram for carbon dioxide that follows, the temperature and pressures for solid, liquid, and gaseous carbon dioxide are shown. At the triple point, solid, liquid, and gas coexist; above the critical point, liquid and gas coexist.

 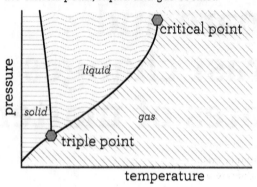

Solid matter has definite volume and shape. Think about a solid block of ice. It has a specific number of molecules (matter) and takes up a specific amount of space. Liquid matter has definite volume but no definite shape, meaning that it will conform to the shape of the container. Gas has no definite volume or shape. Gases are highly compressible and subject to changes in volume, but liquids and solids are generally non-compressible.

Changes Between States of Matter

A change from solid to liquid (melting) requires an addition of heat, which causes the molecules to become more energized, which increases their vibrational and translational motion. Adding heat (energy) causes the forces holding particles together in a solid state to break. Adding heat is also required to change matter from liquid to gas (boiling). Removing heat from matter is required to change gas to liquid (condensation) or liquid to solid (freezing). An unusual phase change called "sublimation" directly converts solids to gas. In deposition, the reverse phase change from gas directly to solid occurs. These occur at room temperature with the element iodine and the molecule carbon dioxide. Solid carbon dioxide (also known as "dry ice") will changed directly from a solid to gas at room temperature.

CHAPTER 51 PRACTICE PROBLEMS

1. Which of the following phase changes requires the loss of heat?

   A. Melting
   B. Evaporation
   C. Freezing
   D. Sublimation

2. Which of the following is true of liquids?

   A. They have definite shape and volume.
   B. They have no definite shape, but they have definite volume.
   C. They have a definite shape but no definite volume.
   D. They have no definite shape and no definite volume.

3. Which of the following is likely to occur after decreasing the pressure of a liquid?

   A. Increase in intramolecular forces between molecules
   B. Increase in boiling point
   C. Decrease in boiling point
   D. Increase in temperature

4. Which of the following best describes the triple point?

   A. Point where temperature, pressure, and volume all equal one another
   B. Point where a substance can exists as a solid, liquid, and gas
   C. Point where no more energy can be absorbed by a substance
   D. Point where a substance starts to lose its shape

5. On a hot summer day, you place a cup of ice water outside. Using your knowledge of states of matter, describe what will likely happen in three to five sentences.

Notes:

_____

_____

_____

_____

_____

_____

_____

_____

_____

_____

_____

_____

_____

_____

_____

_____

_____

_____

_____

_____

_____

_____

_____

_____

CHAPTER

52 Describe chemical reactions

 This objective includes, but is not limited to, the following examples of knowledge, skills, and abilities.

- Identify covalent and ionic bonds.
- Identify simple chemical reactions.
- Describe how conditions affect chemical reactions (e.g., pressure, concentration, temperature).
- Describe how catalysts (enzymes) affect chemical reactions.
- Knowledge of basic molecules (e.g., H_2O, NaCl, CO_2, O_2, $C_2H_2O_2$, KCl).
- Describe acids and bases in terms of pH balance.

Chemical reactions are occurring constantly in nature by creating and breaking bonds between elements and compounds. These reactions occur at varying rates with changing conditions. For this TEAS task, you need to be able to describe chemical bonding and reactions and factors that influence those reactions.

Covalent and Ionic Bonds

Chemical bonds occur when two or more atoms have interactions between electrons. Ionic bonds can only form when the elements involved have a large difference in electronegativity, such as exists between metals and nonmetals. This difference allows for the donation of electrons from one element to the other. These elements then become ions or charged atoms. Metals tend to become positively charged cations, and nonmetals become negatively charged anions. For example, sodium is a metal that easily donates an electron to the nonmetal fluorine. Sodium becomes positively charged because it has lost an electron and fluorine becomes negatively charged. These oppositely charged ions attract one another, forming an ionic bond and making sodium fluoride. Metals can be found toward the left side of the periodic table, and nonmetals can be found toward the right.

Sometimes elements share electrons instead of donating electrons, forming a different type of bond. Covalent bonds require the sharing of electrons and occur between two nonmetals. In covalent bonds, there is not a sufficient difference in electronegativity to gain or lose electrons. However, differences in electronegativity within a covalently bonded molecule cause them to be polar or nonpolar. Polar covalent compounds have a negatively charged side and a positively charged side. Water is a polar molecule; the hydrogen side of the molecule is positively charged, and the oxygen side is negatively charged. This is as a result of the strong electronegativity of oxygen pulling at the shared electrons. These molecules are still neutral in charge.

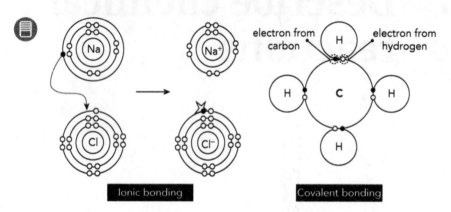

Simple Chemical Reactions

Chemical reactions are represented by chemical equations. Chemical equations have a basic pattern: reactants, reaction sign showing the direction of the reaction ($\rightarrow$), and products. The formation of salt is an example of a chemical equation: $2Na + Cl_2 \rightarrow 2NaCl$. Chemical equations must be shown as balanced equations, meaning there must be the same number of each element on both sides. There are five basic chemical reactions: synthesis, decomposition, single replacement, double replacement, and combustion. Study the following diagram to become familiar with the reactions. The preceding equation is a synthesis reaction; it is taking two substances and combining them into a new substance. Decomposition is the opposite of synthesis; it is a reaction in which a compound is broken down into simpler elements that composed the compound. Water can be broken down into hydrogen and oxygen. Single replacement is a reaction in which an atom or group of atoms is replaced by another. In the single replacement reaction that follows, iron replaces copper in the compound. In a double-replacement reaction, two replacements happen. In the following example, sodium and copper switch places, combining with the one another's original anion. Sodium hydroxide becomes copper hydroxide, and copper sulfate becomes sodium sulfate. The final type of reaction is combustion. In a combustion reaction, oxygen combines with a compound to form carbon dioxide and water. These reactions give off heat and are exothermic. Burning of wood is a combustion reaction.

Conditions That Affect Chemical Reactions

Reaction rates can be altered by changing the conditions of a reaction. Changing factors, such as pressure, concentrations of reactants and substrates, temperature, and the presence of catalysts, will change the speed of a reaction. All of these conditions can be applied to an equation to assess the rate of reaction. For example, when temperature rises, the rate of an endothermic reaction (where heat is required) will increase. However, when temperature rises, an exothermic reaction (where heat is released) will slow down.

Increasing the pressure surrounding a reaction increases the chance of collisions between atoms and molecules. This will increase the reaction rate. Increasing the concentration of reactants increases the probability that reactants will come in contact with each other, thus increasing the likelihood of breaking or creating a bond. If product concentration is increased, the reaction will slow down.

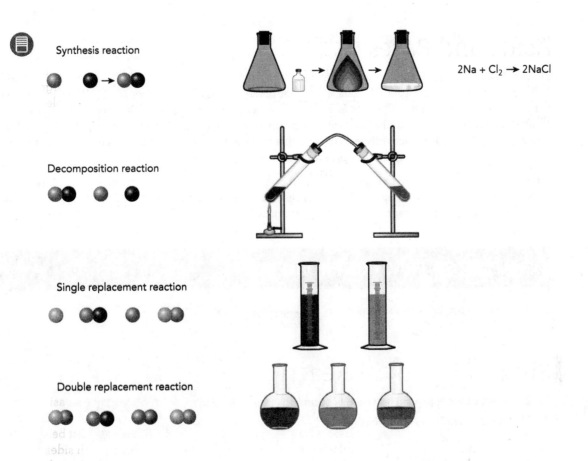

Synthesis reaction

$2Na + Cl_2 \rightarrow 2NaCl$

Decomposition reaction

Single replacement reaction

Double replacement reaction

Catalysts

Catalysts are chemicals that lower the activation energy required for a chemical reaction to occur. Thus, catalysts speed up reactions that would otherwise be extremely slow to occur. The catalyst does not change during the reaction and is reused. In biological systems, catalysts are proteins called "enzymes," which speed up chemical reactions within the body. For example, the enzyme amylase is a catalyst for the breakdown of starch polymers to glucose monomers. This enzyme helps your body digest starches.

Common Molecules

There are some common molecules that you should know. Common ionic compounds include salts like sodium chloride (NaCl) and potassium chloride (KCl). Other common ionic compounds are calcium chloride ($CaCl_2$) and sodium bromide (NaBr). Each includes a metal and a non-metal. Some common covalent compounds include water (H_2O), carbon dioxide (CO_2), and oxygen (O_2). You should also know basic organic compounds such as glucose ($C_6H_{12}O_6$). Ethanol (C_2H_6O) is another common organic compound found in combustion reactions.

Acids and Bases

pH is a measure of the amount of hydrogen ions (H^+) in a solution. Acids are substances that provide hydrogen ions (H^+) or accept OH^- ions, and lower pH. Acids have a pH lower than 7. Bases are substances that provide hydroxide ions (OH^-) or accept H^+ ions and raise pH. Bases have a pH higher than 7. Neutral solutions maintain a pH of 7. Water and human blood are great examples of neutral solutions. Acids mixed with bases react with each other to produce water and salt. When the proper amount of acid and base is used, then the system becomes neutral with a pH of 7.

Cells function in a narrow pH range. The human body uses chemicals called "buffers" to control the pH in the body. Buffers can absorb excess H^+ or OH^-. Buffers maintain the proper pH of the body. Carbon dioxide and bicarbonate are important buffers in the human body.

CHAPTER 52 PRACTICE PROBLEMS

1. Which of the following substances is an example of an ionic compound?

   A. H_2O
   B. CO_2
   C. NH_3
   D. KCl

2. Which of the following reactions is occurring is this equation?

   $AgNO_3 + NaCl \rightarrow AgCl + NaNO_3$

   A. Combustion
   B. Double replacement
   C. Single replacement
   D. Decomposition

3. Orange juice, stomach acid, and coffee are all acids. Which of the following is the pH level for these substances?

   A. A pH lower than 2
   B. A pH less than 7
   C. A pH at about 7
   D. A pH above 7

4. Which of the following would slow down a reaction rate?

   A. Increasing the temperature
   B. Adding enzymes
   C. Decreasing the pressure
   D. Decreasing the substrate

5. Predict the outcome of this decomposition reaction: $2AgCl \rightarrow$

Notes:

Notes:

CHAPTER

53

Identify basic scientific measurements using laboratory tools

 This objective includes, but is not limited to, the following examples of knowledge, skills, and abilities.

- Identify the unit of measurement in a model (e.g., diagram, illustration, photograph).
- Identify the numerical value of a measurement of an object.
- Select the tool necessary to measure volume, mass, or length of an object.
- Choose a scale unit appropriate for the object being measured.

Accuracy in measuring, recording, and diagramming data are important skills. This TEAS task focuses on scientific measurements, scale, and tools. You will need to identify measurement tools and be able to measure volume, mass, and length. You will also need to understand and convert units involved in measuring large and small quantities of objects and substances.

Units of Measurement

Scientists use the metric system, or Système Internationale (SI), to measure and record data. This system uses base units and prefixes to increase or decrease size. The SI base units for mass, length, and time are kilogram, meter, and second, respectively. SI units are also used to measure volume. The volume of a three-dimensional object has length, width, and height, all of which are measured in length units. Thus, the volume of a container 10 cm × 10 cm × 10 cm is 1,000 cm³. This SI base unit for volume is more familiarly called a "liter."

The SI system also uses prefixes to indicate the size of units. For example, the prefix "kilo" means 1,000, so 1 kilometer is 1,000 meters. The prefix "centi" means 0.01, so 1 centimeter is 0.01 meters. The prefixes can be used with any base. One kilogram is 1,000 grams, and 1 centigram is 0.01 grams. The TEAS will cover prefixes including kilo, hecta, deca, deci, centi, and milli. The following table shows some common prefixes and measurements for the SI system.

SCIENCE

Prefix	Meaning
kilo	1000
hecta	100
deca	10
	1
deci	0.1
centi	0.01
milli	0.001

When measuring, it is important to identify the numerical value correctly. Consider the ruler shown here. Each number represents a centimeter (cm). The smaller lines between the centimeter represent 1/10 of a centimeter, or a millimeter. If we were measuring to the first small line after the 2, the length would be 2.1 cm or 21 millimeters (mm).

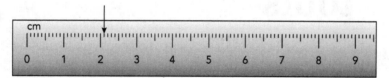

Selecting a Measurement Tool

Tool selection will also be part of this section of the TEAS. Length is typically measured with a ruler or meterstick. Length is the distance from end to end of an object and is used to describe width, height, and length. Be sure to always start measuring length from the 0 point on your measurement tool. Volume can be measured in different ways, depending on the state of matter. Volume is the amount of space an object takes up. The volume of solids can be calculated by multiplying the measurements of length, width, and height, as seen in the following figure. The sides can be measured using rulers or metersticks.

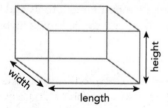

Several types of glassware can be used to measure the volume of liquids. The most accurate tool in measuring large volumes is a volumetric flask, and small volumes are best measured using a volumetric pipette. Graduated cylinders can also be used to measure a range of volumes in the laboratory, but they are less accurate than volumetric flasks or pipettes. Remember that liquids form a meniscus in a measuring tool. A "meniscus" is the curve formed at the top of a liquid in response to its container. The meniscus curve can be upward (concave), downward (convex), or flat, depending on the properties of the liquid and the container. When measuring the volume of a liquid, make sure that the line you are reading is even with the center of the meniscus.

Balances are used to measure the mass of an object. The mass is the amount of matter in an object. There are two types of balances used to measure mass: the triple-beam balance and electronic balance. The electronic balance is more common because it is easier to use.

Choosing an Appropriate Scale

It is important to determine the most appropriate scaled unit to use when measuring items. Large items with a large mass would likely be measured using kilograms (kg). It is more efficient to say a person has a mass of 75 kg than to say a person has a mass of 75,000 grams. Measuring a few drops of water would make more sense in milliliters than liters. For length, small things like insects and fingernails should be measured in millimeters. Objects like the width of a piece of paper can be measured in centimeters, whereas the height of a door or a ceiling should be measured in meters. The distance between two towns can be measured in kilometers (km).

CHAPTER 53 PRACTICE PROBLEMS

1. Which of the following values is appropriate for the height an adult human?
   A. 1.5 mm
   B. 1.5 cm
   C. 1.5 m
   D. 1.5 km

2. Which of the following is the meaning of the prefix "kilo"?
   A. 1,000
   B. 100
   C. 0.01
   D. 0.001

3. Which of the following tools could be used to measure the volume of a liquid sample?
   A. Triple-beam balance
   B. Flask
   C. Meterstick
   D. Ruler

4. A block of ice has height of 10 cm, a width of 5 cm, and a length of 5 cm. Which of the following is the volume of the substance?
   A. 20 cm^3
   B. 50 cm
   C. 250 cm
   D. 250 cm^3

5. Two students measure the distance from one end of the school building to the other. One student measures a length of 2 km, and the other measures a length of 200 cm. Which student most likely measured incorrectly? Why?

Identify basic scientific measurements using laboratory tools **335**

Notes:

CHAPTER

54

Critique a scientific explanation using logic and evidence

 This objective includes, but is not limited to, the following examples of knowledge, skills, and abilities.

- Identify a logical conclusion based on evidence provided.
- Identify the stated cause in a scientific explanation.
- Identify the stated effect in a scientific explanation.
- Evaluate evidence that supports a scientific explanation.

Scientific explanations of the world around us are based on evidence from observation and experimentation. Drawing meaningful conclusions from data is crucial in creating valid scientific explanations. It is also an important skill to be able to analyze scientific arguments for evidence. In this TEAS task, you will read scientific explanations, analyze the content, and evaluate the evidence provided.

Drawing Conclusions

Empirical evidence, or evidence generated through experimentation, is a primary feature of science. Scientists collect data, analyze it, and then draw logical conclusions supported by the data. Conclusions in science are not drawn from just a few observations. Scientists study trends and patterns in large amounts of experimentally reproducible data. To have confidence in the data, scientists repeat experiments with the same variables and procedures. If repeated experiments have similar results, scientists can have confidence in the data and draw valid conclusions. TEAS tasks will ask you to draw conclusions based on data and other evidence. For example, consider a scientist is trying to determine how certain varieties of fertilizer affect the growth of grass. The TEAS task will present you with the scientist's experimental procedure and data. You will be asked to evaluate the scientist's procedure and data and draw a conclusion about the type of fertilizer that produces the most growth.

SCIENCE

Identifying Cause–and–Effect Relationships

Conclusions are often presented as cause-and-effect relationships. Although these relationships can be difficult to establish conclusively, scientists can use this simplified relationship to explain phenomena. Identifying cause and effect in a given scenario is necessary for completing TEAS tasks. For example, consider the scientist studying varieties of fertilizer. You may be asked to identify the effect of different fertilizers on grass growth.

Evaluating Evidence

Conclusions rely on the evidence that supports them. Analyzing the reliability of evidence is important in evaluating the strength of a conclusion. Strong conclusions and theories are produced by reproducible and convincing data. The process of analyzing data includes evaluating the following factors: the presence of bias (either intentional or unintentional), controlled setting (changing only one variable at a time), accurate data collection, and replicable results. Bias sometimes occurs when experimenters influence results. For example, suppose the effectiveness of a new type of medicine is being tested. Experimenters or the people receiving the medicine may believe the medicine is effective, and this bias may influence their observations or conclusions unintentionally. To avoid this, some experiments use placebos to try and eliminate bias. A "placebo" is a substance with no medicinal effect that can be used as a control in an experiment. Common placebos are substances containing water and sugar. Experimenters and subjects do not know who is receiving the medicine and who is receiving the placebo. This helps to eliminate bias.

It is also important to analyze the experimental design when evaluating evidence. Larger sample sizes and repeated trials provide more confidence in the evidence collected. The design should also keep all conditions the same except for the variable being tested, which is called the "independent variable." The conditions being kept the same are called the "controlled variables." Keeping controlled variables the same provides further confidence that the results observed are caused by the variable under consideration. For example, consider the fertilizer experiment. Keeping all conditions such as temperature and amount of water provided the same for all the plants allows the experimenter to have more confidence that it is the fertilizer causing any changes or effects in plant growth.

CHAPTER 54 PRACTICE PROBLEMS

A researcher collected data to measure the effectiveness of a new pain medication in treating chronic pain. Each patient was given a dose of medication every day at 8 a.m. and asked to rate their pain on a scale of 1-10. They were asked to rate their pain at 11 a.m. after the medicine had taken effect. Patient 1 received a placebo medicine containing a saline solution. Patients 2, 3, and 4 received the same doses of the new pain medication. The following table shows the results of the experiment.

Patient number	Patient pain rating (8 a.m.)	Patient pain rating (11 a.m.)
1	9	8
2	8	4
3	9	2
4	5	2

1. Which of the following conclusions can be drawn from the data?

   A. The pain medicine reduces patient pain after 3 hours.
   B. The pain medicine does not affect patient pain levels.
   C. In large doses, the pain medicine is effective.
   D. The correct time to take pain medicine is 9 a.m.

2. Which of the following describes what was done to try and avoid bias in this experiment?

   A. All patients were given the medicine when pain levels were highest.
   B. All patients had similar starting pain levels.
   C. A placebo was given to the patient who did not receive the medication.
   D. The experimenter followed the same directions each time when giving the medication.

3. The experimenter instructed patients to conduct similar activities during the 3 hours of testing. Which of the following is the name for this type of experimental factor?

   A. Data
   B. Independent variable
   C. Dependent variable
   D. Control variable

4. Which of the following experimental practices would strengthen the data supporting the conclusion?

   A. Testing multiple dosages of medicine
   B. Testing the medicine at different times of the day
   C. Testing more patients experiencing similar types of pain to see if the results are reproducible
   D. Removing the placebo group from further testing to prevent bias

5. Many trials of the experiment testing the new pain medication were conducted. Similar results were found among the placebo group and the group of patients who received the medicine. What conclusion would you make based on this data?

SCIENCE

Notes:

CHAPTER

55

Explain relationships among events, objects, and processes

 This objective includes, but is not limited to, the following examples of knowledge, skills, and abilities.

- Compare the magnitude (e.g., size) of events, objects, and processes.
- Determine the causal relationship between events (e.g., smoking and high blood pressure).
- Sequence an event or process.

The natural world—including the human body—is constantly changing. Events such as hurricanes and drought affect many people, whereas specific ailments or disease affect individuals. It is important to distinguish between the magnitude of large- and small-scale events, objects, and processes. This TEAS task focuses on the magnitude of events and processes. You will also be asked to determine causal relationships between events and the sequence of events and processes.

Comparing Magnitude

The human body has many cells, tissues, and organs. Each component of the body is a different size and is reported with a different scale. For example, the diameter of human hair can be measured in micrometers (millionths of a meter), and the height of a human would more commonly be measured in meters. The mass of atoms is measured using atomic mass units, whereas the mass of an elephant is measured in kilograms. Every measurement requires a unit, and the unit identifies the scale of the measurement, such as kilograms, grams, or milligrams. It is important to understand the concept of scale to compare the magnitude or size of objects and processes.

SCIENCE

Determining Causal Relationships and Sequence

Causal relationships are difficult to determine with complete confidence. However, data can suggest a cause-and-effect relationship between two variables. Scientific studies can suggest causal relationships between variables. Examples of causal relationships include smoking and emphysema, high blood pressure and vascular disease, and alcohol consumption during pregnancy and fetal alcohol syndrome.

Determining a causal relationship can also involve determining the sequence of events that leads to a consequence. For example, if your body temperature increases above 37°C (98.6°F), your nerve cells send a signal to the brain. The brain then sends a signal to your sweat glands and you begin sweating. Another example is how the body maintains a proper level of blood glucose. As glucose rises, the pancreas releases insulin. Insulin allows the cells of the body to take in glucose. If blood glucose levels are too low, glucagon is released, causing the liver to break down glycogen into glucose. This TEAS task will ask you to determine causal relationships and sequence of events based on data provided.

CHAPTER 55 PRACTICE PROBLEMS

1. Which of the following units is most appropriate for measuring the height of a giraffe?

   A. Centimeters
   B. Meters
   C. Kilometers
   D. Millimeters

2. Which of the following units is appropriate for measuring the mass of a coin?

   A. Grams
   B. Meters
   C. Kilograms
   D. Kilometers

3. Which of the following can lead to the breakdown of glycogen?

   A. High levels of insulin
   B. High levels of glucose
   C. Low levels of insulin
   D. Low levels of glucose

4. Researchers conducted an experiment on the effects of new antimold product. Which of the following is the dependent variable that should be measured to establish an effect in this experiment?

   A. Amount of antimold product
   B. Amount of mold growth
   C. Humidity
   D. Temperature

5. Research high blood pressure in the human body. Write five to seven sentences describing the possible causes and effects of this condition.

Notes:

Notes:

CHAPTER

56

Analyze the design of a scientific investigation

 This objective includes, but is not limited to, the following examples of knowledge, skills, and abilities.

- Identify a relevant hypothesis based on a given investigation.
- Determine the strengths of a scientific investigation.
- Determine the weaknesses of a scientific investigation.
- Identify dependent, independent, and controlled variables.
- Determine whether a hypothesis is supported by evidence within a case study.

Science is propelled by investigation. Scientists determine hypotheses based on known evidence and then create investigations to test the hypotheses. For information to be validated, scientists submit their ideas for scrutiny by other scientists. This process of investigation is important to society's understanding of the world. This TEAS task will focus on hypothesis and investigations.

Identifying a Relevant Hypothesis

Hypotheses are informed guesses about causal relationships that are generated by observation and initial data collection. In this way, they are not truly guesses about the outcome of an event. Scientists develop hypotheses only after they begin to have ideas about relationships. This could be from observations or background research on a topic. The hypothesis is a guiding idea to develop a strong investigation. During the investigation, the hypothesis will be accepted or rejected based on evidence collected from the investigation. Suppose a scientist wanted to determine the best conditions for germinating seeds. He or she may hypothesize that the seeds need to be in moist soil to germinate. Based on their investigation, the hypothesis will be supported or rejected based on data.

SCIENCE

Variables and the Strength of Experimental Design

Scientific investigations collect experimental data to support or reject hypotheses. A scientific hypothesis is a prediction of what will occur in an experiment based on previous research. To test an hypothesis, an experiment must be set up in such a way that the data is accurate and valid. Scientists must develop strategies in an investigation to control variables. There are three types of variables. Each experiment should manipulate only one variable: the independent variable. Examples of independent variables include type or concentration of a medicine. The independent variable is plotted on the *x*-axis of a graph. The dependent variable is what is measured after the independent variable is changed. It is the observed condition that responds to the manipulation of the independent variable. Examples of dependent variables include growth or response. The dependent variable is plotted on the *y*-axis of a graph. All other variables should be kept the same in a investigation. These are called "control variables," such as temperature and humidity. Controlling all other variables helps to establish a causal relationship between the independent and dependent variable.

Consider the variables in the following experimental design. Scientists ares investigating the effect of water on germinating seeds. Their hypothesis is that water is necessary for seed germination. They have 100 seeds. Fifty seeds receive 25 mL of water each day, and 50 seeds receive no water. The independent variable is the water, and the dependent variable is observing the germination of the seeds. All other variables, such as amount of sunlight, temperature, soil conditions, and type of plant, should be the same or controlled for all seeds in the experiment. It is important to review the methodology of any investigation to determine if it is valid. This experiment only manipulates one independent variable: the water added to the seeds. All other variables that might affect the experiment are kept constant. Another important aspect of an experimental design is sample size and the use of multiple trials. In this experiment, the sample size of each experimental group includes 50 seeds. Imagine if this experiment was only done with 1 seed in each group. Testing on many seeds provides the scientist more data to analyze. The scientist should then repeat the experiment multiple times to make sure she obtains similar results.

Analyzing Data and Drawing Conclusions

After conducting investigations, scientists analyze their data to determine possible conclusions. Scientists accept or reject their hypothesis or prediction based on the data to form a conclusion. Conclusions are thus based on evidence and then subjected to scrutiny by other scientists. Scientists can submit their evidence to professional journals, where the investigation and data are reviewed. Only the most reliable experiments and data will pass the review process and be published. This process is called "peer review." Consider the following data to draw conclusions based on evidence.

Group	Number of Seeds Germinated
No water added	5 seeds
25 mL of water added	27 seeds

One conclusion that can be drawn from this data is that the evidence supports the hypothesis that seeds need water to germinate. This is because more seeds germinated (27 seeds) when water was added than without water (5 seeds germinated). In this TEAS task, be ready to determine if the data presented in a question provides evidence for a given hypothesis.

CHAPTER 56 PRACTICE PROBLEMS

Based on previous research, a group of scientists believe that fruit flies are attracted to rotting fruit. They design an experiment to test this hypothesis. The scientists place 20 fruit flies in a chamber. On one side of the chamber, they place an unripe banana. On the other side of the chamber, they place a rotten banana. After 5 minutes, they count how many fruit flies are on each side of the chamber.

1. Which of the following is the dependent variable in the experiment?

   A. Ripeness of the banana
   B. Size of the chamber
   C. Number of fruit flies placed in the chamber
   D. Number of on each side of the chamber

2. Which of the following statements is the hypothesis in the experiment?

   A. Fruit flies are attracted to any type of fruit.
   B. If presented with an unripe banana, fruit flies will be attracted to it.
   C. Fruit flies live longer when exposed to unripe fruit.
   D. Fruit flies ripen fruit faster than when there are no fruit flies.

Juan Carlos hypothesizes that changing the color of light given to plants will affect their growth. He decides to test his prediction in an experiment. He sets up four groups of plants, giving each a different color of light. Each group has 10 radish plants all about 10 cm tall. He keeps all of them in the same temperature and gives them with the same amount of water each day. After 10 days, he records these results:

Light	Average Starting Height (cm)	Average Height after 10 days (cm)
Blue	10	17
Red	10	16
Green	10	11
Yellow	10	12

3. Which of the following is the independent variable in this experiment?

   A. Color of light
   B. Growth of the plant
   C. Number of plants
   D. Mass of the plants

4. What of the following should be controlled in this experiment?

   A. Color of light
   B. Growth of the plant
   C. Soil conditions
   D. All of the above

5. Reread the experimental design regarding the effect of light color on plant growth. Write a hypothesis that would be supported by the data collected by Juan Carlos.

Notes:

Key Terms

acid. A substance with a pH less than 7.

adaptive immune system. A kind of passive or active immunity in which antibodies to a particular antigen are present in the body.

adrenal. A gland above the kidney that produces hormones to regulate heart rate, blood pressure, and other functions.

alveoli. Microscopic air sacs in the lungs where exchange of oxygen and carbon dioxide takes place.

anatomical position. Standard positioning of the body: standing; feet together; arms to the side; with head, eyes, and palms of hands forward.

anion. A negatively charged ion.

antibody. A specific blood protein produced in response to a specific antigen.

antigen presenting cell (APC). A cell that displays foreign antigens with major histocompatibility complexes on their surfaces.

antigens. A molecule that elicits a response from immune cells.

antimicrobial. A substance that kills or inhibits growth of microorganisms with minimal damage to the host.

anus. The opening of the rectum from which solid waste is expelled.

arteries. Blood vessels that deliver blood from the heart to other parts of the body.

asthma. A lung disease characterized by inflamed, narrowed airways and difficulty breathing.

atom. The most basic complete unit of an element.

autonomic nervous system. The part of the peripheral nervous system that regulates unconscious body functions such as breathing and heart rate.

axon. A nerve fiber that carries a nerve impulse away from the neuron cell body.

B cell. Lymphocytes that mature in bone marrow and make antibodies in response to antigens.

barrier. A divider between parts of the body.

base. A substance with a pH greater than 7.

bias. Prejudice in favor of or against an idea.

boiling point. The temperature at which a liquid boils and turns into vapor.

boiling. The transition of liquid to gas when a substance has acquired enough thermal energy.

bolus. A mass of food that has been chewed and swallowed.

bone. Hard, calcified material that makes up the skeleton

brittle bone disease. A group of genetic diseases that affect collagen and result in fragile bones.

bronchi. The main passageways directly attached to the lungs.

bronchioles. Small passages in the lungs that connect bronchi to alveoli.

canaliculi. Microscopic canals in ossified bone.

capillary. A small blood vessel that connects arterioles to venules.

carbohydrates. Sugars and starches composed of monosaccharides.

cardiovascular system. The system comprised of the heart and blood vessels.

cartilage. Tough, elastic connective tissue found in parts of the body such as the ear and on ends of long bones.

catalyst. A substance that increases the rate of a chemical reaction without undergoing permanent chemical change.

cation. A positively charged ion.

cause. An element that makes something happen.

cell. The basic structural unit of an organism from which living things are created and at which level all life functions can take place.

cellular functions. Processes that include growth, metabolism, replication, protein synthesis, regulation, and movement.

cervix. The passage that forms the lower part of the uterus.

chemical equation. Mathematic representation of a chemical reaction.

chemical properties. Characteristics of a material that present during a chemical reaction or chemical change.

chromatid. One of the two duplicates of a chromosome formed during the cell cycle.

chromosome. A structure made of condensed DNA and histone proteins that contains genetic information.

chyme. The semifluid mass of partly digested food that moves from the stomach to the small intestine.

collagen. The primary structural protein of connective tissue that adds tensile strength to the matrix of bones.

complement. The group of proteins in blood serum and plasma that works with antibodies to destroy particulate antigens.

compound. A substance made of two or more elements.

conclusion. An end judgment based on data.

condensation. The transition of a gas to a liquid.

constrict. To become narrower.

contraction. The process leading to shortening or development of tension in a muscle.

control variable. Something kept constant during an experiment.

covalent bond. A chemical bond in which electron pairs are shared between atoms.

critical point. The temperature at which the liquid and gas phases of a substance have the same density.

cystic fibrosis. A genetic disorder that affects the lungs and other organs, characterized by difficulty breathing, coughing up sputum, and lung infections.

data. A collection of information.

density. The amount of mass per volume.

deoxyribonucleic acid (DNA). Organic molecule with a double-helix structure that contains genetic information for the transmission of inherited traits.

deoxyribose sugar. The sugar portion of a deoxyribose nucleotide.

dependent variable. What is measured in an experiment as a possible effect after another variable is changed in that experiment.

deposition. The transition of a substance from gas to solid without passing through the liquid state.

dermis. The middle layer of skin.

diastole. The portion of the cardiac cycle in which the heart refills with blood.

diffusion. The passive movement of substances from areas of high concentration to areas of low concentration.

dihybrid cross. A cross between parents heterozygous at two specific genes.

dilate. To become wider.

directional terminology. Words used to explain relationships of locations of anatomical elements (distal, posterior, medial, etc.).

dominant. An allele or trait that is always expressed if present.

effect. A result of a cause.

electron. A negatively charged atomic particle.

element. Pure substances that cannot be broken into simpler substances.

empirical. Based on observation.

enzymatic digestion. The breakdown of food by enzymes for absorption.

enzyme. A protein produced by a living thing that acts as a catalyst.

epidermis. The outer layer of the skin

estrogen. Female sex hormones.

evaporation. The transition of liquid to gas that happens with or without the substance acquiring enough thermal energy to reach its boiling point.

excretion. Elimination of metabolic waste from the body.

experiment. A scientific procedure to test a hypothesis.

Fallopian tubes. Tubes that carry eggs from the ovaries to the uterus.

freezing. The transition of a liquid to a solid.

gallbladder. The organ that stores bile

gas. A state of matter that does not have a definite volume or shape and is highly compressible.

gene. The unit of hereditary information; a sequence of nucleotides that occupies a fixed position on a chromosome.

genotype. The set of alleles that determines the trait being studied.

gland. An organ that secretes a substance.

graduated cylinder. A narrow cylinder with measurement marks or gradations that is used to measure liquid volume.

gram. Metric unit of mass.

group. A column of elements in the periodic table with common chemical properties.

Haversian canal. Channels in bone that contain blood vessels and nerves.

heart. The muscle that pumps blood throughout the body.

hemoglobin. The protein in red blood cells that carries oxygen from the lungs to the rest of the body.

hormone. A chemical messenger produced by a gland and transported by the bloodstream that regulates specific processes in the body.

hydrogen bond. A noncovalent bond resulting from the attractive interaction between an electronegative atom and a hydrogen atom bonded to another electronegative atom.

hypothesis. A prediction based on research that states a possible outcome of an experiment.

immunoglobulin. An antibody.

independent variable. An item or aspect of an item that is manipulated or changed in an experiment as a possible cause.

inheritance. Transmission of characteristics to offspring.

innate immune system. A collection of nonspecific barriers and cellular responses that serve as an inborn first and second line of defense against pathogens.

integumentary system. An organ system comprised of skin and its associated organs.

involuntary. Without intentional control.

ion. A positively or negatively charged atom or molecule.

ionic bond. The bond between two oppositely charged ions.

kidneys. The pair of organs that regulate fluid balance and filter waste from the blood.

large intestine. Also known as the colon, where vitamins and water are absorbed before feces are stored for elimination.

length. Measurement of distance from end to end.

leukocyte. White blood cells that protect the body against disease.

lining cells. Flattened bone cells that come from osteoblasts.

lipids. Fats, phospholipids, and steroids made with a high ratio of carbon to hydrogen.

liquid. A state of matter that has definite volume but not definite shape.

liter. Metric unit of liquid volume.

liver. The organ that produces bile, regulates glycogen storage, and performs other bodily functions.

long bones. Long hollow shafts containing yellow bone marrow; the ends are made of spongy bone that contains red bone marrow.

lymph. Clear fluid that moves throughout the lymphatic system to fight disease.

lymphocyte. A subtype of white blood cell found in lymph.

macromolecules. Large biological molecules that are classified as carbohydrates, proteins, lipids, or nucleic acids.

macrophage. A large white blood cell that ingests foreign material.

mass. A measurement of inertia, commonly considered the amount of material contained by an object and causing it to have weight in a gravitational field.

melting point. The temperature at which a solid changes to a liquid.

melting. The transition of a solid to a liquid.

memory cell. A lymphocyte that responds to an antigen upon reintroduction.

Mendelian inheritance. Inheritance of traits that follow Gregor Mendel's two laws and the principle of dominance.

metal. A substance that is a good conductor of electricity and heat, forms cations by loss of electrons, and yields basic oxides and hydroxides.

meter. Metric unit of length.

monohybrid cross. A cross between two organisms with homozygous genotypes for a trait.

monomers. Molecules that can bond to similar or identical molecules to form a polymer.

mouth. The oral cavity at the entry to the alimentary canal.

muscle. Fibrous tissue that produces force and motion to move the body or produce movement in parts of the body.

nephron. The functional unit of the kidney responsible for filtering and reabsorbing various molecules.

nerve. A bundle of nerve fibers that transmits electrical impulses toward and away from the brain and spinal cord.

neutron. An atomic particle with no electric charge.

non-Mendelian inheritance. Inheritance of traits that do not follow Mendelian patterns of inheritance.

non-metal. Any element or substance that is not a metal.

nonpolar. A type of covalent bond in which two atoms share electrons at equal distances from their atomic nuclei.

nucleic acids. Long molecules made of nucleotides; DNA and RNA.

nucleotide. The monomer of DNA and RNA.

nucleus. A large organelle within a cell that houses the chromosomes.

orbital. An area around the nucleus where an electron can be found.

organ. A self-contained part of an organ system that performs a specific job and is composed of several tissue types organ systems. Functional groups of organs that work together within the body: circulatory, integumentary, skeletal, reproductive, digestive, urinary, respiratory, endocrine, lymphatic, muscular, and nervous.

organelle. A specialized part of a cell that has a specific function such as producing adenosine triphosphate (ATP).

organic molecule. A molecule found in a living thing that contains carbon.

osmosis. Passage of fluid through a membrane.

osteoarthritis. Degenerative joint disease in which the cartilage at joints is damaged from injury or by age.

osteoblasts. Cells that make bone.

SCIENCE

osteoclasts. Cells that break down the matrix to release minerals.

osteocytes. Mature bone cells.

osteons. Cylindrical structures that comprise compact bone.

osteoporosis. A disease that causes brittle, fragile bones.

ovary. Organ in which eggs are produced for reproduction.

pancreas. The gland of the digestive and endocrine systems that produces insulin and secretes pancreatic juices.

parathyroid. An endocrine gland in the neck that produces parathyroid hormone.

penis. Organ for elimination of urine and sperm from the male body.

perfusion. The passage of fluid to an organ or a tissue.

period. One of seven horizontal rows in the periodic tables.

periodic table. The table of elements expressed as columns and rows.

peristalsis. A series of muscle contractions that move food through the digestive tract.

pH. The measure of acidity or alkalinity.

phagocytosis. Ingestion of particles by a cell or phagocyte.

phase diagram. A graph of physical states of a substance under varying temperature and pressure.

phenotype. Physical appearance of a trait which is the expression of the genotype at both molecular and organism level.

phosphate group. A phosphorus atom bound to four oxygen atoms.

physical properties. Observable properties of matter.

pineal gland. A small gland near the center of the brain that secretes melatonin.

pituitary. The endocrine gland at the base of the brain that controls growth and development.

plasma cell. A white blood cell that produces a single type of antibody.

plasma. The pale yellow component of blood that carries red blood cells, white blood cells, and platelets throughout the body.

pleura. A membrane around the lungs and inside the chest cavity.

polar. A type of covalent bond in which two atoms share electrons that are not at equal distances from their atomic nuclei. If the geometry of the molecule does not equalize the partial charges created by the polar covalent bond, the region of partial charge remains unbalanced, and the molecule is considered polar.

polymer. A substance composed many similar units bonded together.

prostate. The gland in males that controls the release of urine and secretes a part of semen that enhances motility and fertility of sperm.

proteins. Molecules composed of amino acids joined by peptide bonds.

proton. A positively charged atomic particle.

recessive. Refers to traits that are masked if dominant alleles are also present; also refers to the allele for that trait.

rectum. The last section of the large intestine, ending with the anus.

reference planes. Invisible planes dividing the body to describe locations: sagittal, coronal, and transverse.

reflex. An involuntary action to a stimulus.

relaxation. Release of tension in a muscle.

renal arteries. The two branches of the abdominal aorta that supply the kidneys with oxygenated blood.

renal cortex. The outer layer of the kidney.

renal medulla. The innermost layer of the kidney.

renal pelvis. The center of the kidney where urine collects before moving to the ureter.

renal vein. A vein carrying deoxygenated blood from a kidney to the inferior vena cava.

renin. An enzyme released by the kidney when reduced blood pressure is detected by baroreceptors in aorta and carotid arteries.

rheumatoid arthritis. A progressive autoimmune disease that causes joint inflammation and pain.

saliva. The clear liquid found in the mouth, also known as spit.

salt. A chemical compound formed from the reaction of an acid with a base, with at least part of the hydrogen of the acid replaced by a cation.

scrotum. The pouch of skin that contains the testicles.

sequencing. Organization of cause-and-effect relationships.

SI units. Système Internationale (SI) or International System of units based on meters, kilograms, seconds, amperes, Kelvin, candela, and mole. Commonly known as the metric system.

skin. The thin layer of tissue that covers the body.

small intestine. The part of the gastrointestinal tract between the stomach and large intestine that includes the duodenum, jejunum, and ileum and where digestion and absorption of food occurs.

solid. A state of matter that retains its shape and density when not contained.

stomach. The organ between the esophagus and small intestine in which the major portion of digestion occurs.

subcutaneous. Under the dermis.

sublimation. The transition of a substance from solid to gas without passing through the liquid state.

surfactant. A fluid secreted by alveoli and found in the lungs that maintains surface tension.

sweat. Perspiration excreted by sweat glands through the skin.

synapse. The structure that allows neurons to pass signals to other neurons, muscles, or glands.

systole. The portion of the cardiac cycle in which the heart expels blood.

T cell. White blood cells that mature in the thymus and participate in immune response.

testes (testicles). The organs that produce sperm; also called "testes".

testosterone. The hormone that stimulates male secondary sexual characteristics.

thymus. The lymph organ where T cells mature.

thyroid gland. The gland in the neck that secretes hormones that regulate growth, development, and metabolic rate.

tidal volume. The amount of air breathed in a normal inhalation or exhalation.

tissue. A group of cells with similar structure that function together as a unit but at a lower level than organs.

trachea. The windpipe, which connects the throat to the lungs.

triple point. The temperature and pressure at which solid, liquid, and vapor phases of a pure substance coexist.

urea. The nitrogenous waste found in urine.

ureter. The duct that conducts urine from the kidney to the bladder.

urethra. The tube that connects the bladder to the exterior of the body.

urinary bladder. The structure that stores urine in the body until elimination.

urine. Liquid waste matter excreted by the kidneys.

uterus. The womb.

vagina. The tube that connects the external genitals to the cervix.

valence electron. An electron in an outer orbital that can form bonds with other atoms.

variable. An item or aspect of an item that changes.

vas deferens. The duct in which sperm moves from a testicle to the urethra.

vein. Blood vessels that carry blood to the heart.

ventilation. The movement of air in and out of the body via inhalation and exhalation.

volume. The amount of space taken up by an object.

volumetric pipette. A device used for precise measurement of small amounts of liquid.

voluntary. With intentional control.

SCIENCE

Practice problem answers

Chapter 35

1. Option A is correct. The ribosomes synthesize proteins in a cell. Mitochondria are responsible for energy production; cilia are responsible for movement; and vesicles store molecules.

2. Option B is correct. Mitochondria are involved in energy production. Ribosomes make proteins; the cytoskeleton gives form to a cell; and the cell membrane maintains what enters and leaves a cell.

3. Option A is correct. The nucleus is responsible for storing genetic information. Ribosomes are involved in making proteins; the cell membrane surrounds and protects the cell; and lysosomes are involved in the digestion and recycling of molecules.

4. Option B is correct. Superior refers to above on a human in anatomical position, which would make the trachea superior to the lungs. The stomach is inferior to the lungs; the diaphragm is inferior to the lungs; and the heart is medial to the lungs.

5. Option D is correct. Distal refers to farthest away. The thumb is farthest away from the shoulder of the body.

Chapter 36

1. Option D is correct. The diaphragm is a muscle that increases and decreases the volume in the lungs. The trachea and alveoli function in transporting air and gas exchange. The heart is part of the circulatory system.

2. Option B is correct. The thin walls decrease the distance between the air and bloodstream, increasing the rate of diffusion. Increasing the distance would decrease the rate of diffusion. Small and numerous alveoli increase the surface area, which increases the rate of diffusion.

3. Option C is correct. The respiratory system exchanges oxygen and carbon dioxide. Gas exchange affects the pH of blood, but that is not the primary role of the system. Transporting gases is a role of the circulatory system.

4. Option C is correct. Asthma constricts the airways. The other options are caused by pathogens that affect the respiratory system.

5. Option A is correct. Increasing the tidal volume will increase diffusion of carbon dioxide out of the bloodstream. Oxygen will increase in the bloodstream. Changing the tidal volume will not have a direct effect on heart rate or surfactant.

Chapter 37

1. Option C is correct. The heart is made up of four chambers, two atria and two ventricles.
   - Blood cells travel through the heart chambers.

2. Option A is correct. Red blood cells contain hemoglobin, which transports oxygen.
   - Plasma helps control body temperature and transport substances
   - Dissolved gases can be found in the blood but do not transport substances
   - Leukocytes are white blood cells that help guard against infection.

3. Option D is correct. The right ventricle pumps blood toward the lungs.
   - The left atrium accepts blood from the lungs.
   - The right atrium accepts blood from the body
   - The left ventricle pumps blood to the body

4. Option C is correct. Veins transport blood from the lungs or the body to the heart.
   - Veins can carry oxygenated or deoxygenated blood.

5. Ventricles use a large amount of pressure to push blood to different parts of the body. This puts quite a bit of force on these chambers.

Chapter 38

1. Option A is correct. Digestion begins in the mouth with mechanical and chemical digestion. The other organs play a role but do not start digestion.

2. Option B is correct. With the help of pepsin, protein starts to break down in the stomach.
   - The small intestine also breaks down proteins with the secretion of trypsin from the pancreas, but this is after the food passes through the stomach.

3. Option B is correct. Microvilli absorb nutrients in the small intestine.
   - Enzymes and hormones aid in digestion, but they do not absorb.

4. Option C is correct. Peristalsis refers to the muscle contractions that move food through the digestive tract.

5. Starch begins to breakdown in the mouth. Chewing breaks the molecules into smaller pieces. Amylase also speeds up the process of starches breaking down into smaller molecules. Muscle contractions in the stomach break down food particles into chyme. Then, in the small intestines, more enzymes released by the pancreas break down the starches into simple sugars.

Chapter 39

1. Option A is correct. Walking is controlled by voluntary nerve signals.

    • Breathing, digestion, and heartbeats are controlled by the autonomic nervous system

2. Option C is correct. Synapses allow for the passing of signals to another nerve cell or a muscle cell.

    • Axons are structures that carry nerve impulses away from nerve body.
    • Synapses are just one part of a nerve cell

3. Option A is correct. Skeletal muscles are often voluntary.

    • Smooth and cardiac muscles are often involuntary and control things like heartbeats, breathing, and digestion

4. Option C is correct. Sensory nerves send messages to the brain.

    • Skeletal and smooth refer to types of muscles and not nerves.
    • Motor nerves send messages form the brain to the muscles

5. Sensory nerves send a message to the central nervous system from the hand. Then, motor nerves send a signal to the muscles of the arm to contract.

Chapter 40

1. Option A is correct. Ovaries produce the female gamete (eggs).

    • Testes produce male gametes (sperm)
    • The prostate and uterus are important reproductive structures, but they do not produce gametes.

2. Option D is correct. Sperm is released into the vagina and travels into the uterus and Fallopian tubes. If an egg is present, there is a good chance it will be fertilized by a sperm cell.

    • The vagina is where sperm are release by the penis during sexual intercourse, but it then travels to the uterus and Fallopian tubes.
    • Vas deferens are found only in the male reproductive system.

3. Option B is correct. Estrogen is a hormone that plays a role in egg maturation.

    • Estrogen does not play a role in the male production of sperm cells.
    • Luteinizing hormone plays a role in the release of an egg from an ovary.
    • Fertilization is the fusion of an egg and a sperm cell.

4. Option A is correct. Hormones released during puberty do not lead to bone growth.

    • Hormones released during puberty lead to egg production in females and sperm production in males.
    • Puberty hormones lead to secondary sexual characteristics such as facial hair in men.

5. Male gametes, or sperm, are produced by the testes, whereas female gametes, or eggs, are produced by the ovaries. Sperm are constantly produced, but eggs are developed and matured cyclically. Eggs are typically released one at a time, but many sperm can be released at once during ejaculation.

Chapter 41

1. Option D is correct. The epidermis is the outermost layer that forms a barrier of protection.

    • The dermis is the middle layer of the skin.
    • Sebaceous and sudoriferous refer to glands found in the skin

2. Option B is correct. Melanocytes produce melanin that protects the body from ultraviolet radiation.

    • Secretion occurs in the glands of the skin

3. Option A is correct. Hair follicles are found in the middle layer of skin, the dermis.

    • Sebaceous and sudoriferous glands are also found in the dermis but are not layers of skin.
    • The epidermis is above the dermis and does not contain hair follicles.

SCIENCE

4. Option D is correct. The epidermis has an outer layer of dead cells.

   - The dermis and hypodermis are layers of skin, but they do not form layers of dead cells like the epidermis.
   - Blood vessels are found in skin but do not make up layers of the skin.

5. If the body gets too hot, the integumentary system uses thermoregulation strategies to cool it off. Sweat is produced by the sebaceous glands. As the water in sweat evaporates, the skin is cooled. Blood vessels also dilate and move closer to the skin surface to try and cool off.

Chapter 42

1. Option B is correct. Chemical signals travel through the bloodstream.

   - Electrical signals are part of the nervous system.
   - Physical, audio, and visual signals are received by the nervous system.

2. Option A is correct. The hypothalamus is the endocrine-nervous system integration. It secretes both releasing and inhibiting hormones, which are sent to the pituitary gland.

   - The pituitary secretes a number of hormones sent to other cells.
   - The pancreas secretes hormones to control glucose levels.
   - The liver is not an endocrine gland and is an accessory organ of the digestive system.

3. Option B is correct. The pineal gland secretes melatonin, which helps regulate the body's sleep cycle.

   - Growth hormone is secreted by the pituitary gland.
   - Insulin and glucagon are secreted by the pancreas.
   - Luteinizing hormone is released by the pituitary gland.

4. Option B is correct. The adrenal glands release epinephrine.

   - Although the other glands listed release hormones, only the adrenal gland secretes epinephrine.

5. After eating food, blood glucose levels rise. The pancreas responds by releasing insulin, which promotes glucose being taken up by cells. This leads to a decrease in blood glucose level because glucose leaves the bloodstream and enters the cell.

Chapter 43

1. Option B is correct. The urethra is a tube that empties the bladder. It also transports sperm in males.

   - The ureter is the connecting tubule from the kidney to the bladder.
   - The uterus is a female reproductive structure.
   - The urinary bladder stores urine before it is excreted.

2. Option A is correct. Nitrogen in the form of urea in the urine results from the metabolism of proteins.

   - Sodium chloride levels are regulated, but they do not result from digestion.
   - Protein is not a waste product.
   - Carbon is not a waste product.

3. Option B is correct. Without kidneys that function properly, the human body would not be able to filter out waste in the blood.

   - The capillaries in the lungs, and not in the kidneys, remove carbon dioxide from the blood.
   - Kidneys do not fill with urine. Waste is transported from the kidneys to the bladder.
   - Without functional kidneys, urea would not be produced. Therefore, urine production would not increase.

4. Option C is correct. The nephron is the microscopic tubule system that filters and reabsorbs.

   - Renal capillaries absorb and reabsorb molecules but are not the functional unit.
   - The glomerulus is a part of the nephron.
   - The cortex is the layer where part of the nephron is located.

5. Renin is a hormone that is released by the kidneys and helps to regulate blood pressure.

Chapter 44

1. Option B is correct. Mucus can trap pathogens entering an opening in the body such as in the nasal cavity.

   - Histamines, T cells, and macrophages play roles in the immune response once pathogens have invaded the body.

2. Option B is correct. Histamines are released to stimulate blood flow to the area of the cut, allowing white blood cells to infiltrate the area.

   - Although vaccination, antigens, and T cells are important parts of the immune system, they are not the response to a cut.

3. Option B is correct. Plasma cells produce and release antibodies.

   - T cells, memory cells, and macrophages are all types of white blood cells. Their function is not to produce and release antibodies.

4. Option C is correct. Vaccinations allow the body to recognize and produce antibodies to use in the case of future infection by that pathogen.

   - Vaccinations are not administered to produce an inflammatory response.
   - Vaccinations are active, and not passive, immunity.
   - Vaccinations do not increase macrophage production.

5. Allergies are caused by a substance that enters the body and triggers an immune response even when there is not an invading pathogen. The substance causing the allergy triggers histamine to be released, which can cause sneezing and mucus secretion.

Chapter 45

1. Option A is correct. Osteoclasts break down bone material.

   - Osteoblasts build up bone material.
   - Canaliculi are channels in the matrix.
   - Osteocytes are mature bone cells.

2. Option C is correct. Carpals and tarsals are examples of short bones. They have the same length and width.

   - Skull bones are either irregular or flat bones.
   - Humerus, radius, and ulna are long bones.
   - Scapula is a flat bone.

3. Option D is correct. The covering at the end of long bones where joints form needs hyaline cartilage to reduce the friction of movement.

   - The matrix forms from osteoblasts.
   - Cartilage does not become bone, although it is important in the formation of such.
   - Collagen strengthens the skeletal system.

4. Option C is correct. More bone is being broken down than is being built up, causing bones to weaken and become brittle. Osteoclasts break down bone faster than osteoblasts deposit minerals.

   - Osteoporosis is not caused by pathogens or ligament degradation.

5. The bones of the skeleton connect to the skeletal muscles with a connective tissue known as a "tendon." When the muscle contracts, it shortens, pulling the bone it is connected to.

Chapter 46

1. Option A is correct. Glucose is a carbohydrate monomer.

   - Lipids do not have true monomers but can be made up of fatty acids.
   - Proteins are made up of monomers called "amino acids."
   - Nucleic acids are made up of monomers known as "nucleotides."

2. Option D is correct. Nucleic acids known as "DNA" store copies of genetic information.

   - Carbohydrates perform many functions such as storing sugar (starch) and providing structural support (cellulose).
   - Lipids store energy and can serve as chemical messengers.
   - Proteins have many functions, including controlling the rate of reactions (enzymes), regulating cell processes, and building important cell structures.

3. Option B is correct. Enzymes are proteins, so they are made up of amino acids.

   - Glucose and fructose are carbohydrate monomers.
   - Nucleotides are nucleic acid monomers.
   - Fatty acids are found in lipids.

4. Option B is correct. Oil is made up of lipids.

   - Potatoes are full of starch, which is a carbohydrate.
   - Chicken contains protein.
   - Lettuce is mostly a carbohydrate known as "cellulose."

5. Briefly describe a function of each macromolecule.

   - Macromolecules perform different functions for living things. Carbohydrates are used as a source of energy and for structural purposes.
   - Lipids can store energy and are used as chemical messengers.
   - Nucleic acids store genetic information and help transmit information needed to make proteins.
   - Proteins form many body structures, form enzymes used in metabolism, provide immunity, form cell membrane transport channels, and can even be used as an energy source.

SCIENCE

Chapter 47

1. Option D is correct. Adenine pairs with thymine.

   - Cytosine pairs with guanine.
   - Adenine does not pair with itself.

2. Option C is correct. Humans have 23 pairs of chromosomes.

3. Option C is correct. Nucleotides form strings of DNA that make up genes. Genes make up chromosomes.

   - Nucleotides are the smallest unit.
   - Chromosomes are made up of many genes.

4. Option B is correct. A gene codes for a protein.

5. Genes are segments of DNA that can code for specific proteins. Genes made of DNA are located on larger structures called "chromosomes."

Chapter 48

1. Option A is correct. Capital letters are used for dominant alleles.

   - Homozygous genotypes have two of the same alleles.
   - Ww is heterozygous.
   - ww is homozygous recessive.
   - WX is not a Mendelian configuration.

2. Option D is correct.

   - Performing a Punnett square will reveal that three out of four genotypes will result in green seed phenotypes.

3. Option C is correct. Phenotypes are the expressed traits for a trait.

   - Inheritable is used to describe traits that are passed down from one generation to the next.
   - Genotypes are the two alleles an individual have for a particular trait.
   - P generation is used to define the parent generation in a Mendelian cross.

4. Option C is correct. Monohybrid crosses between heterozygous individuals will result in a 3:1 ratio of phenotypes.

   - Traits must be inheritable and follow the Law of Independent Assortment, which states that traits are inherited randomly.
   - Each trait has one dominant and one recessive allele. If this is not the case, the traits follow non-Mendelian inheritance patterns.

5. The offspring would be 75% tall and 25% dwarf. Heterozygous crosses result in a 3:1 phenotype ratio.

Chapter 49

1. Option A is correct. To determine the type of atom, use the number of protons to determine the atomic number and then find it on the periodic table.

   - Sodium has an atomic number of 11, but that is the number of neutrons in this atom.
   - Calcium has 20 protons.
   - Boron has 5 protons.

2. Option C is correct. The atomic mass is determined by adding the protons and neutrons. Because all carbon atoms have six protons, the number of neutrons must have changed.

   - The charge of an atom will help determine the number of electrons.
   - If the number of protons increased or decreased, the atom would no longer by carbon.

3. Option A is correct. Calcium will give away the two electrons to have a full valence shell.

   - Gaining two electrons will give calcium a valence shell of four. It needs eight to fill it.
   - Changing the protons will not affect the valence shell but would turn calcium into another element.
   - Although gaining six electrons would fill the valence shell, it is easier for calcium to lose two than gain six electrons.

4. Option B is correct. This ion of oxygen has 8 protons and 10 electrons, giving it a charge of –2.

   - Negatively charged ions are called "anions."
   - Use oxygens atomic number to determine the number of protons.

5.

Element Name	Element Symbol	Proton number	Neutron number	Electron number	Atomic number	Atomic mass (amu)
Hydrogen	H	1	0	1	1	1
Nitrogen	N	7	7	7	7	14
Platinum	Pt	78	117	78	78	195
Chlorine	Cl	17	18	17	17	35
Potassium	K	19	20	19	19	39
Helium	He	2	2	2	2	4

Chapter 50

1. Option C is correct. This is the correct ratio of mass to volume: 22.5 divided by 5.

    - Option A is the inverse of density: 5 divided by 22.5.
    - Option B is 22.5 divided by (5 × 3). This is a common error in reading the unit cubed.
    - Option D is 22.5 added—not divided—5.

2. Option B is correct.

    - A chemical property changes the identify of a substance; rust is no longer iron.

3. Option B is correct. Diffusion is the movement of molecules from a region of high concentration to a region of low concentration.

    - Option A does not describe diffusion; it does not change the state of matter.
    - Option C is incorrect because diffusion takes place passively.
    - Option D is incorrect because diffusion is not specific to water; osmosis is specific to the movement of water.

4. Option C is correct.

    - During osmosis, water moves from areas of high concentration to low concentration.
    - Because there are large concentrations of sodium dissolved in water inside the cell, the concentration of water would be lower inside the cell.

5. Density is the ratio mass to volume of a substance. Liquid water has more mass per unit of volume than ice. Because it has more mass, it is denser. The substance with greater density will sink compared to substances that are less dense.

Chapter 51

1. Option C is correct. Freezing is a phase change from liquid to solid as a result of the loss of heat.

    - Melting is a phase change from solid to liquid that requires heat.
    - Evaporation is a phase change from liquid to gas that requires heat.
    - Sublimation is a phase change from solid to gas that requires heat.

2. Option B is correct.

    - Solids have a definite shape and volume.
    - Liquids have no definite shape but definite volume.
    - Gas has no definite shape or volume.
    - No state of matter has a definite shape and no definite volume.

3. Option C is correct. Decreasing the pressure of a liquid would decrease the boiling point.

    - An increase in intramolecular forces would be seen in a change from liquid to solid, which would not seen by decreasing the pressure.
    - Increasing the pressure would lead to an increasing in temperature.

4. Option B is correct. If the temperature is raised above the triple point, the substance can only exist as a liquid and gas.

5. The solid pieces of ice will absorb energy from the hot environment. As heat is added, the forces holding the water molecules together will break, and the water molecules will separate from one another.
    As this happens, the solid ice will lose its shape and turn into water as the molecules move away from one another. As more heat is absorbed, the water molecules will move even more rapidly and spreading further apart as the water evaporates into gas.

SCIENCE

Chapter 52

1. Option D is correct. There is a metal and a non-metal.

   - In the other options, both elements are non-metals, making them covalent bonds.

2. Option B is correct. A double-replacement reaction involves the replacement of two substances. In this example, silver (Ag) and sodium (Na) are taking the place of one another.

   - Combustion involves oxygen and the products water and carbon dioxide; none are found in this equation.
   - A single-replacement reaction would only have one replacement.
   - Decomposition would show products that are broken down.

3. Option B is correct. Acids have a pH lower than 7.

   - Although substances with a pH lower than 2 are all acids, not all these substances are that strong of an acid.
   - Substances with a pH of 7 are neutral.
   - Substances with a pH above 7 are bases.

4. Option C is correct. Decreasing the pressure would decrease the rate of collisions between substances, decreasing the rate of reaction.

   - Adding temperature to an endothermic reaction or enzymes would increase the reaction rate.
   - Less substrate slows reactions because there is less of a reactant to interact with.

5. $2AgCl \rightarrow 2Ag + 2Cl_2$

Chapter 53

1. Option C is correct; 1.5 meters would be the correct height for an adult human.

   - The width of a fingernail is 1.5 mm, which is quite small.
   - The width of a small insect is 1.5 cm, which is also quite small.
   - A measurement of 1.5 km is quite large; 1500 meters is taller than most buildings.

2. Option A is correct.

   - Option B is hecta.
   - Option C is centi.
   - Option D is milli.

3. Option B is correct.

   - Triple-beam balances measure mass.
   - Graduated cylinders measure volume.
   - Rulers measure length.

4. Option D is correct.

   - To find the mass, multiple the length, width, and height.
   - Option A adds the values instead of multiplies.
   - Options B and C do not have the correct unit.

5. The student who measured 200 cm is incorrect; 2 m is about the height of a door, which would be way too small for the width of an entire building.

Chapter 54

1. Option A is correct. All three patients reduced their pain levels after taking the medication.

   - Because patients reported a decrease in pain levels, there is no evidence that the pain medicine does not affect pain levels.
   - The size of the dose was not tested in this experiment.
   - The time the medicine was given was not done in this experiment.

2. Option C is correct.

   - All patients received the medicine at the same time.
   - All patients, except Patient 4, had similar starting pain levels.
   - There is no indication that the experimenter followed the same directions each time, although this would have been useful in setting up a controlled experiment.

3. Option D is correct. Keeping conditions the same is a control variable.

   - The independent variable is the medication.
   - The dependent variable is the pain rating.
   - The data in the experiment is provided in the table.

4. Option C is correct. Increasing the sample size would strengthen the data set.

   - Option A and Option B are ways to test other variables.
   - Option D would weaken the data because there would not be a group to compare with.

5. If the placebo group rated similar losses of pain as those who received the medicine, it would support the conclusion that he medicine does not have an affect on pain levels.

Chapter 55

1. Option B is correct.

   - Centimeters and millimetres are too small to measure the giraffe.
   - Kilometers are too big to measure the giraffe.

2. Option A is correct.

   - Meters and kilometers measure the length of the coin.
   - Kilograms are too large to measure a coin.

3. Option D is correct. Low levels of glucose lead to the release of glucagon, which breaks down glucose.

   - High levels of insulin lead to the glucose being absorbed by cells.
   - High levels of glucose lead to the release of insulin.

4. Option B is correct. The amount of mold growth is the dependent variable. This variable should be measured to determine the is an effect of the new antimold product.

   - The amount of antimold product is the independent variable. This is the variable being changed to determine whether it has an effect on mold growth.
   - Humidity and temperature are control variables. These should be kept the same so that the independent variable is the only aspect being changed.

5. As the cells in the human body release carbon dioxide, the concentration of carbon dioxide rises in the blood. This causes breathing and heart rate to increase. The rise in both of these processes allow more carbon dioxide to diffuse into the lungs and be exhaled, decreasing the carbon dioxide levels in the blood.

Chapter 56

1. Option D is correct.

   - The ripeness is the independent variable.
   - Options B and C are variables, but they are controlled in the experiment.

2. Option B is correct.

   - Options A, C, and D will not be supported or refuted by this experiment.

3. Option A is correct. The light is what the experimenter is manipulating.

   - Option B is the dependent variable.
   - Option C is a controlled variable.
   - Option D is not part of the experiment.

4. Option C is correct. Soil conditions may affect the outcome; therefore, they should be controlled.

   - Option A is the independent variable.
   - Option B is the dependent variable.

5. If plants are grown in blue or red light, they will grow at faster rates than those grown in green or yellow light.

SCIENCE

✅ Unit Quiz

1. Which of the following cell structures contain cristae?
   A. DNA
   B. Smooth endoplasmic reticulum
   C. Mitochondria
   D. Peroxisomes

2. Which of the following terms is used to describe the amount of air in a normal inhalation or exhalation?
   A. Perfusion
   B. Tidal volume
   C. Ventilation
   D. Residual volume

3. Which of the following blood vessels carries deoxygenated blood from the heart to the lungs?
   A. Pulmonary vein
   B. Pulmonary artery
   C. Aorta
   D. Vena Cava

4. Which of the following terms refers to the partially digested food leaving the stomach?
   A. Chyme
   B. Pepsin
   C. Bolus
   D. Lactase

5. In which of the following actions is the autonomic nervous system engaged?
   A. Lifting weights
   B. Holding your breath
   C. Walking
   D. Digestion

6. Which of the following is classified as a carbohydrate?
   A. DNA
   B. Endorphin
   C. Glycogen
   D. Amylase

7. Which of the following best describes the relationship between a chomosome and a gene?
   A. Each gene forms its own chromosome.
   B. Each chromosome contains a single gene.
   C. Each gene contains a specific number of chromosomes.
   D. Each chromosome contains a specific number of genes.

8. A purple-flowered pea plant and a white-flowered pea plant were crossed. The allele for purple flowers is dominant, and the allele for white flowers is recessive. Of 1,000 offspring, 498 were purple-flowered pea plants, and 502 were white-flowered peas plants.

   Based on these results, which of the following can be concluded about the parent plants?
   A. The white-flowered pea plant is homozygous dominant.
   B. The white-flowered pea plant is heterozygous.
   C. The purple-flowered pea plant is heterozygous.
   D. The purple-flowered pea plant is homozygous dominant.

9. Which of the following instruments would most accurately measure 0.1 mL of a liquid?
   A. A 50-mL beaker
   B. A micropipette
   C. A graduated cylinder
   D. An Erlenmeyer flask

10. Joseph and Demarius conducted an experiment on the activity of an enzyme. They tested whether the enzyme activity changed at different temperatures from 10° to 60° C.

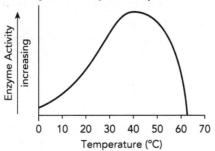

Enzyme Activity vs. Temperature

Based on the graph, which of the following best describes the relationship between enzyme activity and temperature?

A. Enzyme activity is greatest at temperatures below 30° C.
B. Enzyme activity decreases between 20° and 30° C.
C. Enzyme activity is unaffected by temperature changes.
D. Enzyme activity is greatest at 40° C.

11. Which of the following describes the function of the plasma membrane?

A. It provides energy to the cell.
B. It helps to builds proteins.
C. It maintains the cell's internal environment.
D. It produces adenosine triphosphate (ATP) for cells.

12. Which of the following structures is medial to the large intestine?

The Digestive System

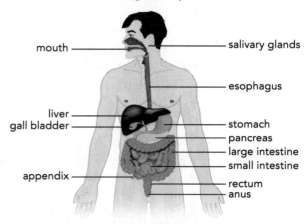

A. Stomach
B. Pancreas
C. Liver
D. Small intestine

13. During inhalation, where would you expect to find a higher concentration of oxygen?

A. In the capillaries
B. In the alveolar air space
C. In the pulmonary artery
D. In the heart

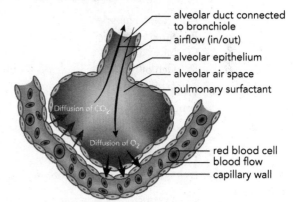

14. Which structure connects the throat to the lungs?

A. Alveoli
B. Trachea
C. Bronchi
D. Surfactant

SCIENCE

15. Where does blood flow next after being oxygenated in the lungs?

    A. Pulmonary artery
    B. Pulmonary vein
    C. Inferior vena cava
    D. Aorta

16. Which type cell helps protect against disease?

    A. Hemoglobin
    B. Stem
    C. Erythocyte
    D. Leukocyte

17. What is the name of the structure that releases an enzyme that breaks down starch in the mouth?

    A. Salivary gland
    B. Pancreas
    C. Liver
    D. Gallbladder

18. Molecules are broken down into smaller pieces by the churning of muscles in the stomach. Which of the following is this an example of?

    A. Mechanical digestion
    B. Chemical digestion
    C. Enzymatic digestion
    D. Peristalsis

19. Which type of tissue would you find in the heart?

    A. Skeletal muscles
    B. Striated muscle
    C. Smooth muscles
    D. Cardiac muscles

20. What proteins are responsible for the contraction of a muscle?

    A. Actin and myosin
    B. Synapse and axon
    C. Peptin and tripsin
    D. Testosterone and estrogen

21. Which structure is where female gametes are produced?

    A. Cervix
    B. Ovary
    C. Fallopian tube
    D. Uterus

22. According to the graph, which of the following identifies when fertilization is most likely?

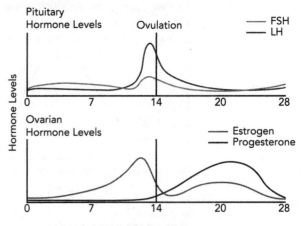

    A. Between day 0 and 7
    B. After luteinzing hormone (LH) levels peak and begin to decline
    C. Before ovulation
    D. When estrogen levels are highest

23. What is the name for the hormone responsible for male secondary sex characteristics?

    A. Luteinizing hormone
    B. Estrogen
    C. Testosterone
    D. Follicle-stimulating hormone

24. A cut reaches the sebaceous glands and hair follicles. This cut has reached which layer(s) of the skin?

    A. Epidermis only
    B. Epidermis and dermis
    C. Hypodermis and dermis
    D. Hypodermis and epidermis

25. Which of the following would result from a decrease in body temperature?

    A. Blood vessels near the surface of the body would dilate.
    B. Blood vessels near the surface of the body would constrict.
    C. Sebaceous glands would excrete water.
    D. Cheeks would become more flush.

26. Which of the following is where melanocytes are found?

    A. Epidermis
    B. Dermis
    C. Hypodermis
    D. Sebaceous glands

27. Which of the following parts of the endocrine system can be found in the brain?

    A. Hypothalamus
    B. Parathyroid
    C. Adrenal
    D. Pancreas

28. Which of the following is a result of the adrenal gland releasing epinephrine into the blood?

    A. Weight gain
    B. Increased muscle growth
    C. Breakdown of glycogen
    D. Increase in heart rate

29. Which of the following structures releases insulin and glucagon?

    A. Adrenal
    B. Hypothalamus
    C. Pancreas
    D. Pituitary

30. Which of the following structures stores waste before it is released from the body?

    A. Kidney
    B. Urethra
    C. Ureters
    D. Urinary bladder

31. Which of the following substances describes the fluid that contains urea, water, and salts that is released through the urethra?

    A. Urine
    B. Filtrate
    C. Blood
    D. Nephron

32. Which of the following parts of the genitourinary system regulates blood pressure?

    A. Ureter
    B. Renin
    C. Bladder sphincters
    D. Heart

33. Which of the following is a nonspecific barrier of the immune system?

    A. Mucus
    B. Antibodies
    C. Interferons
    D. B cells

34. Which of the following diseases is caused by a virus that infects T cells?

    A. Allergies
    B. Asthma
    C. Autoimmune
    D. Acquired immune deficiency syndrome (AIDS)

35. In which of the following body structures are white blood cells produced?

    A. Muscle
    B. Bone
    C. Glands
    D. Skin

36. Which of the following functions is an example of how the skeletal and neuromuscular system work together?

    A. Body movement
    B. Organ protection
    C. Pathogen protection
    D. Calcium storage

37. Which of the following is an example of a long bone?

    A. Tibia
    B. Rib
    C. Skull
    D. Pelvis

38. Which of the following statements best describes the subatomic particles that make up an atom?

    A. Protons and electrons are about the same size and are found in the nucleus.
    B. Protons and neutrons have about the same mass and can be found in the nucleus.
    C. Electrons are found in the nucleus and make up most of the mass of an atom.
    D. Protons are the only particles with mass and can be found in the nucleus.

SCIENCE

39. The diagram shows two substances contained in equal size containers. Which of the following statements best explains the density of the substances?

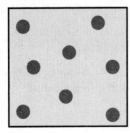 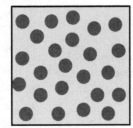

   A. Both substances have equal densities because they have equal volumes.
   B. The first substance is less dense because it has more volume and less mass.
   C. The first substance is less dense because it has less mass in the same amount of volume.
   D. The first substance is denser because it has less mass in the same amount of space.

40. A substance in a solid state is put on a hot plate with a thermometer. Every minute, the temperature of the substance is recorded. According the graph, what is happening to the substance?

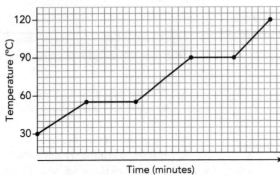

   A. As heat is added, the substance is becoming more and more dense.
   B. As heat is added, the particles holding the substance together are becoming stronger.
   C. As heat is added, the forces holding the particles together are breaking, changing the state.
   D. As heat is added, the substances is maintaining room temperature by absorbing the energy.

41. Which of the following is an example of an ionic compound?
   A. NaCl
   B. CO
   C. $C_6H_{12}O_6$
   D. H_2O

42. This chemical reaction equation is an example of what type of reaction?

   $H_2 + 2O \rightarrow H_2O$

   A. Synthesis
   B. Decomposition
   C. Single displacement
   D. Double displacement

43. What tool and unit would be used to find the volume of a brick?
   A. Ruler and cm^3
   B. Ruler and m^3
   C. Balance and g
   D. Graduated cylinder and mL

An experiment is conducted to test the effects of caffeine on heart rate. Four trials are set up. In each trial, a daphnia, a small water organism, is given different amounts of caffeine. After 5 minutes, the number of heart beats are counted for 1 minute. The results are shown in the table.

Amount of caffeine	Number of heart beats per minute
0 mg	180
0.5 mg	195
1 mg	207
1.5 mg	217
2 mg	0

44. Which of the following explanations states a logical cause and effect of caffeine on the heart beats of daphnia?
   A. Daphnia need caffeine to pump blood throughout their body.
   B. Caffeine causes daphnia to lower their heart rates over time.
   C. Caffeine does not affect daphnia's heart rate.
   D. Daphnia given too much caffeine may die.

45. Based on the data, daphnia that are given too much caffeine may die. Which of the following experimental practices would strengthen the conclusion made about daphnia and caffeine?

    A. The experimenter should test the experiment with other substances besides caffeine.
    B. The experimenter should test the experiment using different organisms.
    C. The experimenter should test each condition more than once.
    D. The experimenter should collect data after 10 minutes instead of 5 minutes.

46. Which of the following is the dependent variable in this experiment?

    A. Length of time measuring heart beats
    B. Amount of caffeine
    C. Number of heart beats
    D. Type of organism

47. Which of the following hypotheses is supported by the data?

    A. All organisms increase their heart beats when given caffeine.
    B. Organisms decrease their heart beats when exposed to caffeine.
    C. When given caffeine, daphnia increase their heart rate.
    D. When given caffeine, daphnia decrease their heart rate.

Unit Quiz Answers

1. Option C is correct. Cristae are the internal, folded membranes of mitochondria where cellular respiration occurs. DNA is a molecule composed of two chains of nucleotides that coil around each other to form a double helix. The smooth endoplasmic reticulum is a series of membranes used in processing cell products such as lipids. Peroxisomes have a single membrane that surrounds the digestive enzymes, which detoxify harmful cell waste products.

2. Option B is correct. Tidal volume is the amount of air in a normal inhalation or exhalation. Perfusion is the movement of fluid to a tissue. Ventilation is a synonym for breathing in any capacity. Residual volume is the amount of air that remains in the alveoli after exhalation.

3. Option B is correct. The pulmonary artery is part of the pulmonary circulation. The pulmonary artery carries deoxygenated blood from the right ventricle, divides into the right and left pulmonary arteries, and delivers deoxygenated blood to the right and left lung. The pulmonary vein brings oxygenated blood from the lungs to the left atrium of the heart. The aorta carries oxygenated blood from the left ventricle to all parts of the body. The vena cava is the large systemic vein bringing deoxygenated blood back to the right atrium of the heart.

4. Option A is correct. Chyme forms after the stomach has churned and mixed the bolus with the stomach's digestive enzymes. Pepsin is a stomach enzyme that starts protein digestion. The bolus is the food mass that forms in the mouth after chewing and mixing food with saliva. Lactase is a pancreatic enzyme that the pancreas secretes.

5. Option D is correct. Digestion is an involuntary action that the autonomic nervous system controls. Lifting weights, holding your breath, and walking are examples of voluntary actions, which are controlled by the somatic nervous system.

6. The correct option is C. Glycogen is a storage form of carbohydrates in animals. Glycogen is found in the liver and in muscles of humans and is used for energy production. DNA is classified is a nucleic acid. Endorphins are neurotransmitters secreted by neurons and amylase is a protein enzyme which breaks down carbohydrates.

7. Option D is correct. An individual chromosome is where specific sequences of DNA called "genes" are found. DNA is the foundational material found in genes and, therefore, in chromosomes.

8. Option C is correct. In Mendelian genetics, homozygous means two of the same allele, and heterozygous means different alleles. A dominant phenotype can be either homozygous or heterozygous. If the purple-flowered plant had been homozygous, the dominant allele would have been expressed in all the offspring, resulting in 1,000 purple-flowered pea plants. For there to be any homozygous recessive white-flowered pea plants, the purple-flowered plant had to contribute a recessive allele.

9. Option B is correct. A micropipette is used to measure extremely small amounts of liquids, starting at 1 microliter. Even a 50-mL beaker is inaccurate for this small amount of liquid because the gradations on this beaker are between 5 and 10 mL. The gradations or marked lines on any size of graduated cylinder or Erlenmeyer

10. Option D is correct. The y-axis indicates enzyme activity, and the highest plot on the y-axis occurs at 40°C. The activity between 20° and 30°C is increasing and not decreasing. The graph shows that enzyme activity changes as temperature changes. flask would also be too large to measure this small amount of liquid accurately.

11. Option C is correct. The plasma membrane is a semipermeable layer that allows only some substances to enter and exit the cell. In this role, it maintains the internal environment of the cell.

12. Option D is correct. Medial refers to structures closer to the medial line of the human body. The small intestine is closer to this line than the large intestine. The stomach, pancreas, and liver are above the large intestine.

13. Option B is correct. During inhalation, the lungs fill with oxygenated air from the environment. The blood in the capillaries will have a low level of oxygen because they just returned from the body. The pulmonary artery and the heart are not directly affected by inhalation.

14. Option B is correct. The trachea is the tubelike structure that connects the throat to the lungs. The primary function is to allow air to enter and exit the lungs. Alveoli are found in the lungs and are small air sacs. Bronchi are the main passageways from the trachea to the other branches of the lungs. Surfactant is a fluid secreted by the alveoli.

15. Option B is correct. The pulmonary vein carries blood back from the lungs. Because the blood recently visited the lungs, it is now oxygenated. The pulmonary artery carries blood to the lungs. The inferior vena cava carries blood back to the heart from the lower part of the body. The aorta carries oxygenated blood to the body after it returns to the heart.

16. Option D is correct. Leukocytes, or white blood cells, help defend the body against disease. Red blood cells transport substances through the blood vessels. Stem cells are cells that generate new types of cells. Hemoglobin is not a cell but a protein found in red blood cells that carries oxygen.

17. Option A is correct. The salivary glands secrete amylase, an enzyme that breaks down starch. The other structures are related to digestion, but they produce or release enzymes that are used in other parts of the gastrointestinal system. For example, another enzyme is lipase, which breaks down fat and is produced in the pancreas.

18. Option A is correct. Mechanical digestion describes the breakdown of food molecules into smaller pieces. Chemical digestion involves breakdown food molecules into simpler molecules. Enzymes are used to speed up chemical digestion. Although peristalsis refers to muscle contractions, these contractions move food down the digestive track and do not further the break down of molecules.

19. Option D is correct. The term "cardiac" refers to the heart. The heart is made up of muscle and connective tissue. The muscle found in the heart is known as "cardiac muscle" and contracts involuntary. When it contracts, it pushes blood throughout the body.

20. Option A is correct. Actin and myosin are proteins found in the sarcomere of muscles. As they move past one another, they create a contraction of the muscle. The synapse and axon are structures found in a nerve cell and not a muscle cell. Peptin and tripsin are both proteins, but they are used in the digestive system to speed up digestion. Testosterone and estrogen are hormones important in the reproductive system.

21. Option B is correct. The ovary is the female structure where eggs, the female gamete, are produced and matured. Once released, they travel through the Fallopian tube and travel to the uterus. The cervix is the narrow passage in the lower end of the uterus.

22. Option B is correct. Luteinizing hormone (LH) levels peak right before ovulation, or the release of a mature egg. After ovulation, LH levels begin to decline. Because ovulation happens, an egg will be in the Fallopian tubes and able to be fertilized if sperm are present. Before ovulation (days 0 to 14), there will not be a mature egg in the Fallopian tubes to be fertilized. Estrogen levels are highest before ovulation, so this answer is incorrect.

23. Option C is correct. Testosterone signals tissues in the body to develop secondary sex characteristics like facial hair and growth of muscles. Although luteinizing hormone, estrogen, and follicle-stimulating hormone send important signals related to the reproductive system, they are not responsible for the development of these characteristics.

24. Option B is correct. Sebaceous glands and hair follicles are found in the dermis layer of the skin. This is the middle layer of the skin, beneath the epidermis. Therefore, the cut must have broke the epidermis and dermis. The cut would not break the hypodermis, the inner layer of skin, without breaking the other two layers.

25. Option B is correct. To prevent heat from leaving through the surface of the skin, blood vessels constrict so that less blood is carried to the surface of the skin. The other responses are what happens when the body temperature rises. Blood vessels dilate, causing flush cheeks, to allow blood to release heat through the skin. Sebaceous glands excrete water. When the water evaporates it has a cooling effect.

26. Option A is correct. Melanocytes are found in the upper layer of skin, the epidermis. These cells release melanin, which helps protect cells below. Melanocytes are not found in lower layers of skin like the dermis and hypodermis. The sebaceous glands excrete waste and do not hold cells.

27. Option A is correct. The hypothalamus, along with the pineal and pituitary gland, are found in the brain and release hormones when signaled by the brain. The other glands also release hormones but are found in various regions of the body. The parathyroid is found in the neck, and the adrenal and pancreas are found in the abdomen.

28. Option D is correct. Epinephrine is released by the adrenal gland during stress and causes an increase in heart rate, blood pressure, muscle strength, and metabolism. Although the other answers can be results of other hormone activity, they are not results in the release of epinephrine.

29. Option C is correct. The pancreas releases insulin when signaled and glycogen to regulate blood sugar. These two substances help regulate the amount of sugar in the bloodstream. The hypothalamus, adrenal, and pituitary regulate other body functions but not blood sugar.

30. Option D is correct. The urinary bladder is a sac that stores waste collected by the kidneys. It is stored here until it is excreted form the body through the urethra. The kidney filters the blood and sends waste through the ureters to the bladder.

31. Option A is correct. Urine is the name for the fluid secreted by the urinary bladder. It contains substances that the body needs to get rid of. Filtrate is a material filtered out of the blood in the nephrons of the kidney; it contains water and urea as well but in different concentrations. While still in the nephron, water and other important molecules are filtered back through and reabsorbed by the body.

32. Option B is correct. Renin is a hormone that helps regulate blood pressure. It does so by changing the concentrations of water and salt in the bloodstream. The ureter and bladder sphincter are part of the genitourinary system but do not regulate blood pressure. Although the heart is responsible for pushing blood through the bloodstream, it is not part of the genitourinary system.

33. Option A is correct. Mucus lines the openings in the body to try and prevent pathogens from entering. For example, mucus can be found in the lungs. Pathogens entering these spaces get stuck in the mucus and pushed out. Antibodies, interferons, and B cells are more specific responses to certain pathogens. B cells release antibodies for particular bacteria pathogens. Interferons are used by the body to stop viruses.

34. Option D is correct. Acquired immune deficiency syndrome (AIDS) is caused by a virus, known as human immunodeficiency virus (HIV), which infects and kills T cells. Without T cells, the body is less competent at fighting other diseases. Allergies and autoimmune are diseases that affect the immune system but do not affect T cells.

35. Option B is correct. Blood cells, including white blood cells, are produced in the bone marrow of long bones. These two systems work together to produce the cells needed to make sure the immune system is working properly.

36. Option A is correct. Although these are all functions of the skeletal system, body movement is the function that needs both the skeletal and neuromuscular system. Bones provide the support and are attached to muscles with tendons. When given a signal from a neuron, these muscles contract or relax causing the bone to move.

37. Option A is correct. The tibia is one of the longer bones of the lower leg. It is longer than it is wide. The ribs are considered flat bones. The pelvis is described as an irregular bone. The skull does not contain any long bones.

38. Option B is correct. Protons and neutrons are found in the nucleus, whereas electrons are found orbiting the nucleus. Protons and neutrons have about the same mass, and electrons have very small amounts of mass. It would be incorrect to say that electrons have mass or can be found in the nucleus.

39. Option C is correct. Looking at the substances in the same containers, the first is less dense. Density depends on the mass divided by volume. Because both containers are of equal size, the volume does not change. The second substance has more particles and, thus, more mass, making it denser than the first substance.

40. Option C is correct. As heat is added to the substance, the molecules break off from one another, causing melting. This continues and eventually causes boiling and leaves the substance as a gas. Although changes of state result in density changes, the graph provides no evidence that density is increasing in this scenario. If the forces between molecules are weakening as heat is added, answer B is incorrect. Answer D states that the temperature is remaining constant, which is not supported by all sections of the graph.

41. Option A is correct. Ionic compounds form when an electron from a metal is donated to a nonmetal atom. This donation causes ions to be formed, which are attracted to one another, and form ionic bonds. NaCl is the only answer choice with both a metal and nonmetal that can form ions. CO, $C_6H_{12}O_6$, and H_2O do not form ionic bonds but share electrons, forming covalent bonds.

42. Option A is correct. In this chemical reaction, hydrogen and oxygen are combining to make water. This is an example of a synthesis reaction because two molecules are combining to form one new molecule.

43. Option A is correct. Volume of a solid object like a brick can be found by measuring the length, width, and height and multiplying these values together. When you multiply these values together, the unit is cubed. A brick is too small to be measured by a unit more than a centimeter, so a meter would not be appropriate. A balance and grams would be an appropriate way to measure the mass of a brick. A graduated cylinder is too small to measure a brick and is better for measuring liquids.

44. Option D is correct. The daphnia in the experiment given the most caffeine had a heart rate of 0. Organisms with a heart rate of zero are no longer alive. Because up to that point, the caffeine had been increasing the heart rate, we can assume that the caffeine was increasing the heart rate up to that point. Daphnia can survive without caffeine, which is supported by the first trial in which no caffeine was given to the daphnia.

45. Option C is correct. The current experiment only has one trial for each condition. To improve this experiment, the experimenter could test each condition multiple times and take the average of each trial. The other changes could be interesting experiments, but they do not help answer this experiment question.

46. Option C is correct. The number of heart beats is the observed condition that is responding to the amount of caffeine given to the daphnia. The amount of caffeine is the independent variable. The type of organism used remained the same and is a constant variable. The number of minutes before collecting heart beats is also the same for each trial, making it a constant variable.

47. Option C is correct. According the data, the daphnia's heart rate was increased when given caffeine. For example, a daphnia given no caffeine had a heart rate of 180 beats per minute, but the daphnia given 1 mg of caffeine had an increased heart rate of 207 beats per minute. The daphnia that was given 2 mg of caffeine had a heart rate of 0, meaning it is no longer alive. This does not necessarily mean the caffeine decreased the heart rate because there is no pattern of this seen in the data.

SCIENCE

English and Language Usage

The following 9 chapters cover the tasks from the ATI TEAS test plan for the English and Language Usage unit. These are focused on assessment of knowledge and understanding of English language and are organized into three sections:

- Conventions of standard English
- Knowledge of language
- Vocabulary acquisition

Each chapter in this unit introduces knowledge, skills, and abilities relevant to the English and Language Usage task and provides an overview of some essential topics, along with specific examples to highlight important concepts. Practice questions at the end of each chapter will allow you to test your knowledge of select concepts. In addition, there are key terms included at the end of each section and a practice English and Language Usage quiz at the end of the unit. This unit quiz includes the same number of questions as the English and Language Usage unit on the ATI TEAS and matches the test plan task allocations (shown below). The quiz will give you a good idea of the number and types of sources you will encounter and the questions that will accompany those sources. Keep in mind that these chapters are a great starting point and guide to your studies, but they are not an exhaustive review of all concepts that might be tested in the English and Language Usage unit of the ATI TEAS. You should use other sources (textbooks, online resources, etc.) for additional study and practice in areas that you haven't mastered.

Conventions of standard English relates to using the conventions of standard English spelling, punctuation, and sentence structure. The knowledge of language section includes items related to applying basic knowledge of elements of the writing process, using grammar to enhance clarity in writing, distinguishing between formal and informal language, and developing a well-organized paragraph.

There are 24 scored English and Language Usage items on the TEAS. These are divided as shown below. In addition, there will be four unscored pretest items that can be in any of these categories.

Section	Number of scored items on the ATI TEAS
Conventions of standard English	9
Knowledge of language	9
Vocabulary acquisition	6

CHAPTER

57

Use conventions of standard English spelling

 This objective includes, but is not limited to, the following examples of knowledge, skills, and abilities.

- Spell words using common rules for English spelling (e.g., "i" before "e," dropping the final "e," changing the final "y" to "i," doubling a final consonant).
- Identify common words that are exceptions to common rules for English spelling (e.g., "receive," "vein," "height," "protein," "neither").
- Identify plural forms of common words found in the English language.
- Reference in-text examples for self-correction of spelling errors.
- Know homophones and homographs (e.g., "their"/"they're," "its"/"it's").

Correct spelling is important to clear written communication. For example, what's the difference between "aural" and "oral"? Not much if you're saying them out loud, but there is a big difference if you're reading them. A prescription might direct you to administer a medication in the ear (aural) or the mouth (oral). Using homophones and homographs correctly is essential to reading and writing accurately. You also need to know common spelling rules, such as those for forming plurals, and the exceptions to those rules. Being able to identify incorrectly spelled words in your writing and correcting them will help you communicate your ideas more effectively.

Spelling Rules

One of the most common spelling rules is taught by the mnemonic: *"'i' before 'e' except after 'c' or when sounding like 'a' as in 'neighbor' and 'weigh.'"* This rhyme helps you remember the rule. It states the rule as well as exceptions to it. There are many more spelling rules that you could learn, but it's best to master the most common ones and to know some common exceptions to those rules. Here are four rules you should know for the TEAS.

"I" BEFORE "E": This rule is well known, but it has plenty of exceptions.

"i" Before "e"	Except After "c"	Sounding Like "a"	Exceptions
believe	ceiling	beige	codeine
fierce	receipt	rein	leisure
friend	receive	sleigh	seize

 DROP THE FINAL "E": When adding a suffix to a word that ends in "e," drop the "e" if the suffix begins with a vowel. Keep the "e" before a suffix beginning with a consonant.

Drop the "e" Before a Vowel	Keep the "e" Before a Consonant	Exceptions
believe	ceiling	codeine
fierce	receipt	leisure
friend	receive	seize

 DOUBLE THE FINAL CONSONANT: In a verb ending in a consonant, double the final consonant when adding a suffix. However, never double "w," "x," or "y." In some cases, though, there isn't a definitive spelling for a word when it comes to this rule.

Double the Consonant	Exceptions	Both Forms Correct
blur + ed =blurred	bleed + ing = bleeding	traveling, travelling
plan + ed = planned	plow + ed = plowed	canceled, cancelled
split + ing = splitting	vomit + ed = vomited	modeled, modelled

 CHANGE THE FINAL "Y" TO "I": When adding a suffix to a word ending in "y" preceded by a consonant, change the "y" to "i" and add the suffix. Don't change the "y" if the suffix begins with "i."

Change the "y" Following a Consonant	Don't Change the "y" Following a Vowel	Don't Change If the Suffix Begins with "i"	Exceptions
believe	ceiling	beige	codeine
fierce	receipt	rein	leisure
friend	receive	sleigh	seize

RULES FOR PLURALS: You should also understand the rules for constructing plurals. Here are some rules to keep in mind.

- For regular plurals, you only need to add "-s." Examples: "apple"/"apples," "car"/"cars," "nurse"/"nurses."
- Add "-es" for words ending in "-ch," "-s," "-sh," "-x," or "-z." Examples: "dash"/"dashes," "lunch"/"lunches," "boss"/"bosses."
- Change to "-ves" for some words ending in "-f" or "-fe." Examples: "elf"/"elves," "life"/"lives," "self"/"selves." Exceptions: "chief"/"chiefs, "proof"/"proofs."

Identifying Homophones and Homographs

You'll need to be able to use context to identify homophones, or words that are pronounced the same but are spelled differently. You also need to correctly use homographs, which are words that are spelled the same but have different meanings. Homographs may be said differently. Here is just a small set of examples often found on the TEAS.

Homophones

bough/bow
its/it's
lead/led
seam/seem
their/there/they're

Homographs

bow: to bend at the waist, the front of a boat, a decoration, or something that shoots arrows
fair: reasonable, an appearance, or an exhibition
lead: to show the way or a metal
perfect: flawless or to make flawless
tear: to rip something or water from the eye

CHAPTER 57 PRACTICE PROBLEMS

The explorers travelled across the desert, and it seemed that it's heat would stop their progress.

1. Which of the following corrects an error in the sentence above?

    A. "Desert" should be "dessert."
    B. "It's" should be "its."
    C. "Seemed" should be "seamed."
    D. Their" should be "they're."

The explorers became thirstier and their vision blurred as they travelled further across the arid desert and tryed to make their way to the oasis.

2. Which of the following corrects a misspelling in the sentence above?

    A. "Blurred" should be "blured."
    B. "Thirstier" should be "thirstyer."
    C. "Travelled" should be "traveled."
    D. "Tryed" should be "tried."

3. Which of the following is spelled correctly, showing an exception to a spelling rule?

    A. recieve
    B. beleive
    C. codeine
    D. feirce

4. Which of the following uses the "double the consonant" rule correctly?

    A. "bleed" to "bleedding"
    B. "vomit" to "vomitted"
    C. "travel" to "travelled"
    D. "plow" to "plowwed"

5. Perform a search and locate two more spelling rules that can support your writing. Write each rule, and then give an example of a word using that rule.

Notes:

CHAPTER

58

Use conventions of standard English punctuation

 This objective includes, but is not limited to, the following examples of knowledge, skills, and abilities.

- Demonstrate knowledge of sentence punctuation patterns (e.g., simple, compound, complex).
- Use a comma to clarify meaning (e.g., placement in compound sentences, after introductory elements, with dependent phrases and clauses, around nonessential elements, in a series, with adjectives).
- Use direct and indirect quotations following standard English rules.
- Use end marks to clarify meaning.

Punctuation is like a system of road signs for written language. Punctuation directs the reader how to read a sentence correctly. Mastering punctuation allows you to read and write with clarity. To successfully answer questions about punctuation for the TEAS exam, you'll need to study the rules for end marks, commas, colons, semicolons, apostrophes, and quotation marks. There are many great websites to reference for rules on using punctuation, but be sure to distinguish between established punctuation rules and matters of opinion. The following concepts are likely to be tested.

ENGLISH

Commas

The comma is used for many purposes, from dividing items in a series to indicating pauses in the flow of a sentence. You'll need to be careful to distinguish between rules and preferences. For example, the serial comma, also known as the Oxford comma, is the comma before the "and" in a simple series of items. It is preferred in many forms of writing but not all. Questions on the TEAS address rules, not preferences, so the omission of a serial comma would not be considered an error. Using a comma without a conjunction to separate two independent clauses, however, is the kind of error that you will need to recognize on the TEAS.

- Place a comma after an introductory phrase or clause.
- Place a comma before and after dependent phrases and clauses that interrupt the main clause of a sentence.
- Place commas after items in a series. The comma before the "and" in a series is a preference.
- Place a comma between two or more adjectives describing the same noun.

Colons

Colons indicate a list, examples, or that a definition will follow. Colons are also used in writing time.

Indirect Quotations

An indirect quotation is when a writer paraphrases what another person has written or said. If a writer writes an idea in her own words, it does not need quotation marks. However, the writer must indicate the person who came up with the idea. The writer must cite the source of the idea.

Direct Quotations

A direct quotation indicates that the words within the quotation marks are exactly what someone else has written or stated. The exact words must be placed within quotation marks, with the end mark within the quotation marks. If a writer uses someone else's words without quotation marks, this is plagiarism.

Apostrophes

An apostrophe shows possession, such as "the writer's style." It can also indicate that a letter is missing, such as in "that's" for "that is."

Sentence Punctuation Patterns

Different sentence types use specific punctuation.

- A simple sentence contains one idea or independent clause and uses only an end mark.
- A complex sentence has an independent clause and a dependent clause. Use a comma following an introductory subordinate clause to separate it from the independent clause. You do not need a comma if the subordinate clause follows the independent clause.
- A compound sentence has two independent clauses. Use a comma before the conjunction that joins the clauses. Use a semicolon between two related independent clauses. Use a semicolon before a transition word that connects two independent clauses and a comma after a transition.

 Punctuation Examples: Punctuation can indicate the type of sentence and how to read the sentence. Consider the comma in the following sentence.

I have been lifting weights for over a year, and I finally set a new maximum bench press.

The comma in this sentence indicates that what follows will be a second independent clause rather than a dependent clause. Commas, along with colons and semicolons, help us identify independent and dependent clauses and interpret how they build compound and complex sentences.

You'll also need to recognize how to use quotation marks, apostrophes, end marks, and other punctuation correctly.

You'll also need to recognize how to use quotation marks, apostrophes, end marks, and other punctuation correctly.

The following example uses a variety of punctuation to convey meaning.

"It's not easy to increase your bench press," she announced. "You've probably heard that there are many different theories for the best approach!"

This example demonstrates a number of concepts. Quotation marks are used for the direct quotation, and a comma is used before the closed quote to indicate that there is additional text in the sentence. An apostrophe is used for a contraction. An exclamation mark is used to indicate both the end of the sentence and strong feeling.

Any concrete rule regarding punctuation is fair game for this task on the TEAS, so be sure to brush up using a variety of sources.

CHAPTER 58 PRACTICE PROBLEMS

1. Which of the following is a correctly punctuated compound sentence?
   A. I've decided to run a 5K race; but running a long race requires training.
   B. I plan on taking two rest days per week and this will help me avoid injury.
   C. I'll run long distances on the weekend, and rest on the following day.
   D. Running a 5K race would be a great accomplishment, and exercise will improve my health.

2. Which of the following uses correct punctuation for a quotation?
   A. "A good laugh and a long run," she said. "Are the two best cures for anything."
   B. "A good laugh and a long run," she said, "are the two best cures for anything."
   C. "A good laugh and a long run are the two best cures for anything." she said.
   D. "A good laugh and a long run are the two best cures for anything," She said.

3. Which of the following uses a correct punctuation pattern for a complex sentence?
   A. Although I enjoy running I would never want to run a marathon.
   B. Although I enjoy running, I would never want to run a marathon.
   C. Although, I enjoy running I would never want to run a marathon
   D. Although I enjoy running I would never want to run, a marathon.

4. Which sentence uses commas correctly to clarify the meaning of the sentence?
   A. In order to begin training as a long-distance runner, you will need high-quality shoes, socks, and running clothes.
   B. In order to begin training as a long-distance runner you will need high-quality shoes, socks, and running clothes.
   C. In order to begin training as a long-distance runner, you will need high-quality shoes socks, and running clothes.
   D. In order to begin training as a long-distance runner you will need high-quality shoes socks and running clothes.

5. Conduct your own research and make a list of rules for the use of a semicolon. Be sure to include only rules, not instances of preferred usage.

Notes:

CHAPTER

Analyze various sentence structures

 This objective includes, but is not limited to, the following examples of knowledge, skills, and abilities.

- Combine dependent and independent clauses.
- Use the "eight parts of speech": noun, pronoun, verb, adjective, adverb, preposition, conjunction, interjection.
- Use sentence parts (e.g., subject, predicate, object, indirect object, complement) to create coherent sentence structures.
- Identify patterns of simple, compound, complex, and compound-complex sentences.

A sentence is a set of words combined to express a complete thought. For this TEAS task, you'll need to be familiar with different types of sentences and how they are built using sentence parts, including subjects, predicates, phrases, and clauses. You'll also need to know the parts of speech and how they are combined within a sentence.

Parts of Speech

Parts of speech refer to how words are used in sentences. There are generally considered to be eight parts of speech: nouns, pronouns, verbs, adjectives, adverbs, prepositions, conjunctions, and interjections. Some grammar experts also consider articles ("a," "an," "the") as parts of speech. These parts of speech combine in various ways to make up sentence parts.

Subject and Predicate

A complete sentence must contain a subject and predicate. The simple subject is the noun (or noun substitute), and the complete subject includes the noun and all its complements and modifiers. The simple predicate is the verb, and the complete predicate includes the verb and all its complements and modifiers. Consider this example.

ENGLISH

The eager, enthusiastic child voiced his story with excitement.

The simple subject is the noun "child," and the complete subject includes the article and modifiers: "the eager, enthusiastic child." The simple predicate is the verb "voiced," and the complete predicate includes the direct object ("his story") and the prepositional modifier ("with excitement").

Clauses and Phrases

Clauses and phrases are also constructions that you should be able to recognize. A clause is a group of words that contains a subject and a verb. An independent clause is basically a simple sentence and can stand on its own. A dependent clause cannot stand on its own because it doesn't finish a complete thought. A phrase is a group of words that doesn't have a subject and a verb, and it is used as a single part of speech. Consider the following examples.

Independent clause: I am studying.
Dependent clause: Although I feel confident in my skills...
Phrase: ...for my TEAS exam.

These can be combined to make a complex sentence with a dependent clause followed by an independent clause.

Although I feel confident in my skills, I am studying for my TEAS exam.

Sentences Types

A good way to enhance your understanding of sentence construction and the parts of speech is to practice identifying sentence patterns. There are plenty of online resources available with information on identifying sentences and opportunities for practice. Here are key elements of each sentence type.

- A simple sentence contains one independent clause.
- A complex sentence has an independent clause and a dependent clause.
- A compound sentence has two independent clauses joined by a conjunction or semicolon.
- A compound-complex sentence has two independent clauses and a dependent clause.

Sentence Diagramming

Another way to enhance your understanding of sentence construction and the parts of speech is to practice diagramming sentences. There are plenty of online resources available with information on diagramming sentences and opportunities for practice. Key rules for diagramming include:

- The key sentence parts of subject, verb, and object are written in a line. They are separated by vertical lines.
- The modifiers of each of these sentence parts extend below them on slanted lines.
- In the case of the prepositional phrase, the preposition extends from the word it modifies and then introduces the prepositional object with its modifiers.

Here's just one example of how to diagram a sentence.

The agile surfer rode that wave with expert balance.

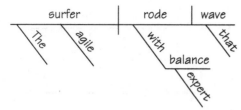

The subject "surfer," verb "rode," and object "wave" are on the straight line separated by vertical lines. "The" modifies "surfer." "That" modifies "wave." "With" is the preposition, and "balance" is the object of the preposition. "Expert" modifies "balance."

CHAPTER 59 PRACTICE PROBLEMS

1. Which of the following examples is a compound-complex sentence?
   A. The large amusement park was packed with people, and they had all come for the opening of a new roller coaster.
   B. Although the weather forecast called for rain, people came to the park to ride the roller coaster.
   C. Just as the roller coaster was about to open, the crowd looked to the cloudy sky.
   D. The sun came out and was surrounded by a rainbow that brought gasps of awe from the crowd.

   Thinking about what you are grateful for is one of the keys to happiness.

2. Which of the following is the simple subject in the sentence above?
   A. Thinking
   B. is
   C. one
   D. keys

3. Which of the following is a dependent clause?
   A. Swimming is a great form of exercise.
   B. Despite the fact that swimming can be difficult.
   C. There are four main swimming strokes to learn.
   D. Although it is time-consuming, everyone should learn to swim.

4. Diagram the following sentence: The parents served their children fresh vegetables.

5. Use a dependent and independent clause to write a complex sentence about one of your hobbies.

Notes:

CHAPTER

60

Use grammar to enhance clarity in writing

 This objective includes, but is not limited to, the following examples of knowledge, skills, and abilities.

- Recognize complete sentences.
- Use transition words (e.g., "but," "and," "next," "however," "therefore") to clarify relationships.
- Be aware of past, present, and future tense.
- Choose precise diction (e.g., "annoyed" or "angry" or "furious").
- Identify and eliminate ambiguous language (e.g., "and stuff").

Clear communication requires a common understanding between the writer and the reader. This is where grammar comes in. Grammar is the set of conventions or rules that allow writers to convey ideas effectively. This TEAS task requires you to recognize both correct and incorrect use of grammar as well as precise versus ambiguous language. To prepare for this task, take note of reading passages you encounter that are unclear. Ask yourself why the passage is unclear and how it could be made more effective. Does the passage use correct grammar and precise diction? How would you change the passage to improve its clarity?

In this TEAS task, you'll be asked to make judgments about sentences and reading passages, using your knowledge of grammar to enhance clarity in writing. The following are conventions that you should know and be able to use.

Complete Sentences

The most fundamental element in grammar is the complete sentence. A sentence conveys a complete thought. It must have a subject and a predicate that communicates what the subject is like or what the subject is doing. Predicates must contain a verb. For this task, you'll need to be able to recognize complete

ENGLISH

sentences. You will also need to recognize incomplete sentences called fragments, which are missing a subject or predicate. You will also identify sentences that are too long, which are called run-on sentences. Study these examples.

- **Finish your homework!** This is a complete sentence with the understood subject "you."
- **Thinking about my weekend.** This is a fragment because there is no subject or predicate.
- **The story had a thrilling ending the plot was built with suspense.** This is a run-on sentence due to the lack of a conjunction or appropriate punctuation. The two ideas ("the story had a thrilling ending" and "the plot was built with suspense") are two complete thoughts that must be separated to be correct.

Transitions

Transition words and phrases are used to connect ideas and clarify the relationship between ideas. You should be able to identify appropriate transitions based on context and recognize when a transition word is misused or another word is needed for clarity. This table provides examples of the types of transitions and specific transition words and phrases.

Transition Type	Examples
Agreement	also, likewise, in addition, similarly
Opposition	but, although, however, conversely
Cause	if, unless, in order to, in the event that
Effect	therefore, consequently, accordingly, as a result
Examples	like, including, in other words, for example
Conclusion	after all, in short, altogether, ultimately
Chronology	before, after, in the meantime, suddenly
Location	here, there, wherever, adjacent to

Tense

Tense refers to the different forms of verbs that express the time an action occurred. The basic tenses are past, present, and future, but tense can also capture whether an action is complete. An action can be progressive, meaning incomplete, or perfective, meaning complete. You'll need to be able to recognize when tenses are misused within a given writing passage. Here is an example of how verbs indicate time.

		Time		
		past	present	future
Aspect	none/simple	walked	walks	will walk
	progressive	was walking	is walking	will be walking
	perfective	had walked	has walked	will have walked

Diction

Word choice, or diction, is also important to clear communication. You'll need to be able to identify which word choices are best for a given context. For example, the words "inaudible," "discreet," and "soft" all could be listed as synonyms for "quiet." But would all of these really be an appropriate replacement for "quiet" in the following sentence?

Florence enjoyed camping because she loves how quiet nature can be.

Language can also be ambiguous. This means that words and phrases can be unclear to the reader. For example, what does the writer mean by "quiet nature"? Does this mean peaceful and serene or soundless? On the TEAS exam, you will need to recognize and replace ambiguous language.

Other Conventions

There are a number of other grammar conventions that you'll need to apply, such as subject-verb agreement and pronoun-antecedent agreement. For this task, any grammar rule is fair game, so be sure to review a number of good grammar resources.

CHAPTER 60 PRACTICE PROBLEMS

1. Which of the following is a sentence fragment?

   A. Go hike a glacier!
   B. According to many experts on Alaska.
   C. Hiking is a great activity for your health.
   D. Maria loves to hike she also enjoys travel.

   Maria was unable to complete her 10-mile hike, _____ she had trained for several months.

2. Which transition word or phrase best completes the sentence?

   A. although
   B. in other words
   C. accordingly
   D. meanwhile

   Maria loved to travel, and no advice about safety is going to keep her from taking a trek across Alaska.

3. Which grammar error appears in the following sentence?

   A. Inappropriate transition word choice
   B. Tense disagreement
   C. Poor diction
   D. Ambiguous word choice

   Navigating the vast wilderness of Denali National Park in Alaska requires that hikers have equipment that can determine their location and other things.

4. Which of the following words in above sentence is an example of ambiguous language?

   A. navigating
   B. requires
   C. hikers
   D. things

5. Practice analyzing diction by reading a passage from your favorite book or a magazine article that appeals to you. Evaluate the author's word choice as you read. Choose a sentence that uses precise diction, and write the sentence below. Explain how two of the words in the sentence enhance the clarity of the sentence.

ENGLISH

Notes:

CHAPTER

61 Distinguish between formal and informal language

 This objective includes, but is not limited to, the following examples of knowledge, skills, and abilities.

- Given several short passages, choose which language fits a scenario.
- Identify language that is formal (e.g., academic, professional, public setting).
- Identify language that is informal (e.g., slang, colloquialisms).
- Be able to identify the narrator's setting/situation from given information (e.g., information provided in audio or in text format).

Good writers choose language that suits their purpose for writing and their intended audience. For example, research papers require formal language. Informal language such as slang and colloquialisms would not be appropriate in an academic paper. In this TEAS task, you will evaluate language and match it to the correct audience.

Formal Language

Certain modes of writing—research papers, business communication, journalism—have conventions beyond simple good grammar. They use formal language, which includes words and phrases that are specific to a profession or situation. The audience for these modes of communication has common expectations that the writer must understand. For instance, a scientific paper should use neutral language in reporting data because an objective approach is expected. Some business acronyms ("CEO," "B2B") can be used without explanation in business communication. Journalistic reporting is expected to address the "who, what, why, when, and where" efficiently. While these conventions can change over time, you can identify the tone and key words that will help you identify the intended audience for a given piece of writing. Formal genres you will be asked to identify include business letters, speeches, textbook articles, science reports, news stories, and essays.

ENGLISH

Informal Language

Informal writing has specific conventions, too. You wouldn't expect a text message from your friend to end with a formal closing such as "Sincerely." Narratives often benefit from informal language to create a feeling of realism or to set a tone. Slang and colloquialisms can provide otherwise unstated information about the time and place in which the communication originated. Consider the following examples.

Decade	Slang	Meaning
1920s	all wet bee's knees a bucket	incorrect or ineffective extraordinary person, place, or thing a car
1960s	cool bug out a gas	hip or very good to leave a good time
2000s	bling bounce word	something fancy to leave agreed or appreciated

Slang can help to create an atmosphere that captures a time and place. Using colloquialisms can make a piece of writing feel more conversational and intimate, which is beneficial in informal communication. You'll be asked to recognize instances of slang and colloquialisms in writing passages for this task of the TEAS. Also, you will need to identify when an author is using the second person (addressing the reader as "you"). This is a good indication that the piece is informal.

Identifying a Scenario Based on Diction

Another task on the TEAS is to identify a situation or type of publication by analyzing the language used. In order to evaluate the language in passages and determine the appropriate scenario, look for key words and phrases that can help identify the setting or the intended audience. When you're reading these passages, ask yourself the following questions.

- Is the author using conventions or language that seems specific to a certain type of audience?
- Does the author use slang or colloquialisms?
- Is the language neutral, or does it imply negative or positive judgments?
- What kind of descriptors does the author use? Do these influence the reader's interpretation of the material?

By analyzing language in a passage, you will be able to identify the time period of a narrative or the type of publication.

CHAPTER 61 PRACTICE PROBLEMS

I think we can take advantage of our organization's vertical synergy to produce a quality proposal by EOD.

1. Which of the following publications would most likely contain this sentence?

   A. Business memo
   B. Scientific journal
   C. Novel
   D. Motivational speech

2. Which of the following sentences contains informal language?

   A. Many people are unaware of the variety of ways they can enhance the privacy settings on their mobile devices.
   B. A recent study found that using a passcode is more secure than using a swipe pattern to unlock a mobile phone.
   C. Write down your 15-digit International Mobile Equipment Identity (IMEI) in case your phone is ever lost or stolen.
   D. Having a phone case with bling may make your phone a target for theft, so don't use too flossy of a cover.

3. Which of the following sentences would indicate that the setting is the United States in the 1920s?

   A. Many people were able to endure the Blitz by the Germans during World War II.
   B. The film critics felt that the new actor was the bee's knees, but the film itself was all wet.
   C. You could feel the tension in the air as the gunslinger entered the room to confront his enemies.
   D. She was a cool cat who had a new hit that she was about to introduce at a gig in Chicago.

Communication skills are important to success in any profession, but effective communication takes practice. First, decide upon the key message you want to convey in clear, straightforward language. Engage your listener by asking questions and soliciting feedback. Then take time to listen carefully and respond to your listener's ideas. The best communicators are the best listeners. If you have not been understood, think of ways to put your ideas in other words, or use examples to make your thoughts more clear to others.

4. Which of the following sentences uses ideas and language that fit the passage?

   A. Maintaining eye contact builds credibility and shows your listener that you care about their ideas.
   B. Bouncing from topic to topic can make your listener feel like they have whiplash.
   C. Talking with your homeskillet will be boss if you cool your jets and really focus on your listener.
   D. Computer skills such as using Excel spreadsheets are critical to success in many jobs today.

5. Perform an Internet search for examples of each of the following and make a list of three conventions or rules for each type of writing.

   A. Business letter
   B. News article
   C. Essay

ENGLISH

Notes:

CHAPTER

62 Apply basic knowledge of the elements of the writing process

 This objective includes, but is not limited to, the following examples of knowledge, skills, and abilities.

- Know elements of the writing process (e.g., planning/preparation/outline, drafting, referencing sources, revision).
- Identify steps necessary to complete a writing task.
- Identify when citation is needed.

Writing is a process that involves several steps, including drafting and revision. Sometimes these steps can move quickly, but sometimes they prove to be challenging. Thankfully, there are plenty of tools and resources available to assist writers in the process. This TEAS task will require you to be familiar with the writing process and the strategies that writers use in that process. What steps do they take? How do they organize the information?

Elements of the Writing Process

There might be nearly as many writing processes as there are writers, but in its basic form the process is made up of three steps: prewriting, writing, and revision. These steps are not necessarily distinct, and each writer will approach them in his or her own way. However, there are elements of each about which you should be knowledgeable.

Prewriting includes all the tasks necessary to start putting pen to paper (or, more likely, fingers to keyboard) and do the actual writing. This can include tasks as basic as determining when and where to write. Most professional writers set schedules to ensure that they are, at the very least, thinking about the piece they want to write. For any given piece, one of the first steps is to determine the thesis. That includes not just the topic but also the purpose for writing about the topic. Brainstorming techniques, such as stream of consciousness writing or mind mapping, can be useful in finding a topic or a purpose.

ENGLISH

Once the topic and purpose have been identified, the writer determines what research is needed. Depending on the type of writing, this could include nothing more than some time alone to think (personal essay), or it could require an assortment of primary and secondary sources that the author will need to cite within the finished piece. The research process will provide the material with which the writer will work. The next challenge is to organize that material into a coherent, engaging framework. Many writers use an outline to assist in organizing thoughts and constructing their pieces. Outlines create a hierarchy of information that allows writers to show coordination and subordination among related topics. In the example below, the writer is describing how to organize your time. The writer is creating coordination between the main points of using a monthly schedule and setting priorities. Each main point then has three examples to support each main point.

 How to Organize Your Time

I. Use a Monthly Schedule
   a. Visualize the month as a whole
   b. Map important deadlines and appointments
   c. Set time to accomplish tasks to meet deadlines

II. Set Your Priorities
   a. Decide which tasks are urgent
   b. Determine the time needed for each task
   c. Determine the resources needed for each task

While brainstorming, researching, and outlining could be considered prewriting, they often occur throughout the writing process. Most writers continue to discover new insights into their topics and purposes as they write.

Furthermore, the writing and revision processes are often indistinguishable. While some writers will complete a full first draft before revising, many writers revise as they write, constantly tinkering with their sentences. Editors can also be involved in the writing process. For a professionally published piece of writing, there typically will be reviews by copy editors, fact checkers, and/or proofreaders with the chance for the writer to revise based on feedback. In some cases, the editors working for a publisher might have the final say regarding whether to revise something.

Citations

Another important part of the writing process is referencing the sources used in the text. Writers must identify the source of a quotation or idea that is not their own. There are different methods used to cite sources, including the guidelines of the Modern Language Association (MLA) and the American Psychological Association (APA). In this TEAS task, you will need to identify when a citation is needed.

CHAPTER 62 PRACTICE PROBLEMS

1. Which of the following is an example of prewriting?

   A. Citing sources
   B. Brainstorming
   C. Proofreading
   D. Editing

2. If all the following tasks are used in writing, which of the following would likely occur last?

   A. Researching potential sources
   B. Mapping possible topics and subtopics
   C. Developing an organizational outline
   D. Editing and proofreading

3. Malik is writing a research paper on a national park near his home. He consulted several reliable sources, created an outline to plan his paper, wrote a rough draft, and then revised his draft. Which element of the writing process does Malik need to add?

   A. Citing sources
   B. Adding an opposition
   C. Developing a writing plan
   D. Adding captions

4. Which of the following situations requires the inclusion of a citation?

   A. The author is stating his or her own ideas.
   B. The author feels that the ideas described are important.
   C. The author is describing a setting in a story.
   D. The author is using a quotation from another person.

5. Locate an article about how to revise your writing. Organize the ideas in the article into an outline with one to three main points. Then write subordinate ideas below each main point. Consider using these ideas when you are revising your next piece of writing!

Notes:

CHAPTER

Develop a well–organized paragraph

 This objective includes, but is not limited to, the following examples of knowledge, skills, and abilities.

- Know the parts of a paragraph (e.g., topic sentence, supporting details, transitions, conclusion).
- Be able to put information in a logical order (e.g., chronological, emphasis, cause/effect).
- Identify information that does not belong.
- Identify where more information/development is needed.

Just as a sentence is the foundational unit of a complete thought, a paragraph is a self-contained unit of discourse. A paragraph is the building block for longer works of writing. A paragraph should convey a coherent message about a topic through all included sentences. In this TEAS task, you will identify the conventions of good paragraph development, including the use of topic sentences, supporting details, and conclusions. You will also analyze paragraph development and identify where revision is required. Focusing on the coherence of the message will be the key to your success for this task.

Parts of a Paragraph

While a paragraph can be as short as a single sentence, we'll focus mostly on longer examples that include the various parts of a well-constructed paragraph. First, the topic sentence introduces the message or idea of the paragraph. A well-constructed paragraph then requires development in the form of supporting details that provide more specific information about the topic. Paragraphs end with a conclusion. A conclusion is used to sum up the message of the paragraph, and often transitions are used to prepare for the introduction of a new idea that will follow. Consider how the following example uses a clear paragraph structure to explain one way to improve your phone photography.

ENGLISH

Topic sentence	To improve the quality of photographs taken with your phone, you can learn to use the gridlines setting for better balance and contrast.
Supporting details	When you switch to "grid on" in your settings, the lines of a grid will appear in your viewfinder. There will be nine boxes.
	According to a photographic theory, you should place the focal points of your image in the intersections or along the grid lines.
	Seeing the grid will help you decide how to balance the images in the photographs that you take. The lines will also help you keep the images level.
Conclusion/ transition	By using this tool, your phone photographs will become more visually interesting, especially if you also use a few strategies for lighting.

Logical Order in Paragraphs

Search online for "types of paragraphs," and you'll quickly find that there are many ways to categorize and organize paragraphs. The key to an effective paragraph is that information about a topic is presented in a logical way. The example above, for instance, demonstrates expository paragraph construction. Expository paragraphs start with a proposition, such as how to improve phone photography using gridlines. They then lead the reader through the supporting details or steps, such as changing settings and placing focal points to complete the task. Paragraphs can also be organized in chronological order, where the order of events is used to support the main idea or message. Other forms are descriptive, narrative, and persuasive paragraphs. Evaluating the various ways that paragraphs can present information coherently is a good exercise to prepare for this TEAS task. You will be asked to put information in paragraphs in logical order.

Identifying Unnecessary and Omitted Information

When you're well practiced at evaluating paragraph construction, you'll be able to notice some common errors that writers make when writing paragraphs. One common trouble spot is the inclusion of information that doesn't support the topic of the paragraph. If the sentence makes you stop and reread, maybe it should not have been included in this particular paragraph. Ask yourself, "How does this contribute to the topic and the rest of the paragraph?"

Another problem is when vital information has been omitted. This also might make you stop to reread. Would a transition have helped? What information would clarify the message of the paragraph? It's often helpful to determine what principle is being used to organize the information and then determine what's required for that principle to work best.

CHAPTER 63 PRACTICE PROBLEMS

1. Which of the following is a key part of a paragraph?

    A. Sources
    B. Topic sentence
    C. Introductory phrase
    D. Opposition

2. Which of the following examples would most likely act as a transition sentence?

    A. When you tap on the screen to refocus, a sun icon appears.
    B. Manually tapping on the subject of your photo adjusts the focus of the camera and also adjusts the exposure.
    C. Another phone camera feature that can improve your photography is manually setting exposure times.
    D. If you make the sun icon brighter, this will increase the light exposure of the photo.

    I. By the time I returned home from vacation, I was starting to get excited about the new courses I would be taking.

    II. I headed to my final exam with a mixture of fear and confidence. I couldn't wait for the exam to be over so I could take a break from my studies.

    III. The exam was difficult, but by keeping to my study schedule, I was well prepared.

    IV. As soon as I completed my exam, our family headed to my grandmother's home for the holiday.

3. Which of the following is the best chronological sequence to construct a paragraph with these sentences?

    A. IV, II, I, III
    B. IV, III, II, I
    C. I, II, III, IV
    D. II, III, IV, I

You might also want to improve your phone photography by setting the focus on your phone camera. Most people don't realize that the automatic focus setting of most phone cameras is on the foreground of the image in the viewfinder. Most people don't bother to read the instruction manual of their phone. This can be a problem if the subject of your photograph is centered or in the background. It is also a problem if there is not a single subject for a photograph. Luckily, you can change the focus feature on your phone camera easily. Open your camera application, and simply tap on the screen where you want to sharpen the view. A square icon will appear on your screen. The focus of your photo will be the images inside the icon.

4. Which of the following sentences contains information that does not belong in the paragraph?

    A. You might also want to improve your phone photography by setting the focus on your phone camera.
    B. Open your camera application, and simply tap on the screen where you want to sharpen the view.
    C. Most people don't bother to read the instruction manual of their phone.
    D. It is also a problem if there is not a single subject for a photograph.

5. Write a paragraph about an experience you had with photography using the following table to organize your sentences.

Topic sentence	
Supporting details	
Conclusion/transition	

ENGLISH

Notes:

CHAPTER

64

Use context clues to determine the meaning of words or phrases

 This objective includes, but is not limited to, the following examples of knowledge, skills, and abilities.

- Recognize synonyms.
- Associate words in a series.
- Be aware of tone.
- Recognize cause and effect.
- Be aware of general ideas of a passage.

Perhaps you've heard the phrase "context is everything." This phrase means that the circumstances surrounding an event often shape it. Context also affects the meaning of words and phrases. The context in which a word is used affects the meaning of a word. Context may refer to surrounding words or ideas within a sentence or passage. Context can also refer to the writer's tone, or attitude toward a topic. For this TEAS task, you'll be asked to evaluate the context of a word and choose its meaning from a list of options.

Synonyms

A straightforward way to determine the meaning of a word or phrase is to evaluate the surrounding text for clues. For example, synonyms, words with identical or similar meanings, can provide clues about intended meaning. Take the word *reservation*, which has different meanings. The sentence below demonstrates how a synonym can provide the meaning of a word.

 Gary was uncertain about what to do next, but Gloria knew his reservations were unfounded.

The word *uncertain* provides a clue that this instance of *reservations* refers to feelings of doubt.

ENGLISH

Words in a Series

Another strategy for using context clues is looking at words in a series. The meaning of each word should fit with the meaning of the other words in the group. Consider the meaning of the word "coach" in the series "*the coach, athletes, and trainers.*" Does the word "coach" mean a horse-drawn carriage or a person working with a team? The terms "athletes" and "trainers" make it clear that here a coach is a person involved in sports. Analyzing the context of a word in a series will help you determine word meaning.

Tone

Another way to determine word meaning is by analyzing the tone of a sentence or passage. Tone refers to the feelings involved in a piece of writing. Setting can provide a context clue to tone that can help you understand the meaning of a word. For example, a passage that takes place in a funeral home uses the word "bereaved" to describe the family. You can guess from the setting that "bereaved" involves sadness and may be an adjective that describes a person in mourning.

Cause and Effect

You also find context clues to word meaning by using logical inferences about the cause and effect of events in a sentence. The following sentence describes a cause and effect that can help you determine the meaning of the word "solution."

 Miguel studied the mechanical failure and came up with a brilliant solution to work around it.

In this sentence, the cause of events is that "Miguel studied the mechanical failure." What effect did this have? We can see that the effect was a "solution." We can infer that in this instance a "solution" refers to a way of solving a problem.

General Ideas of a Passage

Finally, the general ideas of a passage can provide clues to the meaning of a word. If we know, for instance, that the setting of a story is a spaceship, then we can determine that a reference to a "hatch" probably does not refer to an animal emerging from an egg but rather to a small door.

While having a good vocabulary can be helpful on this TEAS task, it's more important to practice reading carefully and finding the clues within the context. You might not even need to know the specific definition of a given word to correctly answer the practice problems. Try each option within the context. Which one seems to work the best? Determine what makes the most sense based on what you know from the passage.

CHAPTER 64 PRACTICE PROBLEMS

Julio decided to try a radical new approach to the stubborn, invasive weeds in his yard.

1. Which of the following best defines the word "radical" based on its use in the sentence?
   A. Politically liberal
   B. Progressive
   C. Carefully planned
   D. Complete and thorough

2. In which of the following sentences does "current" mean "a flow of electricity"?
   A. The current carried the kayak downstream.
   B. Before installing the ceiling fan, David turned off the current.
   C. The air current tossed the leaves on the trees.
   D. Bryan prefers to learn about current events by watching the news.

While the other windows shone with candlelight, the opaque window was completely dark.

3. Which of the following best defines the word "opaque" based on its use in the sentence?
   A. Not transparent
   B. Warmly glowing
   C. Partially broken
   D. Mostly visible

Uncle Bob placed the sandpaper, saw, plane, and T square in his shop.

4. Which of the following best defines the word "plane" based on its use in the sentence?
   A. Model aircraft
   B. Imaginary flat surface
   C. Tool for working wood
   D. Clearly visible

From his harsh, superior voice to his loud and garish clothing, Alan was just obnoxious.

5. Read the sentence carefully and use context to determine the meaning of the word "obnoxious." In one or two sentences, describe how context helped you determine the meaning.

Notes:

CHAPTER

65 Determine the meaning of words by analyzing word parts

 This objective includes, but is not limited to, the following examples of knowledge, skills, and abilities.

- Know common affixes.
- Prefixes: anti-, dys-, inter-, intra-, mid-, pre-, non- sub-, super-, un-
- Suffixes: -ful, -ic, -ation, -ology, -ness, -ous
- Combine affixes with root words.

The English language can be a lot like social networking: knowing one word (or person) easily leads you to countless others. That is especially the case when you familiarize yourself with morphemes. A morpheme is the smallest unit of meaning in a language. Morphemes can be words or word parts. For example, the word "box" is a morpheme. It cannot be broken down into other meaningful units. However, the word "boxes" contains two morphemes. It contains the root word "box" and the affix "es" that means it is plural. Affixes are morphemes that are attached to a word stem, or root, to form either a new word or a variation of the same word. For this TEAS task, you will use your knowledge of word parts to determine the meaning of words.

Most Common Affixes

Adding an affix to a root word forms a word with a new meaning. Prefixes are added to the beginning of a root word such as "do." Adding the prefix "re-" creates the word "redo," meaning "to do again." Adding the prefix "un-" creates the word "undo," which means "to reverse what has been done." Prefixes do not change the type of word. If a prefix is added to a verb, the new word is still a verb. Some common prefixes are shown in the following chart.

Prefix	Meaning	Example	Example meaning
dis-	reverses the meaning of the verb	discredit	to show that someone should not be believed
mis-	badly or wrongly	misinterpret	to analyze incorrectly
out-	more or better	outperform	to complete a task better than another
over-	too much	oversleep	to rest too much
un-	reverses the meaning of the verb	unbend	to remove a change in shape

Suffixes are affixes added to the end of a root word. Suffixes often change the type of word. For example, adding the suffix "-ize" to the adjective "private" will change the word to "privatize," which is a verb. Some common suffixes are shown in the following chart.

Suffix	Meaning	Example	Example meaning
-ate	to cause to be	pollinate	to cause to be fertilized
-en	to cause to be	awaken	to cause to be alert
-ify	to cause or show to be	classify	to put in a group
-ise, -ize	to cause or show to be	characterize	to show the features of something

Prefixes

There are innumerable lists of prefixes available to review on the Internet, and it's a good idea to browse some of these lists. The following prefixes appear in the TEAS objectives, so they are important to be familiar with.

Prefix	Meaning	Example	Example meaning
anti-	against	antiapartheid	against separation of groups
dis-	the opposite of	disinformation	statements that are not true
inter-	between	interstellar	between the stars
intra-	within or through	intravenous	within or through the veins
mid-	indicating a middle part, point, time, or position	Midwestern	in the middle of an area considered west
pre-	before	preorder	to place a request or order before something
non-	not	nonfiction	something based on fact that is not made up
sub-	less than or under	subset	part of a whole
super-	more than or above	superhuman	greater than a usual capability

Another consideration for prefixes is whether to use a hyphen. In most cases, the prefix should be added without using a hyphen, but there are exceptions. Guidelines you should know include the following.

Guideline	Example
Hyphenate prefixes before proper nouns or proper adjectives.	trans-Alaskan highway mid-April
Hyphenate all words beginning with "self-," "ex-," and "all-."	self-sufficient ex-representative all-knowing
Hyphenate when it adds clarity.	re-cover (cover again) versus recover (recuperate)

Suffixes

Suffixes come in two forms: inflectional and derivational. Inflectional suffixes do not change a word's meaning. Instead, they express different aspects of a word such as tense and number. Here's a brief list of inflectional suffixes and what they express.

Suffix	Action
-s, -es, -ies	plural
-ed	past tense
-ing	progressive/continuous
-er	comparative
-est	superlative

You'll also want to be familiar with derivational suffixes, or those that form new words when added to a root word. These suffixes sometimes change the part of speech of a word. The following chart contains suffixes often seen on the TEAS exam.

Suffix	Meaning	Example	Example meaning
-ation	the act of	demonstration	the act of demonstrating or showing something
-ful	having the characteristic of	regretful	having the feeling of regret or remorse
-ic	having the characteristic or form of	melodic	having a pleasing sound or melody
-ness	the state of being	happiness	the state of being joyful or happy
-ology	the study of	anthropology	the study of human beings
-ous	having the characteristic of	porous	having spaces or pores within a substance

Becoming familiar with a range of affixes and roots—particularly those used commonly in medical settings—should help you succeed on this TEAS task. You might not know the exact meaning of a given word, but if you notice that the prefix "anti-" is attached, you'll at least have a clue that this word means "against" something. That might be all the information you need to direct you toward the right answer.

ENGLISH

CHAPTER 65 PRACTICE PROBLEMS

1. In which of the following does the suffix create a word that has a different meaning from the root word?

   A. goodness
   B. demonstrated
   C. running
   D. writes

2. Based on an examination of the word parts, which of the following means "to breathe too quickly or too much"?

   A. hypoventilate
   B. hyperventilate
   C. superventilate
   D. interventilate

3. Based on an examination of the word parts, which of the following means "to stop doing something"?

   A. continuation
   B. continuous
   C. discontinue
   D. anticontinue

4. Using your knowledge of word parts, which of the following means "the act of judging beforehand"?

   A. judged
   B. judicious
   C. postjudgment
   D. prejudgment

5. Perform an Internet search for "medical roots, prefixes, and suffixes" and choose a reliable website that ends in ".edu" or a dictionary website. Choose five medical affixes that are unfamiliar. Write each affix, its meaning, and an example of its use.

Notes:

Notes:

Key Terms

adjective. Word or phrase that describes or modifies a noun.

adverb. Word or phrase that describes or modifies an adjective, verb, or other adverb.

affix. Letters placed at the beginning or end of a word to change its meaning.

apostrophe. Punctuation mark that denotes omission of letters and possessive case.

article. Word ("a," "an," or "the") that refers to a noun.

brainstorming. Discussing as a group to create an idea or solve a problem.

citation. A strictly formatted line of text that provides a source reference.

colloquialism. An informal word or phrase.

colon. Punctuation mark used in introduction of a quote or list, ratio, and time.

comma. Punctuation mark used to separate parts of sentences.

complement. Sentence part that gives more information about a subject or object.

conjunction. A connecting word.

context. Words and phrases that describe the situation in a sentence or text.

dependent clause. A group of words that includes a subject and verb but cannot stand alone as a complete sentence.

derivation. Determining the origin of a word.

diction. The style of writing determined by word choice.

draft. An unfinished version of a text.

emphasis paragraph. A short paragraph that highlights a key point.

end marks. Punctuation marks that end sentences: period, question mark, and exclamation mark.

exclamation mark. End mark that denotes strong feeling.

formal. A style that follows conventional rules.

fragment. An incomplete sentence.

homograph. Words spelled the same but that have different meanings.

homophone. Words pronounced the same but that have different meanings.

independent clause. A group of words that includes a subject and predicate and can stand alone as a complete sentence.

indirect object. The person or thing to whom or which something is done.

inflection. How a word is spoken to modify its tone or meaning.

informal. A relaxed, unofficial style.

interjection. Words or phrases that represent short bursts of emotion.

mind mapping. Visually diagramming ideas around a central concept.

mnemonic. A pattern or other device to help remember something.

modifier. A word or group of words that provides description for another word.

morpheme. The smallest meaningful unit in a word.

noun. A person, place, thing, or idea.

object. A word or group of words that receives the action of a verb.

parentheses. Punctuation marks that set off explanatory material within text.

perfective. A verb for an item that has been completed.

period. End mark that denotes the end of a standard sentence.

phrase. A group of words that work together as a unit.

plural. More than one item.

predicate. The part of a sentence that explains what the subject does or is like.

prefix. An affix that appears at the beginning of a word.

preposition. A word that describes relationships between other words.

prescriptive grammar. Specific rules for using language and grammar.

progressive. A verb that shows something is currently happening.

pronoun. A word that takes the place of a noun.

pronoun-antecedent agreement. Matching like numbers of pronouns and their antecedents: singular with singular, plural with plural.

question mark. End mark that denotes a query.

quotation marks. Punctuation marks that denote spoken or other quoted text.

root. A word to which an affix can be attached.

run-on sentence. A sentence with extra parts not joined properly.

second person. A narrative mode that addresses the reader as "you."

ENGLISH

slang. Informal language usually tied to a specific group of people.

stream of consciousness writing. A narrative device that mimics interior monologue.

subject. The main noun of a sentence that is doing or being.

subject-verb agreement. Matching like numbers of subjects and verbs: singular with singular, plural with plural.

suffix. An affix that appears at the end of a word.

supporting detail. Information that supports the main idea by answering who, what, where, when, or why.

synonyms. Words with identical or similar meanings.

tense. Past, present, and future times.

tone. The implied attitude toward a topic.

topic sentence. The sentence that summarizes the main idea of a piece of text.

transition word. Word that links or introduces ideas.

transition. Words or sentences that lead from one idea to another.

verb. A word that describes an action or state of being.

Practice Problem Answers

Chapter 57

1. Option B is correct. "It's" is a contraction for "it is." The form should be the possessive "its," which means "belonging to it." "Its heat" means that the heat belongs to it (the desert).

   - In Option A, "desert" and "dessert" are homophones. "Desert" is properly used in the sentence, meaning "a hot, arid region."
   - In Option C, "seemed" is properly used in the sentence, meaning "appeared."
   - In Option D, the word "their" means "belonging to them." This is correct for this sentence because "their progress" means the progress belongs to them (the explorers).

2. Option D is correct. The spelling of "tryed" should be corrected to "tried" to follow the "change the final 'y' to 'i'" rule.

   - Option A is incorrect because "desert" is spelled correctly in the sentence. It uses the correct homophone for "desert," meaning "a hot, arid region."
   - Option B is incorrect because "thirstier" is spelled correctly in the sentence. "Thirstier" follows the "change the final 'y' to 'i'" rule: "thirsty" to "thirstier."
   - Option C is incorrect because "travelled" is spelled correctly in the sentence. "Travelled" uses the "double the consonant" rule: "travel" to "travelled."

3. Option C is correct. "Codeine" is spelled correctly and is an exception to the "'i' before 'e'" rule.

   - Option A is spelled incorrectly. "Receive" uses the rule "'i' before 'e' except after 'c.'"
   - Option B is spelled incorrectly. "Believe" uses the rule "'i' before 'e.'"
   - Option D is spelled incorrectly. "Fierce" uses the rule "'i' before 'e.'"

4. Option C is correct. "Travelled" is spelled correctly according to the "double the consonant" rule. It can be spelled "traveled" or "travelled."

   - Option A is spelled incorrectly. It should be spelled "bleeding." It is an exception to the rule.
   - Option B is spelled incorrectly. It should be spelled "vomited." It is an exception to the rule.
   - Option D is spelled incorrectly. It should be spelled "plowed." It is an exception to the rule.

5. Answers will vary. Spelling rules that could be listed include:

   - Double the consonants "f," "l," and "s" at the end of one-syllable words that have just one vowel. Example: "spell."
   - Add "-es" to words ending in "-s," "-ss," "-z," "-ch," "-sh," and "-x" to make them plural. Example: "bus"/"buses"
   - Most words ending in "-f" or "-fe" change their plurals to "-ves." Example: "calf"/"calves"

Chapter 58

1. Option D is correct. This sentence includes two independent clauses, and it is correctly punctuated by including a comma before the conjunction.

   - A comma, not a semicolon, should be used before a conjunction separating two independent clauses.
   - Option B has two independent clauses, so a comma should be used before the conjunction that separates the clauses.
   - Option C is not a compound sentence because there is only one subject ("I"). The comma before the "and" should not be included.

2. Option B is correct. This quotation is correctly punctuated by including a comma before the end quotation mark that leads to non-quotation text and another comma before beginning the quotation again.

   - Option A is incorrect because the period in the non-quotation portion of this text divides the quotation into two fragments.
   - Option C is incorrect because there should be no period before a quotation mark that is followed by additional text.
   - Option D is incorrect because the first word after a quotation ("she") should not be capitalized. It does not start a new sentence.

3. Option B is correct. A comma is required after an introductory dependent clause in a complex sentence.

   - Option A is incorrect because it is missing a comma after the introductory dependent clause.
   - Option B is incorrect because it has misplaced the comma. It should come after the word "running."
   - Option D is incorrect because it has misplaced the comma. It should come after the word "running."

ENGLISH

4. Option A is correct. This sentence has a comma after an introductory phrase ending in "runner." It also has two commas to separate the items "shoes" and "socks" in a series. The comma before the "and" in the series is a preference that is correct.

- Option B is missing a comma after an introductory phrase ending in "runner."
- Option C is missing a comma after the item "shoes" to separate it from the item "socks" in a series.
- Option D is missing a comma after an introductory phrase ending in "runner" and after the item "shoes" in a series.

5. Answers will vary. Semicolon rules that could be listed include:

- Use a semicolon to link two independent clauses in a single sentence that are closely related in thought.
- Use a semicolon between two independent clauses that are connected by conjunctive adverbs or transitional phrases.
- Use a semicolon between items in a list or series if any of the items contain commas.

Chapter 59

1. Option C is correct. This is a compound-complex sentence that includes two independent and one dependent clause.

- Option A is a compound sentence. There is no dependent clause, so it is not complex. There is just one independent clause, so it is not compound.
- Option B is a complex sentence. There is just one independent clause, so it is not compound.
- Option D is a simple sentence with a compound verb and four phrases.

2. Option A is correct. This subject is what's referred to as a gerund, or a verb that takes the form of a noun. It is the "who" or "what" that is the subject of the predicate "is."

- In Option B, the word "is" is the simple predicate.
- In Option C, the word "one" is the object of the sentence.
- In Option D, the word "keys" is the object of the phrase "of the keys."

3. Option B is correct. The clause "Despite the fact that swimming is difficult" is not a complete sentence. It is an introductory dependent clause that needs an independent clause to form a complete sentence.

- Option A is incorrect because it is an independent clause and complete sentence. The subject is "swimming," and the verb is "is."
- Option C is incorrect because it is an independent clause and complete sentence. The subject is "there," and the verb is "are."
- Option D is incorrect because it is a complex sentence. It contains the dependent clause "Although it is time-consuming" and the independent clause "everyone should learn to swim."

4. The following is the correct diagram of the sentence: The parents served their children fresh vegetables.

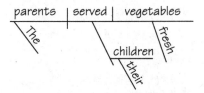

The subject "parents," verb "served," and object "vegetables" are on the straight line, separated by vertical lines. "The" modifies "parents." The indirect object is "children." "Their" modifies "children." "Fresh" modifies "vegetables."

5. Answers will vary but must contain a dependent and independent clause. One example would be: Although I love to swim outdoors, I sometimes swim at an indoor pool.

Chapter 60

1. Option B is correct. "According to many experts on Alaska" is a sentence fragment because there is no subject or verb. This group of words is an introductory phrase.

- Option A "Go hike a glacier!" is a complete sentence with the understood subject "you."
- Option C "Hiking is a great activity for your health" is a complete sentence with the subject "hiking" and the verb "is."
- Option D "Maria loves to hike she also enjoys travel" is a run-on sentence. There should be a period after the word "hike."

2. Option A is correct. The transition word "although" indicates that Maria failed despite training. This is a good choice to indicate that the second idea is opposed to the first idea.

- Option B "In other words" is incorrect because the idea is not repeated.
- Option C "Accordingly" is incorrect because it indicates an effect.
- Option D "Meanwhile" is incorrect because it indicates events happening at the same time. The training occurred before the failure.

3. Option B is correct. The first verb is in the past tense, while the verb for the second independent clause is in the present tense. Tenses must agree.

- Option A is incorrect because using "and" as a transition is an appropriate choice to demonstrate agreement between the ideas of loving to travel and being unable to keep her from taking a trip.
- Options C and D are incorrect because the words selected for use in this sentence fit the context and convey a clear message.

4. Option D is correct. The word "things" does not make clear to the reader what other equipment is needed.

- Option A is incorrect because the word "navigating" clearly describes finding a direction or location.
- Option B is incorrect because the word "requires" indicates that an item is necessary.
- Option C is incorrect because the word "hikers" describes a specific group of people.

5. Answers will vary. An example would be the following sentence and two precise terms explained.

Sentence: Maria decided to increase her chances of completing the hike next spring by practicing walking on ice with crampons and investing in a satellite phone.

Description of Diction: The terms "crampons" and "satellite" are examples of precise diction that helps the reader visualize the steel equipment she will wear on her feet and the type of phone she will carry in the wilderness.

Chapter 61

1. Option A is correct. This sentence contains jargon ("synergy," "EOD") that would be commonly understood within a business setting.

- Option B is incorrect because the sentence does not contain scientific terms likely be found in a scientific journal.
- Option C is incorrect because this sentence would not likely be found in a novel, unless that novel focused on a business setting.
- Option D is incorrect because the sentence does not use persuasion to help people become motivated.

2. Option D is correct. It contains the informal terms "bling" and "flossy."

- Option A states a formal proposition that many people are unaware of ways they can enhance their privacy settings.
- Option B describes the results of a study using formal language.
- Option C provides formal direct instruction to write down your 15-digit IMEI.

3. Option B is correct. The slang "bee's knees" and "all wet" indicates that the setting for this passage is the 1920s.

- The references in option A are about World War II in Europe in the 1940s.
- Option C is incorrect because the reference to a gunslinger indicates that the setting for this was during the "Old West."
- The slang from option D would be more appropriate for the 1960s or later.

4. Option A is correct. "Maintaining eye contact" is an idea that fits the content of the passage, and the sentence uses formal language similar to that of the passage.

- Option B is incorrect because it uses informal language such as "bouncing" which does not fit this formal passage.
- Option C is incorrect because it uses slang like "homeskillet," which does not fit this formal passage.
- Option D is incorrect because "computer skills" are not part of the content in this passage.

5. Answers will vary. Possible conventions for each type of writing include the following examples.

A. Business letter: inside address, date, salutation, closing

B. News article: headline, byline, lead

C. Essay: introduction, thesis, body, conclusion

ENGLISH

Chapter 62

1. Option B is correct. Brainstorming is one way to come up with ideas before you write.

   - The other options are incorrect because citing sources, proofreading, and editing all occur after a draft of a piece of writing is complete.

2. Option D is correct. Editing and proofreading would likely be the last step in a writing process because they occur after revision.

   - Option A is incorrect because research occurs during prewriting and during revision but before editing and proofreading.
   - Option B is incorrect because mapping possible topics and subtopics is part of prewriting.
   - Option C is incorrect because organization would occur during prewriting and sometimes during revision. This is before editing and proofreading.

3. Option A is correct. Malik is writing a research paper and must cite the sources he used in his writing.

   - Option B is incorrect because a research paper does not require an opposition or opposing viewpoint.
   - Option C is incorrect because Malik has already planned his writing with an outline and written a draft.
   - Option C is incorrect because a research paper does not require illustrations and captions.

4. Option D is correct. Quoting a source, whether published or unpublished, requires inclusion of a citation.

   - Option A is incorrect because authors do not need to use citations for their own ideas.
   - Option B is incorrect because the need for citation is not related to emphasis.
   - Option C is incorrect because fictional events do not require citation.

5. Answers will vary. Below is an example of an outline of an article on revision.

   How to Revise Your Writing

   I. Read Your Paper Out Loud

      a. Notice whether each paragraph has a clear key point
      b. Decide whether each key point has enough supporting detail
      c. Listen for grammar errors

   II. Peer Editing

      a. Have a friend listen as you read your paper aloud
      b. Talk over the key points that were clear
      c. Discuss two ways to improve the paper to communicate your key points

Chapter 63

1. Option B is correct. A topic sentence is a key part of a paragraph because it reveals the subject of the entire paragraph.

   - The other options are incorrect because not all paragraphs need a source, introductory phrase, or opposition.

2. Option C is correct. The word "another" lets the reader know that the paragraph is transitioning from one way of improving photography to a different way of improving photos.

   - Option A is incorrect because it is describing an action, not transitioning to a new topic.
   - Option B is incorrect because it is providing a detail about the topic, not transitioning to a new topic.
   - Option D is incorrect because it is describing a cause and effect, not transitioning to a new topic.

3. Option D is correct. This chronological sequence is the most logical order for the paragraph. It starts with going to the exam, then taking the exam, then going on vacation after the exam, and, last, feeling ready to start new courses after the vacation.

4. Option C is correct. The paragraph is about setting the focus of a phone camera. The idea that most people don't bother to read the instruction manual of their phone is not about the focus of the camera.

   - Option A is incorrect because it is the topic sentence of the paragraph.
   - Options B and D are incorrect because they are important details about focusing your phone camera.

5. Answers will vary. The following example uses all parts of a paragraph correctly.

Topic sentence	It is hard to believe that I actually learned how to place photos with the contacts on my phone.
Supporting details	It is pretty simple to do. You just go to your contacts list and select a person. Click on "Edit" in the upper right-hand corner. Under the icon for your contact will be the highlighted phrase "Add photo." Just click on that phrase, and several options for the photo will appear. One of the options is to simply take a photo. One of my friends was in the room when I learned how to do this, so I quickly took his picture.
Conclusion/ transition	Now every time I look at this photo, I remember how easy using some features on my phone can be!

Chapter 64

1. Option D is correct. Cause/effect sets up the meaning of "radical." Option A is an alternate meaning for "radical" that is not related to weeds. Options B and C ignore the fact that the weeds are stubborn and invasive.

2. Option B is correct. Here "current" refers to the electricity used to power the fan. Option A is using "current" to refer to the flow of a river. Option C refers to the flow of air. In Option D, the word means "recent."

3. Option A is correct. The word "dark" provides a synonym for "opaque." Option B describes the other windows mentioned in the sentence. Options C and D have no basis in context clues.

4. Option C is correct. The series of tools listed are all used in woodworking. Choice A refers to an airplane, which is not related to the rest of the series. Choice B is a term from geometry, not woodworking. Choice D is a homonym for "plane."

5. Answers may vary but should be similar to the following example answer. The word "obnoxious" means "extremely unpleasant." The words "harsh," "superior," "loud," and "garish" all set a tone to help the reader understand "obnoxious."

Chapter 65

1. Option A is correct. The suffix "-ness" changes the root "good," to another word indicating the quality of being good. Options B, C, and D are all incorrect because the suffixes do not change the word meaning. They change the tense of each verb.

2. Option B is correct. The prefix "hyper-" means "more than or too much." Option A is incorrect because the prefix "hypo-" means "less than or too little." Option C is incorrect because the prefix "super-" means "beyond." Option D is incorrect because the prefix "inter-" means "between."

3. Option C is correct. The prefix "dis-" means "not." Option A is incorrect because the suffix "-ation" means "the state of." Option B is incorrect because the suffix "-ous" means "to have the quality of." Option D is incorrect because the prefix "anti-" means "the opposite of".

4. Option D is correct. The prefix "pre-" means "before." The suffix "ment" means "the act of." Option A is incorrect because it is the past tense of "judge." Option B is incorrect because it means "the quality of making good decisions." Option C is incorrect because the prefix "post-" means "after."

5. Answers will vary. Examples of medical affixes and their meanings include the following.

"Acanth-" means "thorn or spine." An acanthocyte is a cell that has protrusions.
"Amylo-" means "starch." Amylase is an enzyme that breaks down starches.
"-cardia" means "heart." Tachycardia describes an irregular heartbeat.
"-oma" means "swelling." A blastoma is a type of tumor.
"-phagia" means "swallowing." Dysphagia is the inability to swallow.

ENGLISH

☑ Unit Quiz

They're going to lead the group through the park because it's trails can be confusing.

1. Which of the following corrects a spelling error in the sentence?

   A. "They're" should be "Their."
   B. "lead" should be "led."
   C. "through" should be "threw."
   D. "it's" should be "its."

2. Which of the following words correctly follows the spelling rule to drop the final "e"?

   A. excitment
   B. movable
   C. likness
   D. tracable

3. Which of the following plural words is spelled correctly?

   A. The plural of "self" is "selfs."
   B. The plural of "dash" is "dashs."
   C. The plural of "elf" is "elves."
   D. The plural of "church" is "churchs."

The ice skater trained by lifting weights doing box jumps and stretching to increase flexibility.

4. Which of the following corrects the punctuation errors in the sentence?

   A. The ice skater trained by lifting weights doing box jumps, and stretching to increase flexibility.
   B. The ice skater trained by lifting, weights doing, box jumps and stretching to increase flexibility.
   C. The ice skater trained by lifting weights, doing box jumps, and stretching to increase flexibility.
   D. The ice skater trained by lifting, weights doing, box jumps and stretching, to increase flexibility.

"The movie had an interesting plot" she said. "However, the lack of action made the movie seem too long."

5. Which of the following corrects the punctuation error in the sentence?

   A. "The movie had an interesting plot." she said. "However, the lack of action made the movie seem too long."
   B. "The movie had an interesting plot," She said. "However, the lack of action made the movie seem too long."
   C. "The movie had an interesting plot, she said." "However, the lack of action made the movie seem too long."
   D. "The movie had an interesting plot," she said. "However, the lack of action made the movie seem too long."

Subir and Aisha wanted to play in the snow over the weekend but, the warm weather ruined their plans.

6. Which of the following corrects the punctuation error in the sentence?

   A. Subir and Aisha wanted to play in the snow over the weekend but the warm weather ruined their plans.
   B. Subir and Aisha wanted to play in the snow over the weekend, but the warm weather ruined their plans.
   C. Subir and Aisha wanted to play in the snow over the weekend but. The warm weather ruined their plans.
   D. Subir and Aisha wanted to play in the snow over the weekend, but, the warm weather ruined their plans.

Running for at least twenty minutes three times per week is a great way to get exercise and to stay healthy.

7. Which of the following is the simple subject of the sentence?

   A. Running
   B. is
   C. way
   D. exercise

8. Which of the following is a complex sentence?

   A. We waited for more than two hours.
   B. Although the line was long, it moved rather quickly.
   C. The line was short for me, but it was much longer when I left.
   D. She looked for the shortest checkout line; she did not have much time to waste.

That street runs parallel to Main Street on the other side of the park.

9. Which word in the sentence modifies the simple subject?

   A. That
   B. parallel
   C. Main
   D. other

After she fell, Mikayla was _sad_ because she realized she ripped her favorite jeans.

10. Which of the following is a more precise word that could replace the word "sad"?

    A. unhappy
    B. terrified
    C. dismayed
    D. mournful

Despite donating four boxes of old toys, Keegan still had a lot of stuff in her room.

11. Which of the following words from the sentence should be revised to fix ambiguous language?

    A. boxes
    B. toys
    C. stuff
    D. room

_____ she cooked and enjoyed a wonderful meal, Violet cleaned and put away the dishes.

12. Which transition best completes the sentence?

    A. But
    B. After
    C. In addition
    D. Altogether

---

(1) My friends love to dance. (2) Gwendolyn is a professionally trained ballet dancer who is well versed in classical ballet, neoclassical ballet, as well as contemporary ballet. (3) Timothy recently learned how to line dance, but he also attended dance academy for several years. (4) Jarvis has some groovy moves on the dance floor and loves to create his own music. (5) Marta is a member of her university's dance squad and the team just won a national tournament.

13. Which sentence in the paragraph contains informal language?

    A. Sentence 2
    B. Sentence 3
    C. Sentence 4
    D. Sentence 5.

14. Which of the following sentences contain slang that would indicate that its context is the United States in the 1960s?

    A. Melissa and Suzanne carpooled together to get to work today.
    B. Shaquan and Janell had an exquisite dinner last night at the restaurant.
    C. Joseph and Jamal had a gas last night at the dance hall.
    D. Heidi and Frank are BFFs and are going to see a late movie tonight.

15. Miguel was just assigned a research paper on pollution. He needs to think about different kinds of pollution to narrow his topic for his writing. Which of the following steps of the writing process is being used by Miguel?

    A. proofreading
    B. brainstorming
    C. editing
    D. revising

16. Isabella is finishing an essay that has been through several rounds of revisions. Which of the following steps of the writing process should she complete next?

    A. brainstorming
    B. writing
    C. planning
    D. proofreading

17. Which of the following sentences would most likely act as a topic sentence?

    A. Giraffes are the tallest animals in the world.
    B. Great white sharks have about 300 teeth.
    C. Cheetahs can run at a speed of about 65 to 70 miles per hour.
    D. The tongue of a blue whale can weigh as much as an elephant.

    I. Finally, my mother was able to drop me off at school, just before the bell rang.
    II. We worked together to replace the flat with the spare tire that was in the trunk.
    III. Then we had some more trouble as we discovered that my mother's car had a flat tire.
    IV. This morning, we woke up to realize that the storm overnight had knocked out the power at our house.

18. Which of the following is the best chronological sequence for the sentences?

    A. III, II, I, IV
    B. III, IV, I, II
    C. IV, II, I, III
    D. IV, III, II, I

    Javier wants to <u>chart</u> a career path for success, so he is meeting with his advisor this afternoon.

19. Which of the following is the best synonym for "chart" as used in the sentence?

    A. plan
    B. graph
    C. rank
    D. draw

    The pond was used to <u>retain</u> excess water and often filled after large rainstorms.

20. Which of the following best captures the meaning of "retain"?

    A. remember
    B. hold
    C. maintain
    D. cherish

My soccer team will <u>contend</u> for the regional championship tonight.

21. Which of the following best captures the meaning of "contend"?

    A. debate
    B. compete
    C. declare
    D. cope

22. Based on an examination of the word parts, which of the following means "to treat before or in advance"?

    A. retreat
    B. mistreat
    C. pretreat
    D. overtreat

23. Based on an analysis of the word parts, which of the following means "swelling of the heart muscle"?

    A. amylase
    B. acanthocyte
    C. myocarditis
    D. hydrocephalus

Stephon fell off his bicycle and injured his leg. When he went to the doctor, the doctor told him that he only suffered a hematoma and it would go down in a few days.

24. Based on analysis of word parts, what is the meaning of the word "hematoma" in the sentence?

    A. a severed nerve causing loss of feeling
    B. swelling caused by localized bleeding
    C. a broken bone
    D. a severe laceration

Unit Quiz Answers

1. Option D is correct because it corrects an error. The possessive "its" should be used because the trail belongs to it (the park). "They're" is correctly used because it means "they are". "Lead" is the correct tense of the verb. "Through" is correctly used because it means "across".

2. Option B is correct. The is the correct spelling of "movable" requires dropping the final "e" before adding the suffix. Excitement, likeness, and traceable all are exceptions to the rule. They all keep the final "e" before adding a suffix.

3. Option C is correct. "Elves" correctly uses the spelling rule to change the ending "f" to a "v" and adds "es." The plural of self should also change the "f" to a "v" and add "es" to spell "selves". The plural of dash should add an "es" to form dashes. The plural of church should add an "es" to form churches.

4. Option C is correct. This sentence correctly punctuates the serial comma after "weights" and "jumps." Option A is missing a comma after the word "weights." Options B and D have incorrect commas after the words "lifting" and "doing" that confuse the reader.

5. Option D is correct. This response correctly puts the comma inside the quotation mark following the word plot. Option A is incorrect because it incorrectly puts a period after the word plot. This is not the end of the sentence. Option B incorrectly capitalizes the word "She". Option C incorrectly places quotation marks after "said".

6. Option B is correct because it places a comma before the conjunction "but" that joins two independent clauses. Option A is incorrect because it does not contain the needed comma. Option C is incorrect because even though it separates the two independent clauses into two sentences, it incorrectly keeps the conjunction. Option D is incorrect because it places a comma on either side of the conjunction, when only a comma before the conjunction is needed.

7. Option A is correct because "running" is the topic of the sentence. It is a gerund form of the verb "run" that acts as a noun. The word "is" is the simple predicate. The word "way" is the object of the verb, and "exercise" is the object of the infinitive phase "to get exercise."

8. Option B is correct because it contains an independent clause "it moved rather quickly" and the dependent clause "Although the line was long." Option A is a simple sentence, and Options C and D are compound sentences that contain two independent clauses.

9. Option A is correct because the word "that" modifies the simple subject "street." The word "parallel" is an adverb modifying the verb "runs." The word "Main" is part of the proper noun "Main Street, and the word "other" modifies the noun "side" that is not the subject of the sentence.

10. Option C is correct. "Dismayed" is a more precise word and describes a type of sadness that involves regret. Option A is incorrect because "unhappy" is a synonym for sad but does not describe the type of sadness. Option B is incorrect because "terrified" is not a synonym for sad. Option D is incorrect because "mournful" means a type of deep sadness that involves grief. This is not the type of sadness that fits the context of the sentence.

11. Option C is correct because the word "stuff" is an ambiguous word that is inexact and unclear. Boxes, toys, and room are all nouns that have a clear meaning.

12. Option B is correct. It uses a transition word that refers to chronology. It reveals the sequence of events that first Violet cooked, and "after" this, she cleaned up. Option A is incorrect because it uses an opposition transition word. Option C is incorrect because it uses a transition word to add an idea. Option D is incorrect because it uses a concluding transition word.

13. Option C is correct. The word "groovy" is informal language. Options A, B, and D contain formal language.

14. Option C is correct. The slang phrase "had a gas" identifies the sentence as being from the 1960s. Option A is incorrect because the informal term "carpooled" is from the 1980's. Option D contains the slang term "BFF" from the 2000s. No slang words or phrases appear in Option B.

ENGLISH

15. Option B is correct. Brainstorming by considering different aspects of a topic can help narrow the focus of a paper. Option A is incorrect because proofreading is typically part of the revision step. Option C is incorrect because editing is typically part of the revision step. Option D is incorrect because revising is typically part of the revision step.

16. Option D is correct. Proofreading is the step that occurs after the revision steps. Option A is incorrect because brainstorming is typically done at the beginning of the writing process. Option B is incorrect because Addison has already written and revised her essay. Option C is incorrect because Addison has already planned her essay.

17. Option A is correct because it states a main idea that can be supported by specific facts. Option B is incorrect because it states a specific fact about great white sharks that could be best used as a supporting detail. Option C is incorrect because it states a specific fact about cheetahs that could be best used as a supporting detail. Option D is incorrect because it states a specific fact about blue whales that could be best used as a supporting detail.

18. Option D is correct. Transition words help place the sentences in correct time order from getting up "this morning," "then" having a flat tire, then fixing it, and "finally" going to school.

19. Option A is correct. In this context, "chart a career path" and "plan a career path" mean the same thing. Option B is incorrect because Javier is not "graphing" a career path. Options C and D are incorrect because Javier is not "ranking" or "drawing" career path.

20. Option B is correct. In this context, "retain" means "to hold" excess water. Option A is incorrect because the pond is not used "to remember" the water. Options C and D are incorrect because the pond was not used to "maintain" or "cherish" the water.

21. Option B is correct. In this context, the soccer team will "compete" for the championship. The soccer team will not "debate," "declare," or "cope" for the championship.

22. Option C is correct because the prefix "pre-" means "before." The other options are incorrect because the prefix "re-" means "again," the prefix "mis-" means "badly," and the prefix "over-" means "too much."

23. Option C is correct, because the affix "-cardia" means "heart." The other options are incorrect because the affix "amylo-" means "starch," the affix "acanth-" means "thorn or spine," and the affix "hydro-" means "water."

24. Option B is correct. The root "heme" refers to blood and suffix "-oma" means "swelling." Option D is incorrect because although a cut involves blood, it does not involve swelling. Options A and C are incorrect because they also do not discuss the "swelling" indicated by the suffix "-oma."

ATI TEAS Comprehensive Practice Test

The following practice test matches the ATI TEAS test plan and is composed of questions that have usage data from previous administrations. This data enables ATI to provide the table below that you can use to determine your predicted preparedness*. To ensure the most accurate prediction of your preparedness level, be sure to:

- Take each section in the order in which they are presented. You must complete and score yourself on all four sections.
- Time yourself using the following time limits:
  - Reading – 64 minutes
  - Mathematics – 54 minutes
  - Science – 63 minutes
  - English and Language Usage – 28 minutes
- As much as possible, replicate the proctored testing environment, including:
  - Do not refer to notes or use outside resources other than scrap paper.
  - Do not communicate with others during testing.
  - Do not use electronic devices other than a four-function calculator.
  - Allow yourself a 10-minute break after the Mathematics section.
- Record your responses on a piece of paper and use the answer key to grade your responses after you've completed all four sections. The total number of questions you answered correctly determines your score range for the table below (e.g., 50 total correct answers equals "Basic" preparedness level).

Score Range (total correct answers)	Predicted ATI TEAS Preparedness Level	Academic Preparedness Level Definition
0 to 48	Developmental	Developmental scores generally indicate a very low level of overall academic preparedness necessary to support learning of health sciences-related content. Students at this level will require additional preparation for most objectives assessed on ATI TEAS.
49 to 79	Basic	Basic scores generally indicate a low level of overall academic preparedness necessary to support learning of health sciences-related content. Students at this level are likely to require additional preparation for many objectives assessed on ATI TEAS.

*A score on this practice test does not guarantee that a similar score will be achieved on the ATI TEAS. While the predictive model is based on a broad sample of user data, there are a number of factors that can affect any given test performance and result in an outlier score.

COMPREHENSIVE PRACTICE

80 to 115	Proficient	Proficient scores generally indicate a moderate level of overall academic preparedness necessary to support learning of health sciences-related content. Students at this level can require additional preparation for some objectives assessed on ATI TEAS.
116 to 136	Advanced	Advanced scores generally indicate a high level of overall academic preparedness necessary to support learning of health sciences-related content. Students at this level are not likely to require additional preparation for the objectives assessed on ATI TEAS.
137 to 150	Exemplary	Exemplary scores generally indicate a very high level of overall academic preparedness necessary to support learning of health sciences-related content. Students at this level are not likely to require additional preparation for the objectives assessed on ATI TEAS.

Subscore Comparison Table

If your overall score prediction indicates that you would benefit from additional study before taking the proctored TEAS exam, an indication of your relative strengths and weaknesses on the four subscore areas of the test may help you to effectively focus your study efforts.

The table below accounts for variations in difficulty among the sections of the test and can be used to determine which of your section scores indicates the greatest need for additional study.

Directions:
Find and circle the number of questions you answered correctly in each content area. Which circled score is in the lowest row of the table? We recommend that you start your studying there!

Reading	Mathematics	Science	English
		47	
	32		
			24
47			
		46	
	31		
46			
		45	
			23
	30		
		44	
45			
		43	
			22
	29		
		42	
44			
		41	
	28		
			21
		40	
43			
		39	

Reading	Mathematics	Science	English
	27		
		38	
42			
			20
		37	
	26		
41			
		36	
	25		
		35	
			19
40			
		34	
	24		
		33	
39			
			18
		32	
	23		
38			
		31	
		30	
37			

Reading	Mathematics	Science	English
			17
	22		
		29	
36			
	21		
		28	
			16
35			
		27	
	20		
		26	
34			
			15
	19		
		25	
33			
		24	
	18		
32			
			14
		23	
31			
		22	
	17		
			13
		21	
30			
	16		
		20	
29			
			12
		19	
	15		
28			
		18	
27			
	14		
			11
		17	
26			
		16	
	13		
25			
			10
		15	
24			
	12		
		14	
23			
			9
	11		
		13	

Reading	Mathematics	Science	English
22			
		12	
21			
			8
	10		
20			
		11	
	9		
19			
			7
		10	
18			
	8		
		9	
17			
			6
16			
		8	
	7		
15			
			5
		7	
14			
	6		
13			
		6	
			4
12			
	5		
		5	
11			
10			
			3
	4		
		4	
9			
8			
		3	
	3		
			2
7			
6			
		2	
5			
	2		
4			
			1
3			
		1	
2			
	1		
			0
1			

COMPREHENSIVE PRACTICE

Comprehensive Practice Test

Reading

In school, students are taught that carnivores are meat-eating animals, herbivores are plant-consuming animals, and omnivores eat everything. Now add "locavore" to this list. A locavore is a person who strives to maintain a diet out of locally grown food. Typically, this would include food produced within a 100-mile radius. At a time when there are growing concerns over the safety of our food supply, more and more people are turning to nearby sources of food – whether organic or grown with chemicals – and liking it.

Today it is common for food products to 1,500 "food miles" from a large corporate farm to a consumer's dinner plate. It is entirely possible that some of the produce found at a grocery store in Kansas was grown and harvested in California. This system has evolved to suit industrial scale production and distribution instead of taste or nutrition. This development has led to the worrisome situation in which the average consumer has little chance of knowing where or how the food he or she buys was grown or raised.

There are a number of local alternatives to industrial food, and the variety is growing. Farmers markets are located in nearly every city and town. Some markets operate throughout the year, offering the produce that thrives in the local environment. The organic food movement is thriving to the point that it is the fastest growing sector in the overall food industry, and organic producers often sell their products at local grocery stores. A third alternative is CSA, or community-supported agriculture. A CSA is a subscription service that individuals can purchase from local farms. A subscriber is typically given a weekly supply of whatever the farm produces. Increasingly, it is possible for us to become more and more locavorous.

The following questions are based on this passage.

1. Which of the following is a logical conclusion based on the passage?
   A. People are becoming locavores to avoid food grown with chemicals.
   B. Organic foods are grown within 100 miles of where they are sold.
   C. An increasing number of consumers want to know where their food is grown.
   D. Farmers markets provide a greater diversity of food products than grocery stores.

2. Which of the following is an opinion stated in the passage?
   A. It is worrisome that the average consumer does not know where or how most food is grown or raised.
   B. It is entirely possible that some of the produce found in a grocery store in Kansas was grown and harvested in California.
   C. Some food products travel 1,500 "food miles" from a large corporate farm to a consumer's dinner plate.
   D. Farmers markets offer produce that thrives in the local environment.

3. What is the author's primary argument in the passage?

    A. Consumers should primarily eat organically grown food.
    B. Consumers should take the time to learn where all of their food is produced.
    C. Subscribing to a CSA will promote a healthy diet and support local farmers.
    D. Consuming locally grown food is a viable and beneficial alternative.

4. Which of the following sentences from the passage supports the claim made in the final sentence of the passage?

    A. A locavore is a person who strives to maintain a diet out of locally grown food.
    B. Today, it is common for food products to travel 1,500 "food miles" from a large corporate farm to a consumer's dinner plate.
    C. There are a number of local alternatives to industrial food, and the variety is growing.
    D. It is entirely possible that some of the produce found at a grocery store in Kansas was grown and harvested in California.

5. Which of the following inferences can be drawn from the passage?

    A. Large industrial farms are causing local farms to go out of business.
    B. Organic foods are comprised of fruits and vegetables but not meats and dairy.
    C. Locavores prefer to consume a vegetarian or vegan diet based on local produce.
    D. Industrial scale food production and distribution may affect the quality of foods.

6. A gardener purchased lattice so she could train the grapevine along the side of the house.

    Which of the following defines "train" as used in the sentence above?

    A. to teach so as to make fit or qualified
    B. to direct the growth of
    C. to focus attention
    D. to motivate by discipline

7. A student is writing a research paper about the psychological effects of homework. Which of the following sources should she consult for statistical data?

    A. An encyclopedia entry about the history of homework assignments
    B. An academic study about hours spent on homework each night
    C. A blog detailing a fellow student's experiences with homework
    D. A magazine article by a teacher about the importance of daily homework

Given the media coverage surrounding climate change, most people are aware of this environmental issue. One that is less well known but may become just as crucial is "peak oil." What is peak oil? Simply put, it is the point at which the world production of oil reaches its highest point and begins a steady, irreversible decline. This has been known for some time. Hubbert's Curve (1956), named for the scientist who formulated it, predicted that U.S. production would peak around 1970. He was off by 1 year. Since 1971-2, the oil production of the United States has been gradually declining.

The following questions are based on this passage.

8. Which of the following best describes the author's purpose in the first two sentences of the passage?

    A. To argue that climate change presents a serious danger
    B. To persuade readers to take action on the issue of peak oil
    C. To introduce the subject matter by comparing it to a familiar issue
    D. To provide a definition of the term "peak oil"

9. Which of the following words would the author use to describe the issue of peak oil?

   A. Significant
   B. Confusing
   C.. Reversible
   D. Avoidable

10. Which of the following statements best describes the argument made in the passage?

    A. Peak oil and climate change are directly connected.
    B. Increasing media coverage of peak oil will improve oil production.
    C. Hubbert's Curve provides an example of a way to reverse climate change.
    D. Peak oil is an important issue even if not well known.

Among those who subscribe the self-sufficiency and moving back to the land, Helen and Scott Nearing are a legendary couple. Together, the Nearings exemplified the notion of the good life by living simply in a rural setting.

Scott (1883-1983) came from a wealthy Pennsylvania coal mining family, and Helen Knothe Nearing (1904-1995) was the daughter of an intellectual Ridgewood, New Jersey, family. Together they would travel a path very far away from their rather conventional beginnings. By the time he was in his early 20s, Scott had taken to social activism, speaking out against the unsafe working conditions in the Pennsylvania coal mines. Helen spent a brief period working in a factory before meeting Scott and leaving behind the creature comforts of her former lifestyle.

The two met first in 1921 and again in 1928, and were together from that point. In 1932, they left New York City for rural southern Vermont, where they developed a self-sufficient lifestyle and philosophy. They divided their waking hours in three 4-hour blocks: "bread labor," which was work for food, shelter, fuel, etc.; civic work, such as community service; and recreational or professional pursuits, economics research for Scott and music for Helen. Until 1952, their bread labor in Vermont was primarily maple products; after 1952, when they moved to Maine, it was blueberries. They were prolific builders of stone and concrete structures, completing 21 in all, and all by hand. Since they were cult figures of a sort, they often had the willing help of enthusiastic young volunteers who made the pilgrimage to New England.

The two authored many books, the most famous of which is Living the Good Life (1954). This and other titles by the Nearings are credited with spurring the "back to the land" movement in the 1960s.

The following questions are based on this passage.

11. Scott Nearing was likely involved in which of the following activities the year Helen was born?

    A. Writing Living the Good Life
    B. Harvesting blueberries
    C. Speaking against unsafe coal mines
    D. Building concrete structures by hand

12. Which of the following is a key part of the Nearings' philosophy of a self-sufficient lifestyle?

    A. Dividing time into 4-hour blocks to accomplish goals
    B. Social activism against factory work
    C. Writing books, like Living the Good Life
    D. Moving from New York City to Vermont

13. Which of the following activities might the Nearings have practiced during their civic work based on the passage?

    A. Campaigning to increase coal mining in their area
    B. Shopping for lavish home furnishings
    C. Fundraising for factories that make processed food
    D. Teaching a class on baking bread

14. Which of the following sentences contains an opinion?

    A. In 1932, they left New York City for rural southern Vermont, where they developed a self-sufficient lifestyle and philosophy.

    B. By the time he was in his early 20s, Scott had taken to social activism, speaking out against the unsafe working conditions in the Pennsylvania coal mines.

    C. Together, the Nearings exemplified the notion of the good life by living simply in a rural setting.

    D. The two authored many books, the most famous of which is Living the Good Life (1954).

15. Which of the following is a logical conclusion based on the passage?

    A. The Nearings' writings were their most influential contribution to the culture.

    B. Community service was an example of "bread labor" as defined by the Nearings.

    C. The Nearings inherited their philosophy from the "back to the land" movement.

    D. The Nearings followed in their parents' footsteps in embracing a rural lifestyle.

16. Use the drug facts label below to answer the question.

Drug Facts
Active ingredient: polymyxin B sulfate and bacitracin zinc
Purpose
....Antibiotic Ointment
Uses
Help prevent infection in cuts, scrapes, and minor burns. Relieves itching, burning, and minor irritations.
Warnings
For ecternal use only. Do not use on children under 2 years of age unless directed by a doctor. When using this product, do not get into eyes. If contact occurs, rinse eyes throughly with water. Stop use ask a doctor if irritation occurs or if there is no improvement within 2 weeks. Keep out of reach of children. in case of overdose, get medical help or contact a Poison Control Center right away.
Directions
Wash the affected area and dry thoroughly. Apply a thin layer of the product over affected area four times daily or as directed by a physician. Supervise children in the use of this product. This product is not effective on scalp or nails.
Other information
Inactive ingredients cocoa butter, olive oil, and white petrolatum
Questions comments? Call 1-800-555-5555

Which of the following statements about this product might cause a pharmacist concern?

    A. "I used the ointment on my heat rash."

    B. "I used the ointment for an abrasion on my baby's eyelid."

    C. "I put the ointment on my 4-year-old child's knee scrape."

    D. "I put the ointment on a rash from poison ivy three times today."

17. Read the following before answering the question. A candidate is choosing between job offers 1, 2, 3, and 4. Job 1 offers 2 weeks paid vacation per year and partial health insurance. Job 2 offers 1 week paid vacation per year and partial health insurance. Job 3 offers 2 weeks paid vacation per year and full health insurance. Job 4 offers 2 weeks paid vacation per year and full health insurance. Jobs 1 and 3 pay $5,000 more than Job 4. Job 2 pays $7,000 less than Job 4. What is the best job offer?

    A. 1

    B. 2

    C. 3

    D. 4

18. 1 2 3 4 3 2 1 2 3 4

    Using the number string above, replace every 1 with the letter A, every 2 with the letter B, every 3 with the letter D, and every 4 with the letter E. For letters that appear more than twice, delete the first instance of those letters. Delete the first and the last letter in the string, and replace the vowels with the letter X. Which of the following letter strings corresponds with the directions above?

    A. DBXBD

    B. BXBDX

    C. XDBXBD

    D. BDXDBX

COMPREHENSIVE QUESTIONS

Storytellers known as bards were an important element in sustaining Celtic civilization. They were trained at barding schools where they learned hundreds of poems and different styles of verse. Some bards trained for up to 7 years. In addition to singing memorized poems, they composed poems of their own to celebrate important events or commemorate fallen leaders. Many scholars believe that the bards of Brittany, a region in northwest France, and those of Wales created and passed on the legends of King Arthur and the Knights of the Round Table. Without the oral traditions, these stories would have been lost.

The following questions are based on this passage.

19. Which of the following supporting details best reinforces the argument presented in the first sentence that bards sustained Celtic civilization?

    A. Bards were specially trained at barding schools.
    B. Bards trained for as long as 7 years and learned different styles of verse.
    C. In addition to singing memorized poems, bards would compose poems of their own.
    D. Poems written by bards celebrated important events and commemorated fallen leaders.

20. Which of the following best rephrases the topic of the passage?

    A. The events that led to sustaining Celtic civilization
    B. The history and purpose of bards
    C. The importance of the King Arthur legends
    D. The purpose of barding schools

21. What is the main purpose of the passage?

    A. To inform
    B. To persuade
    C. To entertain
    D. To analyze

22. Use the chart below to answer the question.

Viewership Market Analysis

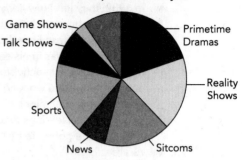

Which of the following television programs might an advertiser use to reach the most viewers?

    A. Game shows, talk shows, and reality shows
    B. Daytime dramas and news
    C. Sitcoms and primetime dramas
    D. Sports and talk shows

23. You encounter the following sentence while reading:

He kept teasing her, not noticing that she was getting frustrated, but when he playfully tossed a pencil at her, she moved to bat it away angrily.

You have not heard of the word "bat" used in this way before, so you look it up in the dictionary and find the following:

Bat n.

    1. the wooden club used in some games to hit the ball.
    2. any of numerous flying mammals of the order Chiropterav.
    3. to strike or hit, as if with a bat or club.
    4. to blink or wink

Which of these definitions best fits the context of the sentence?
    A. Definition 1
    B. Definition 2
    C. Definition 3
    D. Definition 4

24. When she noticed the dust on her running shoes, Jane realized she had become rather complacent about her fitness routine.

Which of following is the closest in meaning to "complacent" as used in the sentence above?

    A. unconcerned
    B. dissatisfied
    C. confident
    D. worried

After the assassination on November 22, 1963, a commission was formed to investigate the circumstances surrounding President Kennedy's death. The Warren Commission determined that no conspiracy was behind the assassination, but conspiracy theorists persisted in their belief that Oswald didn't act alone.

The following questions are based on this passage.

25. Which of the following additional sentences would be appropriate if this passage were found in a United States history textbook?

A. The ambiguous audio recordings and flawed government investigations are proof that there was more to Kennedy's assassination than meets the eye.

B. In spite of the mystery that surrounds the President's death, one thing is clear – American politics was fundamentally changed that November day.

C. Though the nation mourned, no one mourned more than Jacqueline Kennedy.

D. The Kennedy family is still one of the most well-known political families in the United States today.

26. Based on their titles, which of the following articles would provide the most reliable information for a student who wanted to learn more about the Kennedy assassination?

A. "The Political Landscape of Cold War America, 1965-1990"

B. "The Lone Gunman: Lee Harvey Oswald, Sole Conspirator?"

C. "Did JFK Play a Part in His Own Death?"

D. "November 22, 1963: A Brief History"

Baseball has long been known as "the national pastime." But does the name still fit? While baseball's contribution to U.S. culture dates back to the early part of the 19th century, football seems to have supplanted baseball in the U.S. imagination. For instance, in 2007, the top 10 sports broadcasts in television ratings were all games from the National Football League. Meanwhile, participation in youth baseball has fallen, and Major League Baseball teams are now composed of nearly 30% foreign-born players. While the criteria for the status of national pastime are elusive, football fans can make a persuasive argument that there's a new national pastime in the U.S.

The following questions are based on this passage.

27. Which of the following is the author's main purpose in the passage?

A. To argue that football should be considered America's "national pastime"

B. To inform readers about the historical association between baseball and American culture

C. To persuade readers that America should revive the popularity of baseball

D. To express feelings about the importance of football in American culture

28. Which of the following is a supporting detail of the author's main idea?

A. Baseball has long been known as "the national pastime."

B. Baseball's contribution to American culture dates back to the early part of the 19th century.

C. Football fans can make a compelling case that there's a new "national pastime" in America.

D. The top 10 sports broadcasts in television ratings were all games from the National Football League.

COMPREHENSIVE QUESTIONS

29. A nursery has exactly seven types of flowers: 1, 2, 3, 4, 5, 6, and 7. Choose five different types of flowers to plant in a garden, using the following guidelines: If type 1 is chosen, type 5 cannot be chosen. If type 3 is chosen, type 5 must be chosen. If type 2 is chosen, type 6 must be chosen. Which of the following combinations of flowers corresponds with the directions?

    A. 2,3,4,5,6
    B. 1,2,3,6,7
    C. 2,3,4,5,7
    D. 1,4,5,6,7

30. He headed off to the track, where he hoped to make a fast dollar by betting on the races.

    Which of the following dictionary definitions corresponds with "fast" as used in the sentence above?

    A. Distinguished by rapid motion
    B. Having agile mental abilities
    C. Obtained with little effort
    D. Characterized by wild behavior

31. Draw a horizontal line. From the midpoint of this line, draw a perpendicular line extending upward. Write the letter "A" at each end of the horizontal line and the letter "Z" at the end of the vertical line. Rotate the drawing 90 degrees clockwise. Which of the following drawings correctly corresponds with the directions?

A.

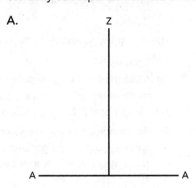

B.

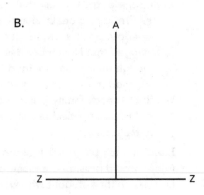

C.

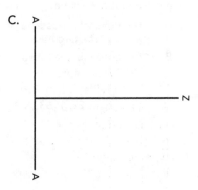

D.

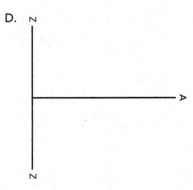

32. Marsupialia (Marsupials)

    Kangaroos
    Koalas
    Wombats

    Primates (Primates)

    Monkeys
    Chimpanzees
    Gorillas

    Rodentia (Rodents)

    Squirrels
    Mice
    Porcupines

    Which of the following statements is correct based on the taxonomy above?

    A. Marsupials are more similar to primates than to rodents.
    B. Rodents are a subcategory of Rodentia.
    C. Wombats are a subcategory of koalas.
    D. Squirrels are more similar to porcupines than to monkeys.

33. I avoided him because he thought he had a score to settle with me.

    Which of the following definitions is correct for "score" as used in the sentence above?

    A. A scratch or mark made on a surface
    B. An action that has a successful outcome
    C. A grudge that one holds against another
    D. The relevant facts related to a situation

34. Phylum Mollusca

    Cephalopoda

    Squids
    Octopuses
    Cuttlefish

    Gastropoda

    Snails
    Sea Slugs

    Pelecypoda
    Clams
    Mussels
    Oysters

    Which of the following statements is correct based on the outline above?

    A. A Pelecypoda is a type of Gastropoda.
    B. An octopus is a type of squid.
    C. Cephalopoda is more closely related to Gastropoda than to Pelecypoda.
    D. Snails are more closely related to sea slugs than to clams.

In the late 1970s, the directors of the Bernard van Leer Foundation invited a team of professors from Harvard University's Graduate School of Education to respond to a daunting challenge: Discover a way for every human being to develop to his or her maximum potential. Out of this collaboration of dozens of esteemed professionals came the theory of multiple intelligences (MI).

In 1983, Howard Gardner, a project team member, published Frames of Mind, which sets out the theory in some detail. In this book, Gardner posits that traditional notions of intelligence, which are largely based on I.Q. testing, do not sufficiently address the range of cerebral engagement. In short, various types of intelligence should be considered because different minds have different strengths. For too long, our notion of intelligence has been too narrow.

Originally, Gardner identified seven areas of human intelligence: verbal-linguistic, musical, logical-mathematical, visual-spatial, bodily-kinesthetic, interpersonal, and intrapersonal. A short time later, Gardner added an eighth intelligence: naturalistic.

Traditional school curriculum in Western culture has heavily emphasized learning through the verbal-linguistic and logical-mathematical intelligences. This has, according to Gardner, left many students poorly served by our educational system. Gifts in other areas of intelligence, such as the arts, should be identified and encouraged as well. Also, different methodologies of conveying information should be used to engage the distinct strengths of students with varying types of intelligence.

COMPREHENSIVE QUESTIONS

Gardner and others, like author Thomas Armstrong, Ph.D., have done much to cause the American educational establishment to rethink the way children learn in school. Many universities include courses about multiple intelligences, and teachers are often encouraged to use the theory of MI in planning their lessons. The result of this re-evaluation of intelligence has begun to transform the way teachers teach.

The following questions are based on this passage.

35. Which of the following is a supporting detail of the author's main idea in the passage?

    A. In this book, Gardner posits that traditional notions of intelligence, which are largely based on I.Q. testing, do not sufficiently address the range of cerebral engagement.

    B. Traditional notions of intelligence have limited the achievement of many students.

    C. Traditional school curriculum in Western culture has heavily emphasized learning through the verbal-linguistic and logical-mathematical intelligences.

    D. Researchers who developed the theory of multiple intelligences have had an effect on education.

36. Which of the following is a logical conclusion based on the passage?

    A. Howard Gardner, at the time of the study, had multiple intelligences.

    B. I.Q. testing focuses mainly on verbal-linguistic and mathematical-logical skills.

    C. Most teachers prefer to use traditional teaching methods in the classroom.

    D. Multiple intelligence principles are excluded from school curricula because they are difficult to test.

37. Which of the following statements best rephrases the key point of Howard Gardner's theory of multiple intelligences as described in the passage?

    A. Verbal-linguistic and logical-mathematical are the two most important types of multiple intelligences.

    B. Cerebral engagement is unrelated to I.Q. testing.

    C. Traditional school curriculum accommodates multiple types of intelligence.

    D. Understanding intelligence effectively requires taking into account overall cerebral engagement.

38. Which of the following changes is appropriate for a teacher who wants to address the theory of MI?

    A. Replacing a history slide show with memorization of names and dates

    B. Replacing written book reports with multimedia collaborations among students

    C. Encouraging more girls to enroll in upper-level mathematics courses

    D. Encouraging classroom competition by using flash card games

39. Which of the following students would most likely benefit the most from an educational system that incorporates MI into its curriculum?

    A. A student who draws intricate portraits on his notebook

    B. A student who excels at taking notes during lectures

    C. A student who likes to take part in spelling bees

    D. A student who reads at a higher level than her classmates

40. A friend calls and says, "Before I pick you up to go to the grocery store, I have to cook breakfast, then shower, so I will see you when I'm done with those two things." When should you expect your friend to pick you up?

    A. After he showers

    B. After he goes to the grocery store

    C. As soon as he hangs up the phone

    D. Before breakfast

41. Which of the following sources will be most helpful for a writer who is trying to use a greater variety of words in an article?

    A. Encyclopedia

    B. Almanac

    C. Style guide

    D. Thesaurus

DD&P Industries is currently seeking friendly, motivated individuals to fill entry-level positions in its call center.

DD&P is an industry leader in the manufacture and servicing of medical equipment. We are committed to providing excellent customer service and dedicated to hiring individuals with top-notch communication skills.

DD&P offers flexible work schedules with daytime, evening, weekend, and holiday shifts. We offer competitive pay and benefits packages, including medical/dental, 401(k), and profit sharing (after a year of employment).

Compensation: Hourly

Responsibilities:

- Providing professional customer service for incoming calls regarding products and services

- Understanding and communicating product and service information

- Routing calls to appropriate sources

- Handling customer complaints

- Qualifications:

- Good communication skills

- Ability to type 60 wpm

- Working knowledge of basic PC applications (Word, Outlook, etc.)

- Previous customer service experience preferred

The following questions are based on this passage.

42. Which of the following statements is a logical conclusion based on the job announcement?
   A. This position will be involved in formulating communications for marketing purposes.
   B. Applicants for this position must have previous experience in the health care industry.
   C. Applicants for this position must have effective telephone communication skills.
   D. This position includes a requirement to work on weekends and during holidays.

43. Which of the following individuals would most likely be interested in this job?
   A. A person who wants a position that provides health insurance
   B. A person who is looking for a salaried position
   C. A person who has previously managed customer service representatives
   D. A person who likes to work with and fix medical equipment

The heroines are in the house. In recent years, there has been a boom of young adult (YA) literature that has taken readers, and bestseller lists, by storm. Though YA novels have existed nearly as long as the novel itself, current YA novels have reinvented the genre. Now they tend to focus on the plight of a central heroine, a young girl tasked with dismantling the oppressive dystopia she lives in to save her friends and her family. The success of these stories is finally making Hollywood sit up and pay attention to the possibility of how lucrative female-led movies can be, and more female-driven films than ever are taking top spot at the box office.

The following questions are based on this passage.

44. Which of the following is the source of this passage?
   A. Young adult novel
   B. Instruction manual
   C. Book review
   D. Entertainment magazine

45. Below are several trends being discussed in the media. Which of the following trends resembles the theme of the passage's description of YA literature?
   A. More students are graduating from college in debt than ever before, and they are flooding the job market.
   B. A new cooking technique is being introduced in culinary schools across the world to great success.
   C. The percentage of people under 30 getting married has decreased greatly in the last 20 years.
   D. An automaker redesigned one of its standard models, and now it is one of their top sellers.

COMPREHENSIVE QUESTIONS

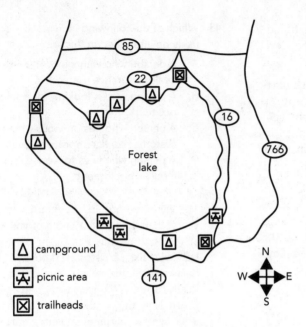

The following questions are based on this art.

46. The majority of the campgrounds are located on what side of the lake?

    A. South
    B. North
    C. East
    D. West

47. What highway runs along the east coast of the lake? (Note: The numbers on the map represent highway names.)

    A. 16
    B. 22
    C. 85
    D. 141

Mathematics

1. Which of the following expresses 425% as a decimal?

   A. 0.0425
   B. 0.425
   C. 4.25
   D. 425

2. The owner of a hot dog stand records the number of hot dogs purchased by each customer on a particular day and obtains the following data:

Number of Hot Dogs Purchased	Number of Customers
1	50
2	27
3	15
4	6
5	2

   Which of the following is the total number of hot dogs purchased during the day?

   A. 15
   B. 100
   C. 115
   D. 183

3. A computer is worth $1,500 at the time of purchase. After 5 years, the computer is outdated and has no monetary value. Assuming the computer's value decreases at a constant rate, which of the following expressions represents the computer's value at any time (t) in years?

   A. $-300t + 1,500$
   B. $-5t + 1,500$
   C. $-300t + 5$
   D. $-5t + 5$

4. $(x^2 + 4x + 4) - (x^2 - 6x + 9)$

   Simplify the expression above. Which of the following is correct?

   A. $10x + 13$
   B. $10x - 5$
   C. $-2x + 13$
   D. $-2x - 5$

5. Which of the following lists the given values from greatest to least?

   $\sqrt{3}, 1, 4, -0.8, -3/5$

   A. $\sqrt{3}, 1, 4, -0.8, -3/5$
   B. $4, 1, -0.8, -3/5, \sqrt{3}$
   C. $4, \sqrt{3}, 1, -3/5, -0.8$
   D. $4, \sqrt{3}, 1, -0.8, -3/5$

6. Which of the following expressions appropriately compares 4.67 and 4 1/3?

   A. $4.67 < 4\ 1/3$
   B. $4\ 1/3 \geq 4.67$
   C. $4.67 = 4\ 1/3$
   D. $4\ 1/3 < 4.67$

7. Which of the following lists the values in order from least to greatest?

   A. $-3, -3/10, 3.3, 3$
   B. $-3/10, -3, 3, 3.3$
   C. $-3, -3/10, 3, 3.3$
   D. $-3/10, 3, -3, 3.3$

8. Estimate the volume of a rectangular box that has a height of 22.1 cm, a length of 98 cm, and a width of 54 cm. The volume of a rectangular box can be calculated by multiplying length × width × height.

   A. $180,000\ cm^3$
   B. $90,000\ cm^3$
   C. $117,000\ cm^3$
   D. $100,000\ cm^3$

9. The data from a study shows that 30 out of every 100 adults surveyed have alcohol use disorder. At this rate, in a town with 2000 adults, how many would be expected to have alcohol use disorder?

   A. 30
   B. 300
   C. 600
   D. 60

10. If five gallons of paint will cover 2,000 square feet, how many gallons of paint are needed to paint 30,000 square feet?

    A. 15
    B. 6,000
    C. 400
    D. 75

11. A typist can type an average of 1,000 words in 15 min. At this rate, how many words can the typist type in 1 hr?
    A. 250
    B. 15,000
    C. 4,000
    D. 60,000

12. The length of an envelope is 21 cm rounded to the nearest whole cm. Which of the following is the smallest possible real length of the envelope?
    A. 20.5 cm
    B. 20.49 cm
    C. 21.44 cm
    D. 20.6 cm

13. In a neighborhood, 5% of the houses have red mailboxes. A student counts 60 red mailboxes in the neighborhood. Which of the following is the total number of houses in the neighborhood?
    A. 120
    B. 300
    C. 1,200
    D. 3,000

14. 9 − 7 3/8

    Find the difference. Which of the following is correct?
    A. 1 3/8
    B. 1 5/8
    C. 2 3/8
    D. 2 5/8

15. Which of the following is 5.4% of 35?
    A. 0.189
    B. 1.89
    C. 18.9
    D. 189

16. L = 2/3k

    This equation is used to determine the length of crutches in inches (L) required for a person of a given height in inches (k). Which of the following statements is true?
    A. Each 1/3 inch of height adds 1 inch to the crutch length.
    B. Each 1 inch of height adds 1/3 inch to the crutch length.
    C. Each 2 inches of height adds 3 inches to the crutch length.
    D. Each 3 inches of height adds 2 inches to the crutch length.

17. Which of the following fractions represents the sum of 0.3, 0.6, 0.04, and 0.02?
    A. 3/20
    B. 24/25
    C. 25/24
    D. 3/2

18. 5/8 + 1 7/9 + 3

    Simplify the expression above. Which of the following is correct?
    A. 4 29/72
    B. 4 12/17
    C. 5 7/18
    D. 5 29/72

19. 8 5/8 − 7 11/16

    Find the difference. Which of the following is correct?
    A. 3/4
    B. 15/16
    C. 11/16
    D. 13/4

20. The attendance at a nursing convention was 400 members, 75% of whom voted for an increase in membership dues. Which of the following is the number of members who voted for the increase?
    A. 75
    B. 100
    C. 300
    D. 325

21. The ratio of students who take the bus to school to the total population of a high school is 2:5. Which of the following is the percent of students who take the bus?
    A. 10%
    B. 20%
    C. 40%
    D. 60%

22. |2x + 1| = 17

    Solve the equation for x. Which of the following solution sets is correct?
    A. {8, 9}
    B. {−8, 9}
    C. {−9, −8}
    D. {−9, 8}

23. $5(x - 2)^2 = 125$

    Solve the equation above for x. Which of the following solution sets is correct?

    A. $\{-3, -7\}$
    B. $\{-3, 7\}$
    C. $\{3, -7\}$
    D. $\{3, 7\}$

24. Nancy ran a distance of 5 km in 30 minutes. What is her speed in meters (m) per hour (h)?

    A. 10,000 m/h
    B. 6,000 m/h
    C. 300,000 m/h
    D. 150 m/h

25. A student leaves college to drive home for the weekend. Along the way he makes one stop to eat lunch. He doesn't make any other stops. Which of the following graphs represents his trip?

    A.

    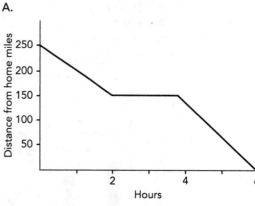

    B.

    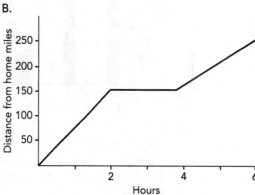

    C.

    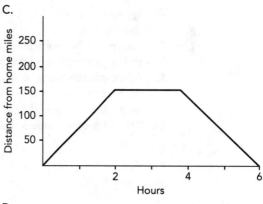

    D.

    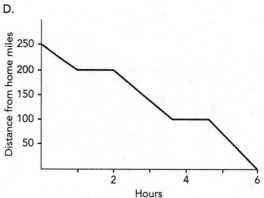

COMPREHENSIVE QUESTIONS

26. The distance from Chicago, IL to St. Louis, MO is 300 miles. Which of the following is the distance in meters (m) between these two cities? (Note: 1 mile = 1.6 km)

    A. 187.5 m
    B. 480 m
    C. 187,500 m
    D. 480,000 m

27. Use the graph below to answer the question.

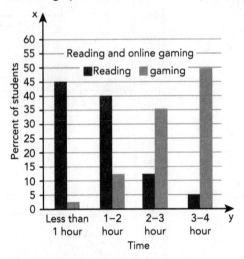

The bar graph shows how long teenagers in high school spend reading and online gaming. Which of the statements below is true about the bar graph?

    A. Teenagers spend more time online gaming than reading.
    B. For up to 1 hr, teenagers spend more time online gaming than reading.
    C. Approximately twice as many teenagers spend 3 to 4 hr online gaming compared to teenagers who spend 1 to 2 hr reading.
    D. About 9% of teenagers read for 3 to 4 hr.

28. Use the graph below to answer the question.

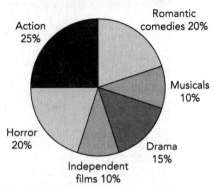

Which of the following statements is true about the circle graph?

    A. Over half of the students prefer horror movies.
    B. More students prefer romantic comedies than independent films.
    C. The percent of students who prefer action is the same as the percent who prefer drama.
    D. Musicals are the most popular movies among the students.

29. Use the scatter plot below to answer the question.

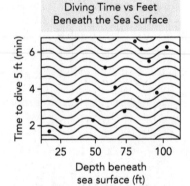

A group of researchers studied the relationship between the depth of a diver beneath the sea surface and the time it takes that diver to descend 5 additional feet. Which of the following statements describes the relationship between the two variables represented in the scatter plot?

    A. As the depth increases, diving time decreases.
    B. There is a positive correlation between depth and 5-foot diving time.
    C. As the depth increases, there is no effect on diving time.
    D. There is a negative correlation between depth and 5-foot diving time.

30. In a certain city, one block equals 0.25 miles. The city's high school is 4 blocks east of a grocery store. The city's library is 6 blocks east of the grocery store. A student walks to the library after school and then walks to the grocery store a few hours later. Which of the following is the number of miles this student has walked?

    A. 1.5 miles
    B. 2 miles
    C. 2.5 miles
    D. 4 miles

31. The distance between A and E in the graphic below represents 10 km. The distance between B and E, as well as A and D, is 8 km. If the distance between A and C is 4.5 km.

    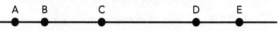

    Which of the following is the distance between B and C?

    A. 2.0 km
    B. 2.5 km
    C. 3.5 km
    D. 6.0 km

32. 10° C = _____ ° F Which of the following completes the equation above?
    (Note: ° F = [° C × 1.8] + 32)

    A. −12.2
    B. −1.2
    C. 33.8
    D. 50.0

Science

1. A person is suddenly frightened. Which of the following reactions occurs next?

    A. Liver cells absorb glucose from the blood stream.
    B. Blood vessels supplying skeletal muscles constrict.
    C. Blood vessels supplying the intestines dilate.
    D. Liver cells release glucose into the blood stream.

2. Which of the following is an example of positive feedback?

    A. Oxytocin causes an increase in uterine muscle contractions, ultimately causing the posterior pituitary to release more oxytocin
    B. An increase in blood glucose level causes the release of insulin, which results in the lowering of glucose levels in the blood and halting the release of insulin.
    C. A drop in body temperature causes the hypothalamus to activate warming mechanisms, which results in the increase of body temperature.
    D. An increase in blood osmolarity causes the release of ADH, which causes urine to become more concentrated and osmolarity to decrease.

3. Demyelinization results in which of the following?

    A. Inhibited detection of a stimulus at the dendrites of a nerve cell
    B. Disrupted propagation of an action potential along the axon of a nerve cell
    C. Inhibited uptake of neurotransmitters at the synapse of a nerve cell
    D. Disrupted ability of the Na+/K+ pumps to depolarize a cell

4. The nephridium in worms has a function most similar to which of the following organs in humans?

    A. Liver
    B. Spleen
    C. Lymph nodes
    D. Kidney

5. Which of the following cell types is responsible for the production of soluble antibodies?

    A. Cytotoxic T-cell
    B. Macrophage cell
    C. Helper T-cell
    D. B-cell

6. Which of the following organ systems is responsible for transporting nutrients, wastes, and other substances throughout the human body?

    A. Respiratory
    B. Immune
    C. Nervous
    D. Circulatory

7. Which of the following is characteristic of the human organism?

    A. Autotrophic with a genome stored in DNA
    B. Heterotrophic with a genome stored in DNA
    C. Autotrophic with a genome stored in RNA
    D. Heterotrophic with a genome stored in RNA

8. Which of the following is the function of the lymph nodes in mammals?

    A. Pump oxygen into tissue spaces.
    B. Store extra glucose for emergencies.
    C. Synthesize hemoglobin for erythrocytes.
    D. Filter debris from intracellular spaces.

9. The bands in muscle sarcomere are formed by actin and which of the following other proteins?

    A. Myosin
    B. Dynein
    C. Keratin
    D. Laminin

10. Which of the following structures within a human cell is responsible for recycling the materials no longer functional or needed within the cell?

    A. Ribosome
    B. Lysosome
    C. Mitochondrion
    D. Nucleolus

11. Which of the following is the correct structure and function of the cell membrane?

    A. A double glycoprotein structure with embedded lipid bodies provides shape and rigidity to the cytoplasm.
    B. A double layer of phosphate proteins with lipid channels allows molecules to pass from the inside to the outside of cells.
    C. Nonpolar phosphate heads and polar lipid tails form a bilayer to control the transport of proteins.
    D. A phospholipid bilayer with embedded proteins regulates molecules entering and leaving cytoplasm.

12. In which of the following areas does protein breakdown begin in the human body?

    A. Mouth
    B. Stomach
    C. Small intestine
    D. Large intestine

13. Which of the following chemical compounds prevents the lungs from collapsing?

    A. Mucus
    B. Surfactant
    C. Enzymes
    D. Buffers

14. Which of these structures diverts food into the esophagus, and prevents it from entering the lungs?

    A. Uvula
    B. Soft palate
    C. Tonsils
    D. Epiglottis

15. Which of these terms related to the respiratory system refers to the "voice box" for sound production?

    A. Pharynx
    B. Trachea
    C. Larynx
    D. Uvula

16. Unlike skeletal muscle, cardiac muscle is highly resistant to lactate-mediated fatigue because cardiac muscle

    A. uses aerobic respiration in mitochondria for energy.
    B. operates with electrical energy supplied by the sinoatrial (SA) node.
    C. primarily metabolizes glucose using the fermentation pathway.
    D. does not need oxygen for the production of energy.

17. Which of the following arteries directly supplies oxygenated blood to the reproductive system?

    A. Common carotid artery
    B. Gonadal artery
    C. Femoral artery
    D. Subclavian artery

18. Which of the following options represents the chromosomal composition of a normal human zygote?

    A. 23 chromosomes
    B. 46 chromosomes
    C. 69 chromosomes
    D. 92 chromosomes

19. Which of the following produces progesterone to prepare the uterus for pregnancy?

    A. Endometrium
    B. Cervix
    C. Corpus luteum
    D. Fallopian tubes

20. Which of the following cell types provides a waterproofing function for the outer layers of skin?

    A. Melanocytes
    B. Keratinocytes
    C. Merkel cells
    D. Langerhans cells

21. Stores of subcutaneous fat can be found in which of the following layers of the skin in the human body?

    A. Epidermis
    B. Dermis
    C. Hypodermis
    D. Dermal papillae

22. Which of the following glands primarily supplies hair shafts and skin with oily secretions?

    A. Eccrine gland
    B. Apocrine gland
    C. Sebaceous gland
    D. Ceruminous gland

23. Which of the following glands is the primary producer of insulin?

    A. Thyroid
    B. Adrenal
    C. Pituitary
    D. Pancreas

24. Type I diabetes is a disease associated with which of the following hormones?

    A. Estrogen
    B. Insulin
    C. Testosterone
    D. Thyroxine

25. Which of the following connects the kidneys to the bladder?

    A. Capillaries
    B. Ureters
    C. Urethras
    D. Arteries

26. Which of the following organs is the site of blood filtration?

    A. Kidney
    B. Heart
    C. Lung
    D. Brain

27. Kidneys remove which of the following from the blood?

    A. Platelets
    B. Salts
    C. Oxygen
    D. Fat

28. In which part of the body do T-cells mature?

    A. Bone marrow
    B. Thymus
    C. Adrenal glands
    D. Thyroid

29. Which of the following is classified as a flat bone?

    A. Tarsal
    B. Vertebrae
    C. Rib
    D. Humerus

30. Which of the following connects two bones together?

    A. Ligament
    B. Tendon
    C. Marrow
    D. Muscle

31. Which of the following are sesamoid bones?

    A. Phalanges
    B. Patellae
    C. Scapulae
    D. Metatarsals

32. The shape of villi and microvilli facilitates which of the following?

    A. Pushing food along the intestine via ciliary motion of villi
    B. Creating barriers to food movement to increase digestion time
    C. Decreasing surface area for absorption
    D. Increasing surface area for absorption

33. $Ca + H_2SO_4$ Which of the following statements correctly describes the product of the reaction above?

    A. Calcium sulfate
    B. Hydrogen sulfide
    C. Calcium sulfide
    D. Hydrogen sulfate

34. Which of the following classes of biomolecules can influence the rate of specific chemical reactions within the living cell?

    A. Nucleic acids
    B. Proteins
    C. Lipids
    D. Carbohydrates

35. Which of the following terms describes a sample composed of particles condensed into a small space and having vibrational, but not translational, motion?

    A. Solid
    B. Liquid
    C. Gas
    D. Plasma

36. An atom has 3 protons, 4 neutrons, and 3 electrons. Which of the following is the atom's mass number?

    A. 3
    B. 6
    C. 7
    D. 10

37. Which of the following substances will dissolve in water?

    A. CH_4
    B. CCl_4
    C. CH_3OH
    D. C_8H_{18}

38. On an imaginary planet called Alpha Vega, purple eyes (F) are dominant over pink eyes (f). Which of the following combinations will produce only offspring with pink eyes?

    A. Ff × ff
    B. Ff × Ff
    C. FF × ff
    D. ff × ff

39. A pregnant woman who is a chain smoker has just been diagnosed with lung cancer. Her biggest concern is if she has passed on the lung cancer to her child. Which of the following statements is correct regarding this situation?

    A. Children do not use their lungs until they are born, so the cancer cannot pass to the child before birth.
    B. The cancer could pass from mother to fetus through blood, but anticancer medications can prevent the child from developing cancer.
    C. If the pregnant mother undergoes treatment for lung cancer, both she and the child can be cured.
    D. The cancer will not be transmitted to the child.

40. In Mendelian inheritance, the dominant allele is for tall plants and the recessive allele is for short plants. Which of the following statements is correct in terms of phenotype and genotype?

    A. Tt is a phenotype that gives 50% short and 50% tall genotype.
    B. TT and Tt are both genotypes for the homozygous recessive phenotype.
    C. TT is the dominant phenotype, and tall plants is the resulting genotype.
    D. TT and Tt are both genotypes for the tall plant phenotype.

41. In a well-controlled experiment, researchers show that a common topical antibiotic called chloramphenicol halts a deadly fungal growth on the skin of amphibians. Which of the following is the best inference for how the antibiotic works to limit a fungal disease?

    A. The antibiotic causes a mutation in the skin tissue that makes it resistant to the fungus.
    B. The antibiotic acts as a physical barrier that interferes with fungal growth.
    C. The antibiotic kills a bacterial partner that is essential in the fungal infection.
    D. The antibiotic activates white blood cell production in amphibians.

42. A defining characteristic of a scientific hypothesis is that it is

    A. testable.
    B. unexpected.
    C. correct.
    D. predictable.

43. The use of an electron microscope would most benefit the study of

    A. the structure of atoms.
    B. the structure of cellular organelles.
    C. the structure of skeletal joints.
    D. chemical bonds in molecules.

44. Which of the following observations refutes the hypothesis that characteristics acquired during the parents' lifetime are inherited by offspring?

    A. Changes in neck length in giraffe populations are due to genetic mutations.
    B. Finches that live on different sources of food become unable to mate with one another after many generations.
    C. Peppered moths turn from gray to white or black depending on the color of the tree bark on which they live.
    D. Primates that have been taught sign language pass that ability to their offspring.

45. In a population that is growing, which of the following must be true?

    A. Immigrants + Births = Deaths + Emigrants
    B. Emigrants + Deaths > Immigrants + Births
    C. Immigrants + Births > Emigrants + Deaths
    D. Emigrants + Immigrants = Births + Deaths

46. Based on the scaled figure of a prairie biomass pyramid below, there is a greater mass of

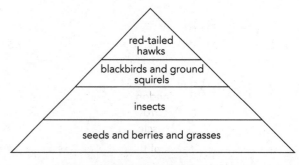

    A. insects than seeds, berries, and grasses.
    B. red-tailed hawks than blackbirds and ground squirrels.
    C. seeds, berries, and grasses than insects.
    D. blackbirds and ground squirrels than insects.

47. Two researchers note that when Weeds A and B grow next to each other, the roots of Weed A stop growing when they enter the root zone of Weed B. Since activated charcoal is known to absorb organic compounds, the researchers apply activated charcoal to the soil around Weed B. They note that the roots of Weed A then grow into the root zone of Weed B. Which of the following hypotheses is being tested by the addition of activated charcoal to the soil?

   A. Weed A absorbs activated charcoal, which enhances root growth for Weed A.
   B. Weed B grows best in soil that contains few organic compounds.
   C. Weed A is attracted to soil that contains activated charcoal.
   D. Weed B produces an organic compound that inhibits root growth for Weed A.

English and Language Usage

1. The director listens to everyone's opinions. She makes up her own mind. She informs us of her decisions.

   Assuming that the sentences in the above passage are in chronological order, which of the following sentences correctly restates the passage?

   A. Prior to making up her own mind and informing us of her decisions, the director listens to everyone's opinions.
   B. Informing us of her decisions, the director listens to everyone's opinions and makes up her own mind.
   C. Since she makes up her own mind and informs us of her decisions, the director listens to everyone's opinions.
   D. Before listening to everyone's opinions, the director makes up her own mind and informs us of her decisions.

2. _____ are a power of the executive branch of our government.

   Which of the following words correctly completes the sentence above?

   A. Vetos
   B. Vetoes
   C. Veto's
   D. Vetoes'

3. He spoke quickly and tried a new method to persuade _____ to concentrate on ways to improve my company's bottom line.

   Which of the following options correctly completes the sentence above?

   A. me, he started
   B. me, He started
   C. me; he started
   D. me; He started

4. The chef compiled a list that included these _____ butter, onions, peppers, and various spices.

   Which of the following options correctly completes the sentence above?

   A. groceries:
   B. groceries,
   C. groceries;
   D. groceries

5. The batter argued with the umpire _____ had called him out.

   Which of the following pronouns correctly completes the sentence above?

   A. that
   B. whom
   C. which
   D. who

6. Accidents do not just _____ are usually caused by a lack of attention.

   Which of the following options correctly completes the sentence above?

   A. happen they
   B. happen, they
   C. happen; they
   D. happen: they

7. Which of the following options is a complete sentence?

   A. Nominating me to serve as secretary of the club.
   B. Nominate me to serve as secretary of the club.
   C. When I am nominated to serve as secretary of the club.
   D. To be nominated to serve as secretary of the club.

8. On our vacation, we explored ancient architectural ruins, viewed astonishing landscapes, and visited many truly historic sites.

   Which of the following words is misspelled in the sentence above?

   A. Ancient
   B. Viewed
   C. Truely
   D. Historic

9. Even in the healthiest of diets, it is permissible to indulge _____ in a favorite dessert.

   Which of the following options is the appropriate spelling of the word that completes the sentence above?

   A   occasionally
   B. ocasionally
   C. occassionally
   D. occasionaly

10. A doctor or a nurse _____ always on duty.

    Which of the following verbs correctly completes the sentence above?

    A. are
    B. is
    C. were
    D. seem

11. The class is nervous about _____ first exam.

    Which of the following options correctly completes the sentence above?

    A. they're
    B. there
    C. it's
    D. its

12. Which of the following sentences would most likely be found in a letter to a friend?

    A. Those involved will meet with you about appropriate protocol for delivery of the message.
    B. There may be some confusion about the correct placement of the message.
    C. We really don't think there should be a bunch of odds and ends just messing up the message.
    D. A message to finalize preparation and the agenda would benefit all concerned.

13. Hi, I wanted to let you know that I can't make the meeting tomorrow. I know this is inconvenient but you'll do an awesome job on your own! Don't sweat it about the handouts. I'll email those to your assistant. See you soon!

    Which of the following is the most likely audience for this passage?

    A. The president of a corporation
    B. A friend at a corporation
    C. A professor at a college
    D. A dean at a college

14. Which of the following sentences in a research paper should include a citation?

    A. This paper summarizes key aspects of supplements to support the immune system.
    B. Numerous studies have been conducted to find ways to improve the immune system.
    C. Several clinics report cases of improved immune system responses.
    D. These results are conclusive of improved immune system, according to Dr. Smith's paper.

15. Kelly is writing a research paper for class. She is keeping a list of the websites and authors from which she is gathering information to include in her paper. Which of the following elements of the writing process is Kelly performing?

    A. Preparing an outline
    B. Writing a draft
    C. Referencing sources
    D. Writing a revision

16. The giant panda or panda bear is described as a rare mammal. It is easily recognizable because of its distinctive black and white marking. The giant panda's diet consists of bamboo stems, leaves, and shoots. It eats about 80 pounds of bamboo every day. Everyone enjoys reading about the giant panda. There are fewer than 1,000 pandas living in the wild.

    Which of the following sentences does not belong in a well-organized paragraph?

    A. The giant panda or panda bear is described as a rare mammal.
    B. It is easily recognizable because of its distinctive black and white marking.
    C. Everyone enjoys reading about the giant panda.
    D. There are fewer than 1,000 pandas living in the wild.

17. Soybean oil contains a high percentage of polyunsaturated fatty acids. Polyunsaturated fats are required for normal bodily functions. Dietitians recommend replacing saturated fats with polyunsaturated fatty acids.

    Which of the following sentences is the best topic sentence for the paragraph above?

    A. Soybeans are grown in many states.
    B. Soybeans are a good source for important fats.
    C. Soybeans are a good source of nutritional fiber.
    D. Soybeans are high in fat and should not be eaten.

18. In the last six months, more than $5 million
_____ spent in this ongoing political
campaign.

Which of the following options correctly
completes the sentence above?

A. are
B. has been
C. were
D. have been

19. Based on the two parts of the word
"circumlocution," which of the following
definitions is correct?

A. Meandering expedition
B. Roundabout way of speaking
C. Type of geometrical pattern
D. Remote destination

20. A can of chemicals has the word "antidote" on
the label providing information and directions.
Which of the following is the definition of
"antidote" in this context?

A. An ingredient that is present in the
chemicals
B. A contraindication for the use of the
chemicals
C. An appropriate place to store the chemicals
when not in use
D. A substance that counteracts the effects of
the chemicals

21. The patient was diagnosed as having dysesthesia.

Which of the following defines the prefix
dys- as used the word "dysesthesia" in the
sentence above?

A. pleasant reaction to touch
B. painful reaction to touch
C. normal reaction to touch
D. no reaction to touch

22. The doctor's message was cryptic because of her
poor handwriting.

Which of the following is the meaning of the
word "cryptic" as used in the sentence above?

A. Rewritten
B. Occult
C. Illegible
D. Terse

23. He typically avoided the local theater
because he found its productions to be banal
interpretations of over-performed plays.

Which of the following is the meaning of "banal"
as used in the sentence above?

A. Confusing
B. Ostentatious
C. Bland
D. Practiced

24. The doctor prescribed physical therapy so that
the muscles in the athlete's injured leg would not
atrophy while she was healing.

Which of the following phrases is an antonym
for the word "atrophy" as used in the sentence
above?

A. Become infected
B. Increase in size
C. Weaken gradually
D. Injure through over-exertion

Comprehensive Practice Test Answers

Reading

1. Option C is correct. The passage indicates that there is an increasing number of people buying local food and that one of the benefits of buying local food is knowing where it is grown. Therefore, it is a logical conclusion that more consumers want to know where their food is grown.

   A. The last sentence of the first paragraph indicates that local food can be grown with or without chemicals.

   B. The definition of organic foods is based on growing methods rather than distribution proximity.

   D. There is no information in the passage to indicate that farmers markets provide a greater diversity of food products than grocery stores.

2. Option A is correct. The notion of what is worrisome is subjective and implies an opinion.

   B. The information in this statement can be factually verified and is not an opinion.

   C. The information in this statement can be factually verified and is not an opinion.

   D. The information in this statement can be factually verified and is not an opinion.

3. Option D is correct. The passage supports the two ideas stated in this option: that locally grown food is more available now and that consuming locally grown food is beneficial.

   A. The passage focuses on locally, not organically, grown food.

   B. While the author indicates that it is worrisome when people do not know where their food comes from, this is a supporting detail rather than the author's primary purpose.

   C. This could be inferred from the passage, but it is not the author's primary purpose.

4. Option C is correct. This explains how we can start avoiding industrial food and become more like a locavore.

   A. This is the definition of locavore, but doesn't tell us how we can become more locavorous.

   B. This is a description of why some people might want to become a locavore, but doesn't tell us how to do it.

   D. This tells us more about the problem of trying to "eat local," but doesn't tell us how to do it.

5. Option D is correct. The third sentence in the second paragraph implies that taste and nutrition are less important than the requirements of industrial food production, which include the use of preservatives and altered harvesting and processing practices.

   A. While this may be true, there is no information in the passage that supports this inference.

   B. This is not true, and there is no information in the passage that supports this inference.

   D. There is no information in the passage that supports this inference.

6. Option B is correct. This definition is most appropriate, as the context of the sentence implies that the gardener wishes to direct the growth of the grapevine along the house.

   A. This definition does not fit the context of the sentence, as one cannot teach a plant to make it qualified.

   C. This definition does not fit the context of the sentence.

   D. This definition does not fit the context of the sentence, as a plant cannot be motivated.

7. Option B is correct. An academic research paper about a specific subject – hours spent on homework each night – is likely to include statistical data.

   A. This would be a good source for obtaining general information about the topic, but encyclopedias do not usually include statistical data.

   C. This would be a good source for gathering anecdotal evidence or an opinion about homework, but is not likely to include statistical data.

   D. This would be a good source for discovering teachers' perspectives on homework assignments, but is not likely to include statistical data.

8. Option C is correct. Readers might not be familiar with peak oil, so the author compares it to an environmental issue with which readers will be familiar. This is a method of engaging readers' interest.

   A. The passage does not focus on climate change, so this is not the author's primary purpose in the first two sentences.

   B. There is no explicit call to action in the passage.

   D. A definition of peak oil is not provided until the fourth sentence in the passage.

9. Option A is correct. In the passage, the author compares peak oil to the widely discussed issue of climate change. The passage also states the effects of peak oil as they began in 1971 to 1972. Both the relevance and immediacy of the issue of peak oil indicate the author's view of peak oil as a significant environmental issue.

   B. The passage does not provide any information that should lead the reader to believe that the issue of peak oil is confusing.

   C. The passage states that peak oil is, by definition, the irreversible decline in possible oil production.

   D. The passage does not provide any information about plans or options for avoiding the effects of peak oil.

10. Option D is correct. The passage discusses the comparative lack of general public awareness of the issue of peak oil. It goes on to provide information about reaching and passing the point of peak oil.

    A. The passage does not make any direct connection between the issues of peak oil and climate change.

    B. The passage does not make a connection to increased media coverage of peak oil and either improved or reduced oil production.

    C. The passage does not make any direct connection between the issues of peak oil and climate change. Hubbert's Curve is defined in the passage as a way to understand the idea of peak oil, but it does not make any connection between this theory and climate change.

11. Option C is correct. Helen was born in 1904. In 1904, Scott would have been 21 years old. The passage states that he was involved in social activism about unsafe working conditions in the coal minds during his early 20s.

    A. Helen was born in 1904. Scott wrote this book with Helen in 1954.

    B. Helen was born in 1904. Blueberries were part of the Nearings' "bread labor" in the years after 1952.

    D. Helen was born in 1904. The Nearings began work on building stone and concrete buildings by hand sometime after they met in 1928.

12. Option A is correct. This division of time is the heart of the philosophy that the Nearings pioneered, because it is what allowed them to be self-sufficient.

    B. This was a part of Scott Nearing's life in his early twenties and was not necessarily a part of his philosophy as stated in the text.

    C. Writing books about their self-sufficient lifestyle was a part of the Nearings' lives. However, it was not a key part of their philosophy as stated in the text.

    D. Moving from New York to Vermont was a part of the Nearings' lives. However, it was not a part of the Nearings' philosophy for a self-sufficient life.

COMPREHENSIVE ANSWERS

13. Option D is correct. The Nearings made their own food at home, so teaching others how to do this would fit into their philosophy.

   A. Scott Nearing protested against coal mining, so he would not campaign in favor of it.
   B. The Nearings believed in a simple lifestyle, so lavish furnishings would not be a part of their home.
   C. The Nearings believed in making their own food at home, so helping to make processed food would not fit into their philosophy.

14. Option C is correct. The notion of what constitutes "the good life" is open to subjective interpretation.

   A. This sentence contains verifiable facts that have been documented.
   B. This sentence contains verifiable facts that have been documented.
   D. This sentence contains verifiable facts that have been documented. For instance, Living the Good Life can be proved to be the most famous of the Nearings' books by the number of book sales.

15. Option A is correct. While many people visited the Nearings to follow their example, it is a logical conclusion that the Nearings' writings were available to a larger number of people and continue to be available. Also, the last sentence states that their books were credited with spurring the "back to the land" movement.

   B. Community service was considered by the Nearings to be civic work, not bread labor.
   C. The passage indicates that the Nearings developed their own philosophy and that they preceded the "back to the land" movement.
   D. There is nothing in the passage to indicate that the Nearings' parents came from a rural lifestyle.

16. Option B is correct. The warnings on the label instruct not to use the ointment on children under 2 years of age and not to get the medicine in the eyes.

   A. One of the uses listed is to treat minor burns. A heat rash is a minor burn and is treatable by this medication.
   C. One of the uses listed is to treat minor cuts and scrapes. A knee scrape is treatable by this medication. Additionally, the child is over 2 years of age, so the medication is acceptable.
   D. The label indicates that the medicine can be applied up to four times daily and can be used to treat minor itching.

17. Option C is correct. Job 3 has the same amount of vacation and pays as much as Job 1, but also offers full health insurance, while Job 1 only offers partial health insurance. Additionally, Job 3 has the same benefits as Job 4, but pays $5,000 more.

   A. Job 1 pays as much as Job 3 and has 2 weeks paid vacation, but only pays partial health insurance coverage.
   C. Job 2 only pays partial health insurance, has the lowest salary, and the least amount of vacation.
   D. Job 4 offers full health insurance coverage and 2 weeks paid vacation, but pays less than the others.

18. Option C is correct. This correctly follows the directions. Replacing every 1 with the letter A, every 2 with the letter B, every 3 with the letter D, and every 4 with the letter E results in ABDEDBABDE. The first B and D should be deleted, resulting in AEDBABDE. The first and last letters, A and E, should be deleted, leading to EDBABD. Replacing the vowels with X results in XDBXBD.

    A. This does not correctly follow the directions. Replacing every 1 with the letter A, every 2 with the letter B, every 3 with the letter D, and every 4 with the letter E results in ABDEDBABDE. The first B and D should be deleted, resulting in AEDBABDE. The first and last letters, A and E, should be deleted, leading to EDBABD. Replacing the vowels with X results in XDBXBD.

    B. This does not correctly follow the directions. Replacing every 1 with the letter A, every 2 with the letter B, every 3 with the letter D, and every 4 with the letter E results in ABDEDBABDE. The first B and D should be deleted, resulting in AEDBABDE. The first and last letters, A and E, should be deleted, leading to EDBABD. Replacing the vowels with X results in XDBXBD.

    D. This does not correctly follow the directions. Replacing every 1 with the letter A, every 2 with the letter B, every 3 with the letter D, and every 4 with the letter E results in ABDEDBABDE. The first B and D should be deleted, resulting in AEDBABDE. The first and last letters, A and E, should be deleted, leading to EDBABD. Replacing the vowels with X results in XDBXBD.

19. Option D is correct. This detail regarding bards' involvement in passing on information about events and people best supports the idea that bards were an important element in sustaining Celtic civilization.

    A. While this is mentioned in the passage, it does not provide the best support for the argument that bards were an important element in sustaining Celtic civilization.

    B. While this is mentioned in the passage, it does not provide the best support for the argument that bards were an important element in sustaining Celtic civilization.

    C. While this is mentioned in the passage, it does not provide the best support for the argument that bards were an important element in sustaining Celtic civilization.

20. Option B is correct. The passage explains the place, purpose, and historical significance of bards and the oral traditions they practiced.

    A. While the passage mentions the bard's importance in sustaining Celtic civilization, the topic of the passage is the history and purpose of bards.

    C. The passage discusses the role of bards in passing on the legends of King Arthur, but this is a supporting detail.

    D. The passage discusses the purpose of barding schools to train bards, but this is a supporting detail.

21. Option A is correct. The passage provides general information about the history and purpose of bards in Celtic culture.

    B. The passage is not attempting to make a persuasive argument but is providing general information about bards.

    C. The passage is not a narrative intended to entertain, but a collection of facts about bards in Celtic culture.

    D. The passage is providing general historical information about bards and does not make critical judgments about bards.

22. Option C is correct. The pie chart shows that the most viewers watch sitcoms and primetime dramas; therefore, advertising on these programs would reach the most viewers.

    A. According to the pie chart, game shows, talk shows, and reality shows do not reach as many viewers as sitcoms and primetime dramas.
    B. According to the pie chart daytime dramas and news do not reach as many viewers as sitcoms and primetime dramas.
    D. According to the pie chart, sports and talk shows do not reach as many viewers as sitcoms and primetime dramas.

23. Option C is correct. It is possible to strike a pencil with one's hand, and this definition makes sense in the context of the sentence.

    A. The word in the sentence is a verb, not a noun, because it is an action she is performing.
    B. The word in the sentence is a verb, not a noun, because it is an action she is performing.
    D. This definition does not make sense in the context of the sentence, as it would be impossible to "blink" a pencil away.

24. Option A is correct. Complacent means self-contented, smug, unconcerned.

    B. This is not a meaning of complacent. Using context clues, if Jane were dissatisfied with her routine, she would still be using her shoes to work out, so they wouldn't have dust on them.
    C. This is not a meaning of complacent. If Jane were confident about her routine, her workout shoes would be in use much more.
    D. This is not a meaning of complacent. If Jane were worried about her routine, she would already be aware of the state of her running shoes.

25. Option B is correct. This sentence is about the big picture and the consequences after the President's death, so it would be appropriate for a history textbook.

    A. Conjecture by conspiracy theorists is not considered proof in an academic textbook, so a history textbook would not include it.
    C. This might be true, but it takes a personal look at the events of the assassination from Jacqueline Kennedy's perspective, while a history textbook would look at how the events affected the nation as a whole.
    D. This might be true, but it changes focus from the assassination of Kennedy to biographical information about the family today and is unlikely to be found in a paragraph about the assassination and the Warren Commission as related to United States history.

26. Option D is correct. This article offers historical information about the day of Kennedy's assassination, so a student can expect the main topic to be the factual events of the assassination.

    A. Kennedy was killed in 1963, so this might tell a student about the after-effects, but not ab out the assassination.
    B. Since this refers to Oswald as a conspirator, it might be about conspiracy theories and not provide objective, reliable information.
    C. This article reveals in its title a bias that Kennedy brought on his own death, so it does not offer an objective view of the events.

27. Option A is correct. The author provides supporting details for the argument that football has supplanted baseball as America's "national pastime."

    B. This is a supporting detail in the passage rather than the author's main purpose.
    C. There are no indications in the passage that the author wants to revive the popularity of baseball.
    D. The author does not express personal feelings about the importance of football in American culture.

28. Option D is correct. This detail supports the main idea of the passage, which is that football could be considered the new "national pastime" in America.

    A. This detail does not support the main idea presented in the passage.
    B. This detail does not support the main idea presented in the passage.
    C. This is the main idea of the passage, rather than a supporting detail.

29. Option A is correct. This combination of flowers corresponds with the directions. Type 5 is chosen, but type 1 is not. Type 3 is chosen, and type 5 is included; type 2 is chosen, and type 6 is included.

    B. If type 3 is chosen, type 5 must also be chosen to conform to the directions.
    C. If type 2 is chosen, type 6 must also be chosen to conform to the directions.
    D. If type 1 is chosen, type 5 must not be chosen to conform to the directions.

30. Option C is correct. One of the definitions of "fast" is something that is obtained with little effort, often by unsavory means. This definition fits the context of the sentence.

    A. This definition does not fit the context of the sentence.
    B. This definition does not fit the context of the sentence.
    D. This definition does not fit the context of the sentence.

31. Option C is correct. This drawing corresponds with all the directions, including the correct rotation of the figure and placement of the letters.

    A. This drawing does not correspond with all of the directions.
    B. This drawing does not correspond with all of the directions.
    D. This drawing does not correspond with all of the directions.

32. Option D is correct. The outline groups squirrels with porcupines within the rodent order. Therefore, squirrels must be more similar to porcupines than to monkeys, which are within the primate order.

    A. The organization of this outline provides no information regarding the relative similarity of marsupials, primates, and rodents. All three are listed at the same level of the hierarchy.
    B. Rodents is another name for Rodentia, which is indicated by the parentheses. If rodents were a subcategory of Rodentia, the term would be listed below Rodentia and indented.
    C. If wombats were a subcategory of koalas, the term would be indented below koalas.

33. Option C is correct. This definition fits with the context of the sentence.

    A. This definition does not fit with the context of the sentence.
    B. This definition does not fit with the context of the sentence.
    D. This definition does not fit with the context of the sentence.

34. Option D is correct. Snails and sea slugs are both within the Gastropoda class; therefore, they are more closely related than clams, which are in the Pelecypoda class.

    A. Pelecypoda and Gastropoda are at the same level in the outline; therefore, Pelecypoda is not a type of Gastropoda.
    B. Octopuses and squids are at the same level in the outline; therefore, an octopus is not a type of squid.
    C. The outline does not provide information on the degree of relation among Cephalopoda, Gastropoda, and Pelecypoda.

35. Option B is correct. This statement is a supporting detail from the passage.

    A. This statement helps determine the topic of the passage but does not support the main idea that Gardner's theory had an impact on education.
    C. This statement helps determine the topic of the passage but does not support the main idea that Gardner's theory had an impact on education.
    D. Every sentence in the passage relates to this main idea, so it is not a supporting detail.

36. Option B is correct. The second sentence of the second paragraph indicates that traditional notions of intelligence are largely based on I.Q. testing. Then, the first sentence of the fourth paragraph states that traditional school curricula emphasized learning through the verbal-linguistic and mathematical-logical intelligences.

    A. There is nothing in the article that suggests Howard Gardner possessed multiple intelligences.
    C. There is nothing in the article to suggest that most teachers prefer to use traditional teaching methods in the classroom.
    D. There is nothing in the article to suggest that multiple intelligences are excluded from school curricula because they are difficult to test.

37. Option D is correct. The key point that the passage makes about Howard Gardner's theory of multiple intelligences is that intelligence cannot be represented by one universal score or measure, but should take into account a broader range of cerebral engagement.

    A. The passage does not identify any types of multiple intelligence as more important than any other.
    B. The passage does not say that cerebral engagement and I.Q. testing are unrelated. Garner is represented as saying that I.Q. testing does not "sufficiently address the range of cerebral engagement."
    C. The passage states that traditional school curriculum in Western culture focuses heavily on verbal-linguistic and logical-mathematical intelligences. This does not represent an accommodation of multiple types of intelligence.

38. Option B is correct. Multimedia collaborations allow students who excel in different types of intelligence to adapt projects to their own strengths.

    A. This does not address the theory of MI.
    C. This does not address the theory of MI.
    D. This does not address the theory of MI.

39. Option A is correct. This student's artistic ability would more likely be identified and nurtured in an educational program that incorporates MI.

    B. This student would likely excel in a traditional educational program, as well as in one that incorporates MI.
    C. This student would likely excel in a traditional educational program, as well as in one that incorporates MI.
    D. This student would likely excel in a traditional educational program, as well as in one that incorporates MI.

40. Option A is correct. Your friend tells you that he has to cook breakfast and shower before he picks you up to go to the grocery store, so you can expect him to pick you up after he showers.

    B. Your friend tells you that he has to cook breakfast and shower before he picks you up to go to the grocery store, so you can expect him to pick you up before he goes to the grocery store.
    C. Your friend tells you that he has to cook breakfast and shower before he picks you up to go to the grocery store, so he will not be ready to leave as soon as he hangs up the phone.
    D. Your friend tells you that he has to cook breakfast and shower before he picks you up to go to the grocery store, so you can expect him to pick you up after he eats breakfast and showers.

41. Option D is correct. A thesaurus is a dictionary of synonyms and antonyms, which would be helpful for a writer trying to use a greater variety of words.

    A. An encyclopedia is a book or a set of books providing information on a range of alphabetically organized topics; it would not be the most helpful source in this situation.
    B. An almanac is an annual publication containing calendar information, information about natural phenomena, and/or interesting facts; it would not be the most helpful source in this situation.
    C. A style guide is a set of standards for writing that is usually specific to an organization or a purpose; it would not be the most helpful source in this situation.

42. Option C is correct. This statement is supported by the fact that this is a call center position, which will include communicating on the telephone, and by the fact that "good communication skills" is listed among the qualifications.

    A. The announcement states that this is an entry-level position in the call center, so it would not include formulating communications for marketing purposes.

    B. While this company sells medical equipment, previous experience in the health care industry is not listed among the qualifications.

    D. The announcement indicates that the company offers flexible work schedules, which include, but do not require, weekend and holiday shifts.

43. Option A is correct. The announcement states that this position includes medical and dental insurance as part of the compensation package.

    B. According to the announcement, this is an hourly, not a salaried, position.

    C. Someone who has previously managed customer service representatives would most likely not want an entry-level position in a call center.

    D. While this company manufactures medical equipment, this particular position would not be involved in working with medical equipment.

44. Option D is correct. Because the passage discusses two different forms of entertainment (books and movies) and has a more casual style, this is the best option.

    A. This passage is about the popularity of YA novels, but it is a nonfiction piece, and novels are fictional.

    B. This doesn't explain how to write a YA novel, or YA movie, so this doesn't fit.

    C. Book reviews focus on just one book, and this passage refers to a type of literature in general without citing specific books.

45. Option D is correct. Since reinventing the existing genre is similar to redesigning an existing car, this answer fits best.

    A. There are more YA novels now than ever before, but that is not the focus of the passage.

    B. The YA novel is not new, so this answer doesn't fit.

    C. YA novels' success has only increased in the last 20 years, so this doesn't fit.

46. Option B is correct. The majority of the campgrounds are on the north shore of the lake along Highway 22.

    A. The south side of the lake only has one campground.

    C. There are no campgrounds on the east side of the lake.

    D. The west shore of the lake has one campground at the junction of Highway 22 and 766.

47. Option A is correct. Highway 16 follows the eastern shore of the lake.

    B. Highway 22 runs along the northwestern side of the lake.

    C. Highway 85 runs across the northern side of the lake.

    D. Highway 141 is on the south side of the lake.

COMPREHENSIVE ANSWERS

Mathematics

1. Option C is correct. When converting a percentage to the numeric equivalent, it is correct to divide by 100.

    A. This is not the correct decimal placement for the numerical conversion of this percentage. 425% is 425 out of 100, which would have a value greater than 1. This decimal is 425 ten-thousandths.

    B. This is not the correct decimal placement for the numerical conversion of this percentage. 425% is 425 out of 100, which would have a value greater than 1. This decimal is 425 thousandths.

    D. This is not the correct decimal placement for the numerical conversion of this percentage. 425% is 425 out of 100, which would have a value greater than 1. This decimal is 425 whole numbers. You would need to divide 425 by 100 to convert to a decimal.

2. Option D is correct. To obtain the total number of hot dogs purchased, the numbers in the rows of the table should be multiplied and then the resulting products should be added.

    $1 \times 50 = 50$
    $2 \times 27 = 54$
    $3 \times 15 = 45$
    $4 \times 6 = 24$
    $5 \times 2 = 10$
    $50 + 54 + 45 + 24 + 10 = 183$

    A. This is the sum of the left column of the table, not the total number of hot dogs purchased.

    B. This is the total number of customers, not the total number of hot dogs purchased.

    C. This number results from adding across the rows and then adding those totals. This is not the correct method to determine the total number of hot dogs purchased.

3. Option A is correct. The value of the computer at the time of purchase was $1,500. Five years later, the computer's value was $0. This means the computer's value decreased by $1,500/5 or $300 each year.

    B. This expression does not yield a value of $0 after t = 5 years.

    C. This expression does not yield an initial value (t = 0 years) of $1,500, nor a value of $0 after t = 5 years.

    D. This expression does not yield an initial value (t = 0 years) of $1,500.

4. Option B is correct. $(x2 + 4x + 4) - (x2 - 6x + 9) = x2 + 4x + 4 - x2 + 6x - 9 = 10x - 5$

    A. This represents an error in simplifying the expression. This the result of adding the 4 and 9, rather than subtracting and finding the difference.

    C. This represents an error in simplifying the expression. Subtracting −6x from 4x is the same as adding 6x and 4x, resulting in a sum of 10x, rather than a difference of −2x.

    D. This represents an error in simplifying the expression. Subtracting −6x from 4x is the same as adding 6x and 4x, resulting in a sum of 10x, rather than a difference of −2x.

5. Option C is correct. This order is correct because √3 is approximately 1.7, which is between 4 and 1. The number 4 is the greatest positive, and therefore the greatest value. The value −0.8 is less than −3/5 because it is further from 0 in the negative direction.

    A. This order is incorrect because 4 is the greatest positive number and should come first.

    B. This order is incorrect because it is not in decreasing order. √3 is a positive number and would have a greater value than −0.8, −3/5, and 1.

    D. This order is incorrect because it is not listed from greatest to least. In comparing the two negative numbers, −3/5 has a decimal value of −0.6. The value −0.8 is less than −3/5 because it is further from 0 in the negative direction.

6. Option D is correct. This is correct. 4 1/3 (≈ 4.33) is less than 4.67.

    A. This is incorrect. 4.67 is greater than 4 1/3 (≈ 4.33), not less than.

    B. This is incorrect. 4 1/3 (≈ 4.33) is less than 4.67. It is neither greater than nor equal to 4.67.

    C. This is incorrect. 4.67 is not equal to 4 1/3 (≈ 4.33).

7. Option C is correct. This is correct. When ordering these values from least to greatest, the negative value that is the furthest from 0 should come first and the positive number that is the furthest from 0 should come at the end of the list.

   A. This order is incorrect. 3.3 is greater than 3.
   B. This is incorrect because −3/10 is greater than −3. With negative numbers, the closer it is to zero, the greater its value.
   D. This is incorrect because −3 is the furthest negative number from zero and has the least value; therefore, it should appear first in the list, ahead of other negative values.

8. Option D is correct. This is correct. If 22.2 is rounded to 20, 98 is rounded to 100, and 54 is rounded to 50, $20 \times 100 \times 50 = 100,000$.

   A. This is incorrect because it is obtained by rounding all values up instead of applying rounding rules.
   B. This is incorrect because it is obtained by rounding all values down instead of applying rounding rules.
   C. This is incorrect because it is obtained by rounding all values down instead of applying rounding rules.

9. Option C is correct. This is correct. A correctly set up proportion might look like 30 alcohol users/100 adults = x/2000 adults. Multiplying both sides by 2000 adults will give (30 alcohol users x 2000 adults)/100 adults = x. Simplifying the left side leads to x = 600 expected alcohol users.

   A. This is incorrect. This is the numerator of the rate of alcohol use disorder.
   B. This is incorrect. This is 30% of 1000, not 30% of 2000.
   D. This is incorrect. Instead of multiplying the results by 20, because the new population is 20 times greater than the original survey population, this incorrect answer is found by doubling the numerator of the rate of alcohol use disorder.

10. Option D is correct. This is correct. This can be calculated by 5 gallons/2,000 ft² × 30,000 ft².

    A. This is incorrect. The larger area is 15 times greater; therefore, the paint quantity needs to be 15 times larger.
    B. This is incorrect. This number does not take into account the number of square feet 5 gallons of paint can cover.
    C. This is incorrect. This is the number of square feet 1 gallon covers.

11. Option C is correct. This is correct. 1,000 words/15 min = x words/60 min; x = 4,000 words. This can also be calculated by multiplying 1,000 by 4, because the time duration is 4 times longer.

    A. This is incorrect. The number of words per hour must be larger than the number of words in 15 min.
    B. This is incorrect. This is the product of 15 min and 1,000 words.
    D. This is incorrect. This would be true if the typist could type 1,000 words per min.

12. Option A is correct. This is correct. The value 20.5 rounded to the nearest whole cm is 21 cm and is the smallest possible length.

    B. This is incorrect. The value 20.49 rounded to the nearest whole cm is 20 cm.
    C. This is incorrect. The value 21.44 rounded to the nearest whole cm would be 21 cm; however, this is the largest possible length.
    D. This is incorrect. The value 20.6 rounded to the nearest whole cm is 21 cm; however, this is greater than 20.5 cm and is not the smallest possible length.

13. Option C is correct. To determine the total number of houses, take the number of red mailboxes, 60, and divide by the numerical equivalent of the percent, 0.05. The total is 1,200 houses.

    A. This is less than the actual total and represents an incorrect method for determining the total based on a percent. This results from doubling the amount of red mailboxes, or assuming that they represented 50% of the neighborhood.
    B. This is less than the actual total and represents an incorrect method for determining the total based on a percent. The amount of red mailboxes, 60, represents 5% of the total number of houses in the neighborhood. There are 20 groups of 5% in 100%, or the total number of houses. Multiplying 60 by 5 only results in 25% of the neighborhood.
    D. This is more than the actual total and represents an incorrect method for determining the total based on a percent. This results from dividing 60 by 0.02, which would only be 2% of the houses in the neighborhood.

14. Option B is correct. This expression can be rewritten as: 9 − (7 + 3/8) = 9 − 7 − 3/8 = 2 − 3/8 = 16/8 − 3/8 = 13/8 = 1 5/8

    A. This represents an error in the subtraction of mixed numbers. The value 9 can be written as 8 8/8. So, 8 8/8 − 7 3/8 = 1 5/8.
    C. This represents an error in the subtraction of mixed numbers. The value 9 can be written as 8 8/8. So, 8 8/8 − 7 3/8 = 1 5/8.
    D. This represents an error in the subtraction of mixed numbers. The value 9 can be written as 8 8/8. So, 8 8/8 − 7 3/8 = 1 5/8.

15. Option B is correct. To calculate the percent of a number, multiple 35 by the decimal equivalent of 5.4%, 0.054. This product equals 1.89.

    A. This represents incorrect placement of the decimal. The correct multiplication is 0.054 × 35.
    C. This represents incorrect placement of the decimal. The correct multiplication is 0.054 × 35.
    D. This represents incorrect placement of the decimal. The correct multiplication is 0.054 × 35.

16. Option D is correct. According to the equation, each 3 inches of height adds 2 inches to the crutch length (2/3 × 3 = 2).

    A. According to the equation, each 1/3 inch of height adds 2/9 inch to the crutch length.
    B. According to the equation, each 1 inch of height adds 2/3 inch to the crutch length.
    C. According to the equation, each 2 inches of height adds 11/3 inches to the crutch length.

17. Option B is correct. The total of these numbers is 0.96, which is equivalent to 96/100. This fraction can be simplified to 24/25.

    A. This is less than the actual amount and represents improper addition of the decimals.
    C. This is more than the actual amount and represents improper conversion from a decimal to a fraction.
    D. This is more than the actual amount and represents improper addition of the decimals.

18. Option D is correct. When adding mixed numbers, first find the least common denominator for the fractions. This produces the following expression: 4 5/72 + 1 56/72 + 3. This equals 4 101/72, which can be simplified to 5 29/72.

    A. This represents an error in simplifying a mixed number.
    B. This represents an incorrect method for adding mixed numbers.
    C. This represents an error in simplifying a mixed number.

19. Option B is correct. When subtracting mixed numbers, first find the least common denominator for the fractions. This produces the following expression: 8 10/16 − 7 11/16. Since 10/16 is less than 11/16, change the mixed numbers to improper fractions and subtract (138/16 − 123/16 = 15/16).

    A. This represents an incorrect method for subtracting mixed numbers. 8 5/8 is equal to 7 26/16. So, 7 26/16 − 7 11/16 = 15/16.
    C. This represents an incorrect method for subtracting mixed numbers. 8 5/8 is equal to 7 26/16. So, 7 26/16 − 7 11/16 = 15/16.
    D. This represents an incorrect method for subtracting mixed numbers. 8 5/8 is equal to 7 26/16. So, 7 26/16 − 7 11/16 = 15/16.

20. Option C is correct. To find the number of members who voted for the increase in dues, take the total number (400) and multiply by the numerical equivalent of 75% (0.75). This equals 300.

    A. This represents an error in determining the number of members who voted for the increase in dues.
    B. This represents an error in determining the number of members who voted for the increase in dues.
    D. This represents an error in determining the number of members who voted for the increase in dues.

21. Option C is correct. To convert from a ratio to percent, divide the first number, 2, by the second number, 5. This equals 0.4, which is the equivalent of 40%.

    A. This represents a misinterpretation of the ratio.
    B. This represents an improper method for converting this ratio to a percent.
    D. This represents an improper method for converting this ratio to a percent.

22. Option D is correct. Both of these numbers can be substituted for x to make the equation true.

    A. These numbers do not both make the equation true.
    B. These numbers do not both make the equation true.
    C. These numbers do not both make the equation true.

23. Option B is correct. Either of these numbers makes the equation true:
    $(x - 2)^2 = 125/5$
    $(x - 2)^2 = 25$
    $x = 7$ or $x = -3$

    A. This is not the correct solution set.
    C. This is not the correct solution set.
    D. This is not the correct solution set.

24. Option A is correct. This is correct. To determine the rate per hour, 5 km per 30 minutes is multiplied by 2, resulting in 10 km/hr. Multiplying this by 1,000 m/km converts the units to m/hr, resulting in 10,000 m/hr.

    B. This is incorrect. This results from dividing 30 minutes by 5 km, finding an incorrect rate of 6 minutes per kilometer. This was then multiplied by 1,000 m/km, to correctly convert kilometers to meters.
    C. This is incorrect. This results from correctly converting kilometers to meters by multiplying 5 km by 1,000 m/km, resulting in 5,000 meters per half hour. This value is then multiplied by 60 minutes, without considering that the rate is per half-hour, and not per minute.
    D. This is incorrect. This results from multiplying 5 km by 30 min, without considering the unit conversion of kilometers to meters.

25. Option A is correct. This graph shows that at the beginning of the trip, the student had 250 miles to travel. After 2 hours, he stopped for 2 hours. Then he finished the drive home.

    B. This graph indicates that the student did not end up at home.
    C. This graph indicates that the student's net distance traveled is zero miles.
    D. This graph indicates that the student's net distance traveled is zero miles.

26. Option D is correct. 300 miles / x = 1 mile / 1.6 km
    x = 480 km = 480,000 m

    A. This represents an incorrect method for setting up the proportion.
    300 miles / x = 1 mile / 1.6 km
    x = 480 km
    B. The value of x is not given in the requested units.
    C. This represents an incorrect method for setting up the proportion.

27. Option A is correct. This is correct. The blue bars get taller as more hours apply and the red bars get smaller as more hours apply. This means teenagers spend more time online gaming than reading.

    B. This is incorrect. The opposite is true.
    C. This is incorrect. For this to be true, because 50% of teenagers spend 3 to 4 hr online gaming, 25% of teenagers would have to spend 1 to 2 hr reading. The graph shows that 40% of teenagers spend 1 to 2 hr reading.
    D. This is incorrect. About 5% of the teenagers spend 3 to 4 hr reading.

28. Option B is correct. This is correct because 20% is greater than 10%.

    A. This is incorrect. Only 20% of the students prefer horror films, which is less than half.
    C. This is incorrect because 15% is less than 25%.
    D. This is incorrect. Musicals are preferred by the smallest percent of students.

29. Option B is correct. This is correct. As the depth increases, diving time also increases. A positive correlation means that as one variable increases, the other one does as well.

    A. This is incorrect. As the depth increases, diving time also increases.
    C. This is incorrect. As the depth increases, diving time also increases.
    D. This is incorrect. As the depth increases, diving time also increases. A negative correlation means that as one variable increases, the other variable decreases.

COMPREHENSIVE ANSWERS

30. Option B is correct. The student first walks two blocks east to the library, and then walks six blocks west to the grocery store for a total of eight blocks. Eight blocks times 0.25 miles per block equals 2 miles. The street is laid out as follows:
    Grocery store _____(4 blocks)_____ High school __(2 blocks)__ Library

    A. This distance corresponds to six blocks, which is not the correct number of blocks that the student walked.
    C. This distance corresponds to 10 blocks, which is not the correct number of blocks that the student walked.
    D. This distance corresponds to 10 blocks, which is not the correct number of blocks that the student walked.

31. Option B is correct. Since the distance between A and E is 10 km and the distance between B and E is 8 km, then the distance between A and B is 2 km. Since the distance between A and C is 4.5 km and the distance between A and B is 2 km, the distance between B and C must be 2.5 km.

    A. Although this is the distance between A and B, as well as D and E, it is not the distance between B and C.
    C. Although this is the distance between C and D, it is not the distance between B and C.
    D. Although this is the distance between B and D, it is not the distance between B and C.

32. Option D is correct. $(10°C \times 1.8) + 32 = 18 + 32 = 50.0°F$

    A. This value does not correctly complete the equation.
    B. This value does not correctly complete the equation.
    C. This value does not correctly complete the equation.

Science

1. Option D is correct. Epinephrine causes liver cells to break down glycogen, which causes an increase in sugar in the blood stream.

    A. Epinephrine causes liver cells to break down glycogen, which causes an increase in sugar in the blood stream, not the absorption of sugar from the blood.
    B. Epinephrine causes blood vessels supplying skeletal muscles to dilate, which increases blood flow to muscle cells.
    C. Epinephrine causes blood vessels supplying the intestines to constrict, restricting blood flow to the organs of the digestive system.

2. Option A is correct. When a response reinforces a stimulus, causing an even greater response, positive feedback is occurring.

    B. This is an example of negative feedback. The response of lower glucose levels reduces the initial stimulus and stops the pancreas from releasing insulin.
    C. This is an example of negative feedback. The response of increasing body temperature reduces the initial stimulus and stops the hypothalamus from activating warming mechanisms.
    D. This is an example of negative feedback. An osmolarity increase causes a response that decreases osmolarity and reduces the release of ADH.

3. Option B is correct. The myelin sheath, which is a lipid-based structure, insulates the axon, allowing rapid electrical conduction of the action potential down the axon. Deterioration of the myelin sheath disrupts this process.

    A. The myelin sheath does not directly affect the reception of a stimulus at the dendrites.
    C. The myelin sheath covers the axon and does not function in the reabsorption of neurotransmitters.
    D. Na+/K+ pumps still function even if the myelin sheath has deteriorated.

4. Option D is correct. Nephridia in segmented worms operate similarly to the nephron of the kidneys. Nephrons in the kidneys contain a collecting tubule that aids in urine production.

    A. Liver cells make bile and help regulate blood sugar levels. They do not contain collecting tubules used to collect and concentrate filtrate.
    B. The spleen functions to remove old, fragmented red blood cells and pathogens from the blood. Spleen cells do not contain collecting tubules used to collect and concentrate filtrate.
    C. The lymph nodes filter out pathogens from interstitial fluid (lymph). The cells of the lymph nodes do not contain collecting tubules used to collect and concentrate filtrate.

5. Option D is correct. The production of antibodies by B-cells is part of the humoral response to antigens.

    A. Cytotoxic T-cells destroy pathogens and infected cells.
    B. Macrophages ingest and digest both non-self cells and dead cells.
    C. Helper T-cells help cytotoxic T-cells and other immune cells.

6. Option D is correct. The heart pumping blood through the arteries, capillaries, and veins provides the means of transporting substances throughout the body.

    A. The respiratory system exchanges gases with the outside environment, bringing oxygen in and letting carbon dioxide out.
    B. The immune system protects the body from pathogens (infectious agents) using a combination of white blood cells and antibodies.
    C. The nervous system, which includes the brain, spinal cord, and peripheral nerves, controls the actions of other body systems.

7. Option B is correct. Humans consume rather than manufacture nutrient molecules (heterotrophic), and human genes are encoded in DNA.

    A. Humans consume rather than manufacture nutrient molecules.
    C. Humans consume rather than manufacture nutrient molecules, and human genes are encoded in DNA.
    D. Human genes are encoded in DNA.

8. Option D is correct. Lymph nodes filter debris, lymphocytes, and pathogens from intracellular fluid.

    A. This is not a function of the lymph nodes. Oxygen diffuses to these areas from capillaries of the circulatory system.

    B. This is not a function of the lymph nodes. Glucose is stored as glycogen in the liver and muscles of mammals.

    C. This is not a function of the lymph nodes. Hemoglobin is synthesized in the red blood cells.

9. Option A is correct. Myosin contains "heads" that contact actin and pull the actin fibres together in an ATP-dependent mechanism that causes muscles to contract.

    B. Dynein is an ATP-dependent molecule that "walks" along microtubules, causing them to move, but it is not part of the sarcomere.

    C. Keratin is the fibrous protein of hair and nails and is not part of the sarcomere.

    D. Laminin is a protein of the nuclear envelope and is not part of the sarcomere.

10. Option B is correct. Lysosomes are specialized vacuoles containing digestive enzymes.

    A. The ribosome is not involved in recycling materials that are no longer functional or needed.

    C. Mitochondria function in cellular respiration, facilitating the production of ATP.

    D. The nucleolus functions in the assembly of ribosomes.

11. Option D is correct. The cell membrane consists of a phospholipid bilayer with polar phosphate heads, nonpolar lipid tails, and embedded proteins, which permit the movement of molecules across the membrane.

    A. The double structure is not composed of glycoprotein.

    B. The double layer is not composed of phosphate proteins.

    C. The heads are polar and the tails are nonpolar; molecules pass through protein channels.

12. Option B is correct. The stomach is the first place in the digestive system in which proteinases are produced.

    A. Carbohydrate digestion starts in the mouth, but protein breakdown does not.

    C. Protein breakdown continues in the small intestine, but it does not start here.

    D. Protein is generally digested by the time it enters the large intestine.

13. Options B is correct. Surfactants are lipopolysaccharides that have a hydrophobic and hydrophilic layer. They keep the lungs inflated.

    A. Mucin is a type of mucus produced by lung cells that absorbs water.

    C. Enzymes are a catalytic protein and do not prevent the lungs from collapsing.

    D. Buffers maintain acid-base balance and are not involved in lung function.

14. Option D is correct. The epiglottis shuts off the tracheal opening, diverting food into the esophagus.

    A. The uvula is found in the back of the throat and prevents food entry into the nasal passages.

    B. The soft palate is found in the back of the buccal cavity. It helps in swallowing and prevents food entry into the nasal passages.

    C. The tonsils are made of lymphatic tissue that does not typically interfere with food movement.

15. Option C is correct. The larynx is a cartilaginous structure containing the vocal chords, which is used to generate sound.

    A. The pharynx is the muscular region at the intersection of the respiratory and digestive systems, not the voice box.

    B. The trachea is the large tube containing cartilaginous rings through which air passes into and out of the lungs.

    D. The uvula is a fleshy extension of the back of the soft palate, hanging above the throat. It does not function in the production of sound.

16. Option A is correct. Aerobic respiration (oxidative respiration) is almost exclusively used by the heart. The byproducts of this type of respiration are water (H_2O) and carbon dioxide (CO_2), not lactate.

    B. The sinoatrial (SA) node, also known as the pacemaker, produces electrical impulses for heart contraction. It does not provide energy to the heart.

    C. The lactose-producing fermentation pathway operates during oxygen deprivation in the skeletal muscle. It does not primarily operate in the heart.

    D. The heart is highly sensitive to oxygen deprivation, and requires a steady oxygen supply for adenosine triphosphate (ATP) production by oxidative phosphorylation during aerobic respiration.

17. Option B is correct. The gonadal artery is the primary artery that supplies oxygenated blood to the gonads and male reproductive system. It is called the testicular artery in males and the ovarian artery in females.

    A. The common carotid artery supplies oxygenated blood to the head.

    C. The femoral artery supplies oxygenated blood to the lower limbs.

    D. The subclavian artery supplies oxygenated blood to the upper limbs.

18. Option B is correct. The fusion of a sperm with 23 chromosomes and an egg with 23 chromosomes would result in a zygote with 46 chromosomes.

    A. The unfertilized egg and the sperm each contain 23 chromosomes. This is the haploid chromosome number for a human.

    C. 69 chromosomes represent the fusion of a diploid human cell with a haploid human cell. This is not the diploid chromosome number for a normal human zygote.

    D. 92 chromosomes represent the fusion of two diploid human cells. This is not the chromosome number for a normal human zygote.

19. Option C is correct. The corpus luteum refers to the remnant of the graafian follicle. It secretes progesterone to prepare the uterus for the pregnancy.

    A. The endometrium is the highly vascularized tissue of the uterine lining. It does not produce progesterone following ovulation.

    B. The cervix is the external opening of the uterus and does not produce progesterone.

    D. The fallopian tube carries the egg from the ovary to the uterus and does not produce progesterone.

20. Option B is correct. Keratinocytes contain the protein keratin. They are produced in the epidermis and migrate upwards. The tight junctions between cells prevent water entry. They eventually form a layer of dead cells on the skin surface, which produces a waterproofing effect.

    A. Melanocytes are pigment cells found in lowest layer of the epidermis of skin, the basal layer. They produce melanin, a pigment that absorbs UV light. They do not provide a waterproofing function for the skin.

    C. Merkel cells are integumentary cells that work as mechanoreceptors and sense touch and pressure. They do not provide a waterproofing function for the skin.

    D. Langerhans are dendritic cells of the immune system and are found in the lower layers of the epidermis. They immunologically process material that enters through the skin. They do not provide a waterproofing function for the skin.

21. Option C is correct. The hypodermis contains stores of subcutaneous fat as well as deeper blood vessels.

    A. The epidermis contains living and dead keratinocytes, melanocytes, as well as dendritic and tactile cells. It does not contain stores of subcutaneous fat.

    B. The dermis is a layer of skin that contains blood capillaries, hair shafts, nail roots, and sweat glands. It does not contain stores of subcutaneous fat.

    D. Dermal papillae are wavy projections of the dermis into the epidermis that lock the two layers together. It does not contain stores of subcutaneous fat.

22. Option C is correct. Sebaceous glands produce sebum, which supplies hair shafts and skin with oily secretions.

    A. Eccrine, or merocrine, glands are distributed across the surface of the skin and produce a dilute, salty sweat. They do not supply hair shafts and skin with oily secretions.
    B. Apocrine glands are usually found in groin and armpits and produce sweat and scent. These glands do not supply hair shafts and skin with oily secretions.
    D. Ceruminous glands produce a waxy secretion in the ear canals. Although they produce sebum, they do not primarily supply hair shafts and external skin with oily secretions.

23. Option D is correct. The pancreas produces insulin.

    A. The thyroid gland produces thyroid hormone.
    B. The adrenal glands produce cortisol and stress hormones.
    C. The pituitary gland secretes hormones that control other glands.

24. Option B is correct. Type I diabetes is a disease that is caused by the absence of insulin.

    A. Estrogen production is affected by diseases that harm the uterus and ovaries.
    C. Testosterone production is affected by diseases that harm the testes.
    D. Thyroxine production is associated with goiters and diseases that affect the thyroid gland.

25. Option B is correct. Ureters connect the kidney to the bladder.

    A. Capillaries connect veins to arteries.
    C. Urethras connect the bladder to the outside of the body.
    D. Arteries carry blood away from the heart.

26. Option A is correct. The kidneys filter blood.

    A. The heart pumps blood but does not filter it.
    B. The lung oxygenates blood but does not filter it.
    C. Some drugs can cross the blood-brain barrier, but it does not actually filter the blood.

27. Option B is correct. Salts are removed by the kidneys.

    A. Platelets are removed by the spleen and liver.
    C. Oxygen is used in every cell in the body, not filtered by the kidneys.
    D. Fat in the blood is taken up by cells or metabolized in the liver.

28. Option B is correct. The thymus is the location of maturation for T-cells.

    A. T-cells are produced in the bone marrow, but they are not matured there. B-cells are matured in the bone marrow.
    C. Adrenal glands produce several hormones, but they do not produce parts of the immune system.
    D. The thyroid produces the thyroid hormone.

29. Option C is correct. The rib is a flat bone.

    A. The tarsal is a short bone.
    B. The vertebrae are irregular bones.
    D. The humerus is a long bone.

30. Option A is correct. Ligaments connect bones together.

    B. Tendons connect muscle to bones.
    C. Marrow is inside the bone and does not connect to other bones.
    D. Muscle is not typically a connective tissue.

31. Option B is correct. Patellae are sesamoid bones, which develop in response to strain. Patellae are also considered short bones.

    A. Phalanges are long bones because their length is greater than their width.
    C. Scapulae are flat bones because they do not have a bone marrow cavity.
    D. Metatarsals are long bones because their length is greater than their width.

32. Option D is correct. The folds increase the surface area, allowing more nutrients to be absorbed and delivered to the blood stream.

    A. Movement of food is aided by smooth muscle contractions, not by villi projections.
    B. Movement of food is aided by smooth muscle contractions, not impeded by villi projections.
    C. The folds increase the surface area, allowing more nutrients to be absorbed and delivered to the blood stream.

33. Option A is correct. Calcium and sulfuric acid react to produce calcium sulfate and hydrogen gas.

    B. Hydrogen sulfide is not produced by this reaction. Hydrogen sulfide is produced by iron sulfide reacting with hydrochloric acid.

    C. Calcium sulfide is not produced by this reaction. Calcium sulfate can be reduced to calcium sulfide using carbon.

    D. Hydrogen sulfate is not produced by this reaction. Hydrogen sulfate (bisulfate ion) is the conjugate base of sulfuric acid.

34. Option B is correct. Some proteins fold into shapes that allow them to function as biochemical catalysts or enzymes within a cell.

    A. These contain genetic information for the synthesis of proteins.

    C. These molecules, which repel water, function in cellular membranes and in the storage of excess energy.

    D. These "sugar and starch" molecules function in energy input and storage, as well as in some structural capacities.

35. Option A is correct. Solids have little space between particles, and the particles vibrate within a fixed lattice structure.

    B. Liquid particles move about in a fluid manner due to translational motion.

    C. Gas particles are widely separated by empty space and move about randomly due to translational motion.

    D. Atoms in a plasma state move so rapidly that their electrons separate from the rest of the atom; it is as fluid as a gas.

36. Option C is correct. The mass of an atom is the sum of protons and neutrons in its nucleus.

    A. This is the atomic number of the atom, not its mass.

    B. The sum of protons and electrons in an atom is not the atomic mass number.

    D. The sum of protons, neutrons, and electrons is not the atomic mass number.

37. Option C is correct. CH_3OH is a polar molecule, because oxygen is highly electronegative and draws electrons towards itself. Because water molecules are polar, water acts as a solvent for polar molecules.

    A. CH_4 is a nonpolar molecule. Because water molecules are polar, water does not act as a solvent for nonpolar molecules.

    B. CCl_4 is a nonpolar molecule. Because water molecules are polar, water does not act as a solvent for nonpolar molecules.

    D. Octane is a nonpolar molecule. Because water molecules are polar, water does not act as a solvent for nonpolar molecules.

38. Option D is correct. Since there is no F, all the offspring will have pink eyes.

    A. Since the F is dominant, half the offspring will have purple eyes.

    B. Since the F is dominant, three quarters of the offspring will have purple eyes.

    C. Since the F is dominant, all the offspring will have purple eyes.

39. Option D is correct. Only germline mutations are transmitted, so the lung cancer, a somatic mutation, will not be passed to the child.

    A. Somatic mutations, such as lung cancer, are not passed on in this manner.

    B. Somatic mutations, such as lung cancer, are not transmitted through the blood.

    C. Somatic mutations, such as lung cancer, are not passed on in this manner. The child does not require treatment for lung cancer.

40. Option D is correct. The T allele is dominant and encodes the tall plant phenotype, and it requires only one dominant allele to express the dominant trait.

    A. The use of the terms phenotype and genotype is incorrect. Phenotype refers to physical attributes and genotype refers to genetic makeup.

    B. TT and Tt both code for dominant phenotypes. Phenotype refers to physical attributes and genotype refers to genetic makeup.

    C. The use of the terms phenotype and genotype is incorrect. Phenotype refers to physical attributes and genotype refers to genetic makeup.

41. Option C is correct. If an essential bacterial partner is killed by the antibiotic, then the disease-causing potential will be reduced. This is the best inference.

    A. Mutations occur in DNA, and antibiotics do not cause mutations in DNA.
    B. Antibiotics work on cellular action rather than by creating a physical barrier.
    D. White blood cell production is increased by infection, not by antibiotics.

42. Option A is correct. A testable and falsifiable hypothesis is the hallmark of scientific investigation. Experiments can only be used to accept or discard hypotheses.

    B. Unexpected experimental results lead to the formulation of new, different hypotheses.
    C. However, this is not adefining principle of scientific hypotheses.
    D. A scientific hypothesis will either be supported or refuted by the evidence, but it is never considered correct or incorrect.

    Only some scientific predictions are supported by evidence; other predictions are refuted by testing.

43. Option B is correct. Electron microscopy has significantly improved the ability to see and understand the workings of these organelles because electron wavelengths are short enough to resolve the structure of organelles, which are around 100 times larger than the wavelengths of an electron.

    A. Electron wavelength in electron microscopy is of the same order of magnitude as the size of an atom. This is too small to visualize because electron waves cannot resolve particles that are of the same order of magnitude.
    C. The structure of skeletal joints can be effectively examined using an X-ray machine, rather than an electron microscope.
    D. The bonds between atoms use electrons, which cannot be visualized with an electron microscope because they cannot resolve particles that are of the same order of magnitude.

44. Option A is correct. The neck length of giraffes was once thought to be an acquired characteristic (due to stretching to reach food) that was passed on to offspring. Further study determined that mutations in DNA actually caused the increase in neck length, which was preferentially passed on to offspring through selection.

    B. While this is an example of natural selection, it does not present any evidence that would dismiss the possibility that acquired characteristics can be passed on to offspring.
    C. While this is an example of natural selection, it does not present any evidence that would dismiss the possibility that acquired characteristics can be passed on to offspring.
    D. This observation would support, not refute, the hypothesis that acquired characteristics are passed on to offspring. Inherited aptitude is a better indicator of learning language than parental training.

45. Option C is correct. If immigration (people joining a population) and births are greater than emigration (people leaving a population) and deaths, then the population will grow.

    A. This equation describes a stable population.
    B. This equation describes a decrease in population.
    D. This equation describes a stable population.

46. Option C is correct. In a biomass pyramid, the greater mass is at the lower levels. According to the pyramid, there is a greater mass of seeds, berries, and grasses than insects.

    A. According to the pyramid, there is a greater mass of seeds, berries, and grasses than insects.
    B. According to the pyramid, there is a greater mass of blackbirds and ground squirrels than red-tailed hawks.
    D. According to the pyramid, there is a greater mass of insects than blackbirds and ground squirrels.

47. Option D is correct. Since activated charcoal is known to absorb organic compounds, its use indicates that the hypothesis being tested is that Weed B produces an organic compound that inhibits root growth for Weed A.

    A. This is not the hypothesis being tested.
    B. This is not the hypothesis being tested.
    C. This is not the hypothesis being tested.

English and Language Usage

1. Option A is correct. This construction reflects the same chronology of the original passage, with the director listening to everyone's opinions before making up her mind and informing people of her decisions.

   B. This sentence construction implies that the director is simultaneously informing people of her decisions while listening to everyone's opinions and making up her own mind, which does not reflect the order of events in the passage.

   C. The word "since" implies a cause-and-effect relationship that is not evident in the original passage.

   D. This construction does not reflect the chronology of the original passage.

2. Option B is correct. This is the correct spelling of the plural version of "veto."

   A. When making a word plural that ends in a vowel, it is necessary to add "e" before the final "s."

   C. An apostrophe indicates possession or a contraction; it does not create a plural.

   D. An apostrophe indicates possession; it does not create a plural.

3. Option C is correct. Using a semicolon to separate two independent clauses is appropriate, and the first word following the semicolon should not be capitalized unless it is a proper noun.

   A. Using a comma to separate two independent clauses in this manner is an error known as a comma splice.

   B. Using a comma to separate two independent clauses is an error known as a comma splice. Also, only proper nouns are capitalized within an independent clause.

   D. The first word following a semicolon should not be capitalized unless it is a proper noun.

4. Option A is correct. A colon should be used to introduce a list.

   B. A comma is not appropriate for introducing a list.

   C. A semicolon is not appropriate for introducing a list.

   D. Punctuation is required to introduce the list in this sentence.

5. Option D is correct. The pronoun must be subjective case because it is functioning as the subject of the clause.

   A. The pronoun "that" should refer to a thing or things, rather than a person.

   B. This pronoun is in the objective case, which is incorrect in this context.

   C. The pronoun "which" should refer to a thing or things, rather than a person.

6. Option C is correct. "Accidents do not just happen" and "they are usually caused by a lack of attention" are both independent clauses and require some form of separation. Because there is no coordinating conjunction present, such as "and," "but", or "yet," the two clauses should be separated by a semicolon.

   A. "Accidents do not just happen" and "they are usually caused by a lack of attention" are both independent clauses and require some form of separation. Because there is no coordinating conjunction present, such as "and," "but," or "yet," the two clauses should be separated by a semicolon.

   B. "Accidents do not just happen" and "they are usually caused by a lack of attention" are both independent clauses and require some form of separation. Because there is no coordinating conjunction present, such as "and," "but," or "yet," the two clauses should be separated by a semicolon, rather than a comma.

   D. "Accidents do not just happen" and "they are usually caused by a lack of attention" are both independent clauses and require some form of separation. The first independent clause is not an introductory statement; therefore, a semicolon should be used, rather than a colon.

COMPREHENSIVE ANSWERS

7. Option B is correct. This is a complete sentence. A complete sentence has a subject and a verb and presents a complete thought. This is an example of an imperative sentence, where the subject is the understood "you" and the verb is "nominate."

   A. This is not a complete sentence. A complete sentence has a subject and a verb and presents a complete thought. The pronoun "me" in this option serves as the direct object of the verb "nominating," and a subject is missing.

   C. This is not a complete sentence. A complete sentence has a subject and a verb and presents a complete thought. This clause does not present a complete thought, because the conjunction "when" at the beginning makes it a relative clause, which is used to modify a noun or noun phrase. The noun or noun phrase that is being modified is missing from this option.

   D. This is not a complete sentence. A complete sentence has a subject and a verb and presents a complete thought. This option is missing a subject and a verb: the phrases "to be nominated" and "to serve" are infinitives that require an auxiliary verb to function as verbs.

8. Option C is correct. The word "truly" is an exception to the rule to drop the final e before a suffix beginning with a vowel (a, e, i, o, u), but not before a suffix beginning with a consonant.

   A. This is the correct spelling of the word meaning "old." This is a spelling exception to the rule of "I before E, except after C."

   B. This is the correct spelling of the word meaning "to look at." This is the past tense of the word "view."

   D. This is the correct spelling for the word meaning "significant."

9. Option A is correct. When adding "-ly" to a word ending in "-al," keep the original "l" and add "ly." When forming an adverb, an "-ly" is added to an adjective without changing the original spelling of the word, except in cases where the root word ends "e" or "y." These exceptions do not apply to the word occasional.

   B. There is no need to remove a letter "c" from occasional when adding an "ly." The addition of a suffix to a root word rarely changes the spelling of the root, except in cases where the root word ends "e" or "y." These exceptions do not apply to the word occasional.

   C. There is no need to insert an additional "s" into the word occasional when adding an "-ly." The addition of a suffix to a root word rarely changes the spelling of the root, except in cases where the root word ends "e" or "y." These exceptions do not apply to the word occasional.

   D. This spelling does not follow the rule for adding "-ly" to a word ending in "-al." When adding "-ly" to a word ending in "-al," keep the original "l" and add "ly."

10. Option B is correct. This verb is in the singular form, which agrees with the singular subject. The word "or" in the phrase "A doctor or a nurse" makes the subject singular.

    A. This verb is in the plural form, which does not agree with the singular subject.

    C. This verb is in the plural form, which does not agree with the singular subject.

    D. This verb is in the plural form, which does not agree with the singular subject.

11. Option D is correct. The subject of the sentence is "the class," which is singular and requires the singular pronoun "it." Additionally, the pronoun should be possessive. "It" is an exception to the usual grammar rule to add an "apostrophe s" to indicate possession, and is instead written as "its."

    A. The subject of the sentence is "the class," which is singular, and the plural "they" would not be an appropriate pronoun. Additionally, the pronoun should be possessive, whereas "they're" is a contraction of the phrase "they are."

    B. The subject of the sentence is "the class," which is singular and requires a singular pronoun. The adverb "there," denoting a place or position, would not be appropriate.

    C. While it is true that the subject of the sentence is "the class," which is singular and requires the singular pronoun "it," the pronoun must also be possessive. "It's" is a contraction of the phrase "it is."

12. Option C is correct. The use of the contraction "don't" is appropriate in a personal letter. Contractions should be spelled as two separate words (i.e., do not) in a formal letter. The use of the phrase "bunch of odds and ends just messing up the message" is colloquial and is indicative of informal writing.

    A. The tone and language in this sentence are formal and appropriate for a business letter.

    B. The tone and language in this sentence are formal and appropriate for a business letter.

    D. The tone and language in this sentence are formal and appropriate for a business letter.

13. Option B is correct. This passage is informal and is appropriate for a friend. The use of the informal greeting "hi"; the use of contractions, such as "can't," "you'll," and "don't"; the use of exclamation points; and the use of informal phrases, such as "don't sweat it," are all examples of informal language.

    A. This passage is informal and is not appropriate for a president of a corporation.

    C. This passage is informal and is not appropriate for a professor at a college.

    D. This passage is informal and is not appropriate for a dean at a college.

14. Option D is correct. This sentence does require a citation. It refers to a specific point from Dr. Smith's research and requires a citation for her work.

    A. This sentence does not require a citation. It summarizes the purpose of the paper.

    B. This sentence does not require a citation. It is a general statement introducing a supporting detail of the paper.

    C. This sentence does not require a citation. It is a general statement introducing a supporting detail of the paper.

15. Option C is correct. Kelly is referencing sources found on the internet. Keeping a list of these references will enable her to include citations for each source.

    A. Kelly is not preparing an outline. An outline is an organizational tool used to create a summary of the key points and supporting details that will be included in a paper.

    B. Kelly is not writing a draft. During this stage, the writer collects ideas and begins to write.

    D. Kelly is not writing a revision. This is the final element of the writing process, where the writer rereads a completed draft of the paper and makes any necessary changes.

16. Option C is correct. This sentence does not belong in this paragraph. It is an opinion that does not support the topic sentence about the rarity of Giant Pandas.

    A. This is the topic sentence and introduces the topic of the paragraph.

    B. This sentence is a supporting detail about the topic sentence.

    D. This sentence is a supporting detail about the topic sentence.

17. Option B is correct. This sentence establishes soybeans and fats as the topic of the paragraph.

    A. This sentence does not introduce the topic of soybeans and fats.

    C. This sentence does not introduce the topic of soybeans and fats.

    D. This sentence gives the opposite information of the supporting sentences.

18. Option B is correct. Since the campaign is "ongoing," the present perfect tense "has been spent" is appropriate. An indeterminant amount of money, "more than $5 million," should be treated as a singular noun, which requires a singular verb.

    A. The word "are" makes the verb phrase present perfect tense, which is incorrect for the context of this sentence.

    C. The word "were" makes the verb phrase past tense, which is incorrect for the context of this sentence.

    D. Using "have been" is incorrect for the context of this sentence. When the subject of the verb phrase is plural, using "have been" is appropriate; however, an indeterminant about of money, such as "more than 5 million," should be treated as a singular noun.

19. Option B is correct. The Latin root "circum" means "around," and the Latin root "loqui" means "to speak."

    A. The Latin roots "circum" and "loqui" do not combine to mean "meandering expedition."

    C. The Latin roots "circum" and "loqui" do not combine to mean "type of geometrical pattern."

    D. The Latin roots "circum" and "loqui" do not combine to mean "remote destination."

20. Option D is correct. An antidote is a substance that "acts against," or counteracts, the effects of another substance, such as the chemicals in the example above. The prefix anti- means against.

    A. The prefix anti- indicates opposition. Rather than referring to an ingredient in the chemicals, the word antidote is mostly likely referring to a substance that counteracts the effects of the chemicals.

    B. An antidote is a substance that counteracts the effects of another substance, while a contraindication is a condition or situation that prohibits the use of a substance.

    C. An antidote is a substance, not a place.

21. Option B is correct. The definition of dys- is difficult or painful. A patient who has dysesthesia feels pain when touched.

    A. The definition of dys- is difficult or painful. A patient who has dysesthesia feels pain, not pleasure, when touched.

    C. The definition of dys- is difficult or painful. A patient who has dysesthesia does not have a normal reaction to touch.

    D. The definition of dys- is difficult or painful. A patient who has dysesthesia feels pain when touched.

22. Option C is correct. The context clue "because of poor handwriting" suggests that "illegible" is the correct synonym for this context.

    A. While "rewritten" could fit the context of the sentence, it is not a synonym for "cryptic."

    B. While "occult" is a synonym for "cryptic," it does not fit the context of the sentence.

    D. While "terse" is a synonym for "cryptic," it does not fit the context of the sentence.

23. Option C is correct. Bland is a synonym for banal, and it fits the context of the sentence because it makes sense that one would avoid bland plays.

    A. Confusing is not a synonym for banal.

    B. Ostentatious is not a synonym for banal.

    D. Practiced is not a synonym for banal.

24. Option B is correct. Atrophy means "to waste away," so this is an appropriate antonym.

    A. The phrase "become infected" is not an antonym for atrophy.

    C. The phrase "weaken gradually" is not an antonym for atrophy.

    D. The phrase "injure through over-exertion" is not an antonym for atrophy.

Index